OXFORD MEDICAL PUBLICATIONS

Oxford Handbook of
Trauma and
Orthopaedic Nursing

T0177580

Published and forthcoming Oxford Handbooks in Nursing

Oxford Handbook of Adult Nursing 2e
Edited by Maria Flynn and Dave Mercer

Oxford Handbook of Cancer Nursing, 2e
Edited by Mike Tadman and Dave Roberts

Oxford Handbook of Cardiac Nursing, 3e
Edited by Kate Olson

Oxford Handbook of Children's and
Young People's Nursing, 2e
Edited by Edward Alan Glasper, Gillian
McEwing, and Jim Richardson

Oxford Handbook of Clinical Skills in
Adult Nursing, 2e
Edited by Frank Coffey, Alison Wells, and
Mark Fores

Oxford Handbook of Clinical Skills for
Children's and Young People's Nursing
Paula Dawson, Louise Cook, Laura-Jane
Holliday, and Helen Reddy

Oxford Handbook of Critical Care
Nursing, 2e
Sheila Adam and Sue Osborne

Oxford Handbook of Dental Nursing
Elizabeth Boon, Rebecca Parr, Dayananda
Samarawickrama, and Kevin Seymour

Oxford Handbook of Diabetes Nursing
Lorraine Avery, Joanne Buchanan, Anita
Thynne

Oxford Handbook of Emergency
Nursing, 2e
Edited by Robert Crouch, Alan Charters,
Mary Dawood, and Paula Bennett

Oxford Handbook of Gastrointestinal
Nursing, 2e
Edited by Jennie Burch and Brigitte Collins

Oxford Handbook of Learning and
Intellectual Disability Nursing
Edited by Bob Gates and Owen Barr

Oxford Handbook of Mental Health
Nursing, 2e
Edited by Patrick Callaghan and Catherine
Gamble

Oxford Handbook of Midwifery, 3e
Janet Medforth, Susan Battersby, Maggie
Evans, Beverley Marsh, and Angela
Walker

Oxford Handbook of Musculoskeletal
Nursing
Edited by Susan Oliver

Oxford Handbook of Neuroscience
Nursing 2e
Edited by Sue Woodward and Catheryne
Waterhouse

Oxford Handbook of Nursing Older
People, 2e
Edited by Marie Honey, Annette Jinks, and
Lauren Hanson

Oxford Handbook of Trauma and
Orthopaedic Nursing 2e
Rebecca Jester, Julie Santy, and Jean
Rogers

Oxford Handbook of Perioperative
Practice
Suzanne Hughes and Andy Mardell

Oxford Handbook of Prescribing for
Nurses and Allied Health Professionals
Sue Beckwith and Penny Franklin

Oxford Handbook of Primary Care and
Community Nursing 3e
Edited by Judy Brook, Caroline McGraw,
and Val Thurtle

Oxford Handbook of Renal Nursing
Edited by Althea Mahon, Karen Jenkins,
and Lisa Burnapp

Oxford Handbook of Respiratory
Nursing
Terry Robinson and Jane Scullion

Oxford Handbook of Surgical Nursing
Edited by Alison Smith, Maria Kisiel, and
Mark Radford

Oxford Handbook of Women's Health
Nursing, 2e
Edited by Sunanda Gupta, Debra
Holloway, and Ali Kubba

OXFORD HANDBOOK OF

Trauma and Orthopaedic Nursing

SECOND EDITION

EDITED BY

Rebecca Jester
Professor of Nursing
Institute of Health
University of Wolverhampton
UK

Julie Santy-Tomlinson
Adjunct Associate Professor
Orthopaedic Nursing
Odense University Hospitals
University of Southern Denmark
Denmark

Jean Rogers
Practice Teacher
Open University
UK

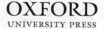

OXFORD
UNIVERSITY PRESS

OXFORD
UNIVERSITY PRESS

Great Clarendon Street, Oxford, OX2 6DP,
United Kingdom

Oxford University Press is a department of the University of Oxford.
It furthers the University's objective of excellence in research, scholarship,
and education by publishing worldwide. Oxford is a registered trade mark of
Oxford University Press in the UK and in certain other countries

© Oxford University Press 2021

The moral rights of the authors have been asserted

First Edition published in 2011
Second Edition published in 2021

Impression: 2

All rights reserved. No part of this publication may be reproduced, stored in
a retrieval system, or transmitted, in any form or by any means, without the
prior permission in writing of Oxford University Press, or as expressly permitted
by law, by licence or under terms agreed with the appropriate reprographics
rights organization. Enquiries concerning reproduction outside the scope of the
above should be sent to the Rights Department, Oxford University Press, at the
address above

You must not circulate this work in any other form
and you must impose this same condition on any acquirer

Published in the United States of America by Oxford University Press
198 Madison Avenue, New York, NY 10016, United States of America

British Library Cataloguing in Publication Data
Data available

Library of Congress Control Number: 2020944548

ISBN 978–0–19–883183–9

Printed and bound by
Ashford Colour Press Ltd.

Oxford University Press makes no representation, express or implied, that the
drug dosages in this book are correct. Readers must therefore always check
the product information and clinical procedures with the most up-to-date
published product information and data sheets provided by the manufacturers
and the most recent codes of conduct and safety regulations. The authors and
the publishers do not accept responsibility or legal liability for any errors in the
text or for the misuse or misapplication of material in this work. Except where
otherwise stated, drug dosages and recommendations are for the non-pregnant
adult who is not breast-feeding

Links to third party websites are provided by Oxford in good faith and
for information only. Oxford disclaims any responsibility for the materials
contained in any third party website referenced in this work.

Preface

Welcome to the second edition of the *Oxford Handbook of Trauma and Orthopaedic Nursing*. Since the publication of the first edition in 2011 nurses in the speciality have continued to develop specialist and advanced practice roles to support the needs of patients, their families and service provision and reflect the way orthopaedic and trauma nurses are leading the way in nurse-led and interdisciplinary working. There has continued to be a gradual shift of service delivery away from the acute hospital setting to community and primary care services as well as towards streamlined pathways of care.

This second edition continues the original focus on providing comprehensive information for students and practitioners caring for patients in orthopaedic and trauma settings with a focus on both fundamental and specialist practice. The information has been expanded and updated to include up-to-date evidence to facilitate the best effective care. There are several new and updated sections within the book which aim to reflect changes in practice, social and professional context, and national and global policy.

The inclusion of a dedicated topic about providing support for people with a learning disability (PWLD) who require trauma and orthopaedic services reflects the need for an approach to practice that embraces diversity of patient need. There is also a dedicated section considering the public health and health promotion role of those working with people with and at risk of musculoskeletal disease and injury; for example, relating to the care and management of obesity in orthopaedic and trauma patients. Chapter 3 includes updated information regarding the assessment of the trauma patient reflecting current professional guidelines. Other additional topics include enhanced recovery pathways and fast-track and virtual clinics in the elective surgery setting. The inclusion of more detailed discussion of the needs of the older person being cared for in the orthopaedic trauma setting reflects the increasing average age of the orthopaedic and trauma patient. The global epidemic that is fragility fracture is also given deeper consideration.

As with the first edition, the book has been designed to be a user friendly easy to read resource to dip in and out of in busy clinical areas as well as to reflect interdisciplinary approaches and promotion of evidence-based practice. Up-to-date recommendations are provided for further reading to support practitioners in taking individual responsibility for extending their learning in areas beyond that which can be provided in a handbook.

Rebecca Jester
Julie Santy-Tomlinson
Jean Rogers
February 2020

Preface

Contents

Contents

List of contributors

Dr Mary Drozd
Senior Lecturer
Institute of Health
University of Wolverhampton, UK

Beverley Gray Linnecor
Clinical Editor,
International Journal of Orthopaedic
and Trauma Nursing
Guernsey

Sarah Ryan
Nurse Consultant in Rheumatology
and Professor of Rheumatology
School of Nursing and Midwifery
Keele University;
Staffordshire and Stoke on Trent
Partnership NHS Trust
Haywood Hospital, UK

Symbols and abbreviations

●	cross-reference
ℬ	website
~	approximately
>	greater than
<	less than
ACT	autologous chondrocyte transplantation
AHP	Allied Health Professional
AIMS	Arthritis Impact Measurement Scale
AMTS	Abbreviated Mental Test Score
ANP	Advanced Nurse Practitioner
AP	anteroposterior
ARA	American Rheumatism Association
ARDS	adult respiratory distress syndrome
AS	ankylosing spondylitis
ASA	American Society of Anesthesiologists
ATLS ®	Advanced Trauma Life Support
BCG	Bacillus Calmette–Guérin
BDI	Beck Depression Inventory
BMD	bone mineral density
BMI	body mass index
BOA	British Orthopaedic Association
BP	blood pressure
CAM	complementary and alternative medicine/therapy
CBT	cognitive behavioural therapy
CCP	cyclic citrullinated peptide
CRP	C-reactive protein
CSF	cerebrospinal fluid
CT	computed tomography
DASH	disabilities of arm, shoulder, and hand
DIP	distal interphalangeal
DMARD	disease-modifying antirheumatic drug
DoH	Department of Health
DVT	deep vein thrombosis
DXA	dual-energy X-ray absorptiometry

EA	enteropathic arthritis
ECG	electrocardiogram
ED	emergency department
ESR	erythrocyte sedimentation rate
EUA	examination under anaesthesia
EWS	early warning score
FBC	full blood count
FES	fat embolism syndrome
FRASE	Fall Risk Assessment Scale for the Elderly
GCS	Glasgow Coma Scale
GP	general practitioner
HADS	Hospital Anxiety and Depression Scale
HaH	Hospital at Home
HDP	high-density polyethylene
HLA	human leucocyte antigen
IA	intra-articular
ICP	integrated care pathway
IM	intramuscular
IP	interphalangeal
IV	intravenous
JIA	juvenile inflammatory arthritis
KSS	Knee Society Score
LFT	liver function test
LMWH	low-molecular-weight heparin
LRTI	lower respiratory tract infection
MCP	metacarpophalangeal
MDT	multidisciplinary team
MEWS	modified early warning score
MMSE	Mini Mental State Examination
MOF	multiple organ failure
MoM	metal-on-metal
MRI	magnetic resonance imaging
MRSA	meticillin-resistant *Staphylococcus aureus*
MSU	midstream urine
MT	metatarsal
MTP	metatarsophalangeal
NEWS	National Early Warning Score
NHS	National Health Service (UK)

NICE	National Institute for Health and Care Excellence	RA	rheumatoid arthritis
NJR	National Joint Registry	RCN	Royal College of Nursing
NSAID	non-steroidal anti-inflammatory drug	RF	rheumatoid factor
		RICE	rest, ice, compression, and elevation
NWB	non-weight-bearing	SC	subcutaneous
OA	osteoarthritis	SCI	spinal cord injury
OCD	osteochondritis dissecans	SIP	Sickness Impact Profile
OI	osteogenesis imperfecta	SMP	self-management programmes
PARS	patient at risk score	SSI	surgical site infection
PBD	peak bone density	TB	tuberculosis
PCA	patient-controlled analgesia	TENS	transcutaneous electrical nerve stimulator
PE	pulmonary embolism		
PIP	proximal interphalangeal	THR	total hip replacement
PMP	Pain Management Programme	TJR	total joint replacement
PMR	polymyalgia rheumatica	TKR	total knee replacement
POP	plaster of Paris	U&Es	urea and electrolytes
POUR	postoperative urinary retention	UKCC	United Kingdom Central Council for Nursing, Midwifery and Health Visiting
PROM	patient-reported outcome measure	URTI	upper respiratory tract infection
PTH	parathyroid hormone	UTI	urinary tract infection
PTSD	post-traumatic stress disorder	VTE	venous thromboembolism
PU	pressure ulcer	WBC	white blood cell
PV	plasma viscosity	WOMAC	Western Ontario and McMaster Universities Arthritis Index
PWB	partial weight-bearing		
PWLD	people with learning disability		

Chapter 1

Introduction

The orthopaedic patient

Introduction

The term orthopaedics derives from two Greek words: *orthos* (straight) and *paedios* (child). Indeed, originally the specialty of orthopaedics focused on correcting bony deformities in children such as club feet, scoliosis, and hip dysplasia. However, in contemporary orthopaedic and trauma services, treatment is given across all age groups. The demography of the UK and other countries such as the USA, Canada, and Australia indicates that there will be an increasing number of older people within society which will result in an ever-increasing demand for orthopaedic and trauma services. Disease processes affecting orthopaedic and trauma patients are generally classified as:

- Acute onset, e.g. ruptured ligaments and fractures
- Gradual onset/relapsing course, e.g. rheumatoid arthritis (RA)
- Acute onset/constant course, e.g. spinal cord injury and traumatic amputation
- Gradual onset/progressive course, e.g. osteoarthritis (OA) and osteoporosis
- Congenital, e.g. congenital dislocation of the hip and club feet.

Most individuals will require treatment and care for at least one of these types of pathologies. Some patients will access trauma and orthopaedic services as a one-off episode; others will require ongoing treatment and care throughout their lives. It is important to remember that the vast majority of patients (especially older patients) will have other comorbid conditions besides their musculoskeletal problem, such as heart failure, diabetes, and enduring mental health problems. As nurses, we must remember to focus on the patient as a whole and not just their disease, and adopt holistic approaches to care which include physical, social, psychological, and spiritual aspects.

Characteristics of the orthopaedic/trauma patient

The manifestations of the specific orthopaedic or trauma problem will vary depending on the pathology of the condition. However, there are some common problems that the majority of patients present with, including:

- Pain—localized and/or diffuse
- Reduced movement/mobility/function
- Deformity.

Pain

The clear majority of patients who present to orthopaedic services will have a chief complaint of pain which is usually localized to a limb segment or joint, but occasionally is diffuse and/or multicentred. Pain can be classified as acute or chronic/long term. Acute pain has a clearly defined onset and physiological responses and is present in cases such as traumatic soft tissue injury, fracture, and in the immediate postoperative period. Acute pain is considered to last up to 7 days, with prolongation to 30 days being common.[1] Chronic pain is defined as lasting >3 months and not manifesting with the same physiological responses as acute pain and typically presents with patients with low back pain or OA. Pain is often defined as follows: 'Pain

is what the experiencing person says it is and exists whenever he says it does'.[2] This definition highlights the individualized and subjective nature of pain and that patients' responses to pain and their coping strategies will vary depending on many factors, including:
- Age
- Gender
- Culture
- Previous experience of pain
- Anxiety levels
- Level of knowledge and control.

Unrelieved or ineffectively managed pain can have a major negative impact on patients' physical, social, and psychological well-being, including:
- Immobility and reduced function
- Inability to work
- Withdrawal and isolation
- Anxiety and depression.

Evidence-based pain assessment and pain management are essential components of the nursing role and are discussed in detail in Chapter 4 (see ➔ p. 117).

Reduced movement/mobility and function

Many patients will present with reduced movement, mobility, and function due to musculoskeletal pain and/or deformity. For example, patients with RA of the joints of the hands may have greatly diminished grip strength and dexterity of their fingers and patients with injury to the ligaments/cartilage of the knee may complain of reduced walking distance, difficulty in ascending/descending the stairs, and not being able to participate in sporting and recreational activities. Again, it is important to remember that reduced movement, mobility, and function will impact the physical, psychological, and social aspects of the patient's life. Examples include:
- Pressure ulcers
- Increased risk of deep vein thrombosis (DVT)
- Weight gain
- Constipation
- Social isolation
- Inability or reduced ability to work—resulting in reduced income
- Altered body image
- Low self-esteem
- Depression
- Lack of independence.

Reduced movement, mobility, and function have a major impact on the quality of life of orthopaedic patients and can have life-threatening consequences in terms of DVT and pulmonary embolism (PE). The multidisciplinary team (MDT) needs to work together to assess the patient's abilities and to optimize independence.

There are two basic approaches to treatment/care: restoration of function and adaptation. Whenever possible, treatment should aim to restore function, either through improving muscle strength and tone, pain management, pharmacological treatment of the disease process, or surgery.

However, for some patients restoration to full function is not possible and the MDT needs to develop a collaborative plan to focus on adaptation to the disability. This will include adaptations to the home/work environment, provision of suitable mobility aids, retraining or deployment to alternative forms of work, access to social service support and benefits advice, psychological support around life change and adaptation, and information and advice about minimizing the risk of complications of reduced activity.

Deformity

Orthopaedic and trauma patients may develop or indeed be born with a deformity of the musculoskeletal system. Examples of congenital deformity include club foot and spina bifida. Deformities may develop through the life course due to conditions such as RA or developmental spinal deformities such as kyphosis and scoliosis. Such deformities will have physical, social, and psychological implications, including reduced mobility, function, and movement; pain; altered body image; poor self-esteem and problems with sexual relationships; stigma; and negative responses from society which can result in bullying, non-integration into peer group, and social isolation. Many types of musculoskeletal deformity can be corrected or improved by surgery and/or therapy and orthotics. However, for some patients deformity cannot be totally corrected and they need support and treatment from the MDT to maximize their independence and to cope with the social and psychological impact of the deformity.

Orthopaedic and trauma patients with special needs

It is important to remember that a significant number of people accessing orthopaedic and trauma services may have special needs because they have a disability that makes verbal communication difficult, e.g. people with hearing and/or speech impairment, people with learning disability (PWLD), mental health problems, or cognitive disorders such as dementia. Often people with special needs do not have the same quality of access and treatment within healthcare as those without disability. The evidence for this since the first edition of this handbook has increased and therefore a dedicated topic on supporting PWLD has been added (see ➔ People with a learning disability or cognitive impairments, p. 22). It is important that nurses in orthopaedic and trauma services work collaboratively with people with special needs, their family, carers, and specialist learning disability, mental health, and dementia services to provide care and treatment that meet their needs. Effective communication is the most important factor in providing sensitive and individualized care. Use of clear lay language, use of sign boards, speaking directly to the patient so they can see your facial expressions, and use of non-verbal communication are simple steps that can help.

Cultural diversity

People accessing orthopaedic and trauma services will be from a wide range of cultural and religious backgrounds. Culturally sensitive care and treatment is about respecting people's individual beliefs and customs. Always talk to the individual and find out what their particular needs are; it can be as simple as a female patient not being examined by a male nurse or doctor, or using interpreters to make sure communication is effective.

Conclusion

Most of the population will access healthcare for a trauma or orthopaedic problem at some point in their lives and for a significant number of people with chronic musculoskeletal diseases this will be a long-term relationship. Increasingly, people will be assessed and treated within the primary care setting with referral to hospital-based services for major surgery or complex trauma cases only. The most important message is to consider each person as an individual and respect their cultural, religious, and social backgrounds and be cognisant and responsive to people with special needs. Patients should be involved as active partners in their care and treatment. Nurses have a key role in advocating for patients and to ensure they are consulted with about their preferences for the type of treatment and care they receive. The needs of patients through the lifespan from birth to very old age are discussed on ➲ p. 24.

References

1. Kent ML, Tighe PJ, Belfer I, et al. (2017). The ACTTION–APS–AAPM Pain Taxonomy (AAAPT) multidimensional approach to classifying acute pain conditions. *Pain Med* 18:947–58.
2. McCaffery M, Beebe A (1989). *Pain: Clinical Manual for Nursing Practice*. St. Louis, MO: Mosby.

Orthopaedic nursing in the twenty-first century

Introduction

The first national orthopaedic course for nurses was established in 1937 and Dame Agnes Hunt, Mary Powell, and Edith Prosser are some of the key nurses instrumental in establishing orthopaedic nursing as a specialism. In the twenty-first century, orthopaedic nurses will find themselves dealing with patients of all ages from the newborn infant with a congenital disorder such as club foot or developmental displasia of the hip to the very old with degenerative conditions such as OA and fragility fractures. Increasingly, the role of the orthopaedic nurse is spanning the primary/secondary interfaces of care with an increasing shift towards care in the community and hospital length of stay being as short as possible. The development of nurse-led services in both hospital and primary care services has developed rapidly over the last decade with roles such as Advanced Nurse Practitioner (ANP) and nurse consultant roles being well established in the UK and USA and an international move towards developing these roles. There is a shortage of registered nurses globally and some countries including the UK are developing support roles such as associate nurses to address this. There is an increasing need for public health and health promotion roles for nurses working in the specialism. Increasing rates of obesity, morbid obesity, and sedentary lifestyles throughout the lifespan are resulting in increased challenges to musculoskeletal health such as earlier onset OA in weight-bearing joints, lower peak bone density (PBD) at skeletal maturity, and back pain. Nurses need to ensure they address these issues with patients and offer them evidence-based advice and support for weight loss/management and active lifestyles (see ➔ pp. 184–187).

Specialist and advanced practice roles in trauma and orthopaedic nursing

A global study commissioned by the International Council of Nursing (ICN) reported 17 titles describing specialist/advanced nursing roles across 31 participating countries and great variability in regulation and educational preparation.[1] Advanced/specialist nursing roles in trauma and orthopaedics make a significant contribution to patient services and patient satisfaction and are cost-effective, but it is important to ensure public protection by appropriate training, education, and professional regulation. Advanced practitioners should be educated to master's degree level in advanced practice, be assessed as competent in expert knowledge and skills, and have the autonomy to make decisions about the assessment, diagnosis, and treatment of patients.[2,3] In orthopaedics and trauma, ANPs have developed roles and nurse-led services in the following:

- Preliminary assessment and triage of patients presenting with musculoskeletal problems in primary care settings
- Postoperative review and surveillance of patients following joint replacement surgery (both face-to-face clinics and telephone services)
- Preoperative/anaesthetic assessment
- Preoperative information sessions and preparation for surgery

- Hospital outreach/Hospital at Home (HaH) schemes facilitating early discharge and admission prevention
- Minor surgical procedures, e.g. joint injection and release of carpal tunnel
- Support and follow-up of patients with external fixators
- Fast-track trauma coordination for older hip-fracture patients
- Initial assessment of patients referred to orthopaedic services including decision to treat and obtaining informed consent for surgical procedures
- Specialist falls clinics
- Bone health and fracture prevention.

This list is not meant to be exhaustive, but illustrative of the type of nurse-led services that have been and continue to be developed in trauma and orthopaedic services. It is important that the development of nurse-led services is based upon a sound business case to improve quality and efficiency of patient services. The legal, ethical, and professional implications of taking on roles previously carried out by other healthcare professionals such as doctors or therapists must be carefully considered, and appropriate training, education, and organizational indemnity provided to protect the individual practitioner, the patient, and the healthcare organization.

The health promotion role of nurses in orthopaedics and trauma

One of the key global health challenges in the developed world is the rising rates of obesity coupled with sedentary lifestyles, both of which impact negatively on musculoskeletal health. Obesity (body mass index (BMI) ≥ 30 kg/m^2) is known to be a risk factor contributing to OA due to increased weight load and altered mechanical axis on weight-bearing joints.[4] Smoking, poor diet, and sedentary lifestyle impact negatively on achieving PBD at skeletal maturity and increase the risk of osteoporosis in older age. Every nurse has a responsibility to provide evidence-based advice and to promote health and support changes in health behaviours. Making Every Contact Count (MECC)[5] was introduced by NHS England with an aim to capitalize on the opportunities presented every time a patient has contact with a healthcare professional in any setting and to receive support and guidance on improving aspects of their health including:

- Smoking cessation
- Drinking alcohol only within the recommended limits
- Healthy eating
- Being physically active
- Keeping to a healthy weight
- Improving mental health and well-being.

Skills such as brief interventions to produce and sustain changes to health behaviours and approaches such as motivational interviewing are essential for nurses to support patients in improving their health. For further information on this topic see ℬ http://www.makingeverycontactcount.com/.

Competence in orthopaedic and trauma nursing

Competence and skill are essential aspects of providing safe and effective care to the orthopaedic patient. Underpinning this competence is an understanding of the nature, core values, and beliefs of orthopaedic nursing. This includes application of knowledge and understanding of the musculoskeletal system, orthopaedic and trauma conditions, and injury to the holistic care of individuals who suffer from musculoskeletal disease, injury, or disorder.

Domains of practice

A national consensus project to determine the domains of trauma and orthopaedic nursing in the UK revealed trauma and orthopaedic nursing practice is categorized into five domains or sub-roles[6]:
• Comfort enhancer
• Coordinator
• Partner/guide
• Risk manager
• Technician.

Levels of competence

In addition to the domains of practice there is also a range of levels of competence. Competence and confidence are developed through both formal learning and experiential or workplace learning. Inherent within increasing competence is diagnostic and clinical decision-making skills. Although there may be variation in levels of competence between countries, generally it is acknowledged there are four levels of practice:
• Healthcare support worker
• Associate practitioner
• Competent registered practitioner
• Experienced/proficient practitioner.

For further reading on this topic see *A Competence Framework for Orthopaedic and Trauma Practitioners.*[7]

References

1. International Council of Nursing (2008). *The Scope of Practice, Standards and Competencies of the Advanced Practice Nurse.* Geneva: International Council of Nursing.
2. Royal College of Nursing (2018). *Royal College of Nursing Standards for Advanced Level Nursing Practice.* London: Royal College of Nursing.
3. Health Education England (2017). Multi-Professional Framework for Advanced Clinical Practice in England. ✂ https://www.hee.nhs.uk/our-work/advanced-clinical-practice/multi-professional-framework
4. Jiang L, Tian W, Wang Y, et al. (2012). Body mass index and susceptibility to knee osteoarthritis: a systematic review and meta-analysis. *Joint Bone Spine* 79:291–7.
5. Public Health England (2018). *Making Every Contact Count Implementation Guide.* London: PHE Publications.
6. Drozd M, Jester R, Santy J (2007). The inherent components of the orthopaedic nursing role: an exploratory study. *J Orthop Nurs* 11:43–52.
7. Royal College of Nursing (2019). *A Competence Framework for Orthopaedic and Trauma Practitioners.* London: Royal College of Nursing. ✂ https://www.rcn.org.uk/professional-development/publications/pub-007036

Orthopaedics and trauma along the lifespan: childhood and adolescence

Orthopaedic and trauma care are often viewed as a healthcare specialty that is active along the full span of life. Models of nursing highlight the role of the nurse in relation to the dependency of the child at birth, the increasing degree of independence as human life progresses, and the increasing dependency as we reach old age and near death. All age groups are affected by musculoskeletal conditions, disease, and injury and these can lead to decreased independence at any time of life. The musculoskeletal system is dynamic and constantly changes throughout the lifespan, meaning that a variety of conditions and diseases are more likely to appear in different stages of life while some are a feature for any age group. Orthopaedic care, although based on the same principles whatever the age of the patient, must adapt to changing needs throughout the lifespan. In some countries such as the UK, nurses are trained at pre-registration level to work with children or adults; however, in many countries, nurses' pre-registration courses prepare them to work with patients across all age groups and fields such as mental health, adult and child. The trauma and orthopaedic nurse needs to have the skills and knowledge to provide evidence-based care to all age groups, although it is preferable to have specialist education and training with specific age groups such as children and older people.

The newborn

The newborn has approximately 300 cartilaginous structures that ossify and turn into bone after birth and some fuse together to make longer bones. The musculoskeletal system grows and develops rapidly following birth, particularly during the first year. Because of complex developmental issues, the musculoskeletal system sometimes fails to develop in a completely normal manner *in utero*. Problems during birth can also cause skeletal problems. Depending on genetic and congenital influences, a baby may have one or more skeletal problems at birth, such as developmental hip dysplasia and talipes equinovarus (club foot). Immediately after birth there is a need for those caring for the newborn to be skilled in recognizing such problems so that specialist orthopaedic assessment and treatment can begin as rapidly as possible. Delays in diagnosis and treatment can result in poorer outcomes and the need for more complex and costly interventions.

Early childhood

There are many factors which affect the development of bones and joints during childhood. Genetic conditions such as osteogenesis imperfecta and achondroplasia are relatively uncommon, but are important aspects of orthopaedic care in the child. Very few other musculoskeletal problems affect babies who are not of walking age. Children generally begin to walk at around 1 year of life. Any injury that occurs before this must lead the healthcare professional to consider the possibility of non-accidental injury. Walking is an important development step as it means that the child can start to move around independently and interact with others and the environment in new ways. Once they are mobile, however, children become significantly more prone to accidental musculoskeletal injury. The rate of healing for bone and soft tissue injury in the child is much faster than the adult. For example, a simple fracture of a long bone in a child will generally heal completely in 4–6 weeks compared to 8–12 weeks in an adult. The challenge of caring for very young children and babies who may be immobilized due to musculoskeletal problems and injuries is ensuring that their development is not affected by separation from parents and that they continue to learn about and interact with their surroundings. Family-centred care and ensuring the child's parents are active partners in all aspects of care and treatment will minimize the detrimental effects of hospitalization for the child and their family. Healthy normal development of the musculoskeletal system of children requires good nutrition and regular weight-bearing exercise. Avoiding prolonged hospitalization is important when treating young children and many treatments and care can safely be delivered within the child's home environment and the primary care setting and will minimize disruption to their education, family life, and play with their peers.

Later childhood

As children become more independent in life and begin to expand their social circles they begin to need the care of their family in less obvious ways. Children often learn by taking risks and experimenting with the world around them. Long bones increase in length as the child becomes taller and there is much activity at the epiphyseal plates a few centimetres from the ends of long bones while this happens. The largest spurt in growth occurs in early adolescence and usually results in a significant increase in height as bone length increases from the epiphyseal plates. Damage to epiphyseal plates through trauma can cause significant problems throughout childhood. Increased exposure to risk of injury as the child becomes more independent means that trauma is by far the most common reason for children to need orthopaedic care. Perthes disease of the hip and scoliosis of the spine are examples of the few non-traumatic conditions which may lead to a need for orthopaedic care. This age group, as well as adolescents and young adults, are affected by bone and soft tissue tumours, either benign (osteoma, osteochondroma, chondroma, and osteoclastoma) or malignant (osteosarcoma, chondrosarcoma, and Ewing's sarcoma). Bone tumours are extremely rare and for this reason can often be misdiagnosed or there are significant delays before referral to a specialist centre is made. Again, wherever possible, treatment and care of this age group should be focused at home to avoid disruption to their education, family life, and socialization with their peers.

Adolescence

The adolescent years (normally considered as 13–18 years) are linked to puberty and are a period of rapid growth and development in the musculoskeletal system. The outward changes we see as the child becomes an adult, such as change in facial structure, are often related to the maturation of skeletal structures. For adolescent boys in particular, growth spurts are quite common and associated with activity at the epiphyseal growth plates at this time. Traumatic injury remains the most significant issue, although non-traumatic conditions such as idiopathic adolescent scoliosis and slipped capital femoral epiphysis can lead to the need for hospitalization and orthopaedic surgery. Adolescence is a time at which education and consideration of the physical and psychological features of puberty are important aspects of care.

Conclusion

Nurses working within the trauma and orthopaedic setting must liaise with colleagues who have specialist training and education in children's services to ensure that the physical, psychological, and social needs relevant to the child's stage of development are met. Also, nurses must have an understanding that musculoskeletal trauma may be the result of non-accidental injury, and if this is suspected, prompt referral to the child protection team is needed.

Orthopaedics and trauma along the lifespan: adulthood

The stages of adulthood are complex and more difficult to define than those of childhood. The following phases are intended to help to demonstrate the progression of the lifespan after childhood. Humans age at varying rates and the age groups described here are not chronological classifications.

Early adulthood

Between the ages of 16 and 18 years, many young people feel that they have reached adulthood. In developed countries, people reach their optimum skeletal maturity around the age of 16 years although the density of bone continues to increase into the early to mid-20s—tending to increasingly decline after that period. Between the ages of 16 and 25 years, accidental injury is the greatest threat to musculoskeletal integrity. This is largely because of lifestyle choices and the increase in risk-taking related to issues such as road traffic collisions, alcohol and drug use, and engagement in sports. This age group are also entering the world of employment and can present with occupational injuries. Young adults are at greatest risk of severe trauma and multiple fractures. Spinal cord injury is most common in this age. Primary tumours of bone and soft tissue are very rare but if they do occur it tends to be in early adulthood, adolescence, or childhood.

Middle adult years

As adulthood progresses, traumatic injury remains relatively common. The years between the approximate ages of 30–55 years are often seen as a period of relative social stability when the adult has made partnerships, become a parent, and stabilized in employment and social networks. In deprived areas and developing countries, and for many individuals, this is not necessarily the case. Many adults in every community live in poverty and/or social deprivation. In this phase of adulthood there is often the greatest degree of responsibility in terms of parenthood, employment, and social arrangements. Such responsibility can be a significant issue for individuals who cannot work or carry out other responsibilities due to musculoskeletal disease or injury and orthopaedic practitioners need to consider these issues as an important part of the care process. Throughout life, behaviour and lifestyle choices can impact the health of the musculoskeletal system. For example, smoking, excessive alcohol consumption, and lack of weight-bearing exercise impact adversely on bone density and muscle, ligament, and tendon strength and tone.

Later life

Increasing life expectancy in the developed world means that the majority of adult orthopaedic patients are over the age of 60 years. The later years of human life are often portrayed as a period of declining mobility and musculoskeletal heath. Conditions such as OA may begin to appear in the middle years of adulthood, but the impact of these tends to be greatest over the age of 55 years. The decline in bone density increases with age. Osteoporosis is more common in women than in men by a ratio of 3:1 and is a significant problem in developed countries, leading to an increase in fragility fractures, e.g. of the hip, spine, and wrist. The increasing prevalence of multiple health problems in later life means that recovery from injury and orthopaedic surgery is more problematic for the older adult. Regaining mobility and returning to previous levels of independence can be problematic. Older people are also more prone to the complications of surgery and immobility. Providing care which is sensitive to the specific needs of older people is an essential aspect of the practitioner's role.

End of life

Musculoskeletal injury and orthopaedic surgery carry a risk of death due to complications of surgery, particularly in patients with associated comorbidities and haemorrhage following major trauma. Also, patients present with pathological fractures due to bone metastases from a primary tumour. Supporting patients and their families through end of life care is an important aspect of the nursing role. End of life issues and care are discussed in more detail later within this chapter (see ➔ End of life and palliative care, p. 24).

The older orthopaedic patient

Most adult orthopaedic patients are over the age of 60 years, a sign of the way in which ageing impacts the musculoskeletal system. Deciding to work in this specialty is a conscious decision for nurses who find the challenge of caring for older members of society with musculoskeletal problems both a joy and a privilege. The complex health and social care needs of older adults mean that all orthopaedic care practitioners need a commensurate range of specialized knowledge, skills, and education as well as sound motivation to work with older people.

Life expectancy and the proportion of the world's population who are older are both increasing. In the coming decades, the pace of growth in older adult populations is likely to be greatest in Asia and South America as living standards and healthcare continue to improve. This will continue to create increasing demand for health and social care services.

The ageing process is universal and unavoidable, but it varies in its impact on individuals. Advancing age has physical, psychological, and social effects on both older people and wider society, depending on social and cultural norms. The physical effects of ageing have a significant impact on health and are thought to be related to a combination of two factors:

- Primary ageing—the effects of advancing age that cannot be avoided and which reflect the way the human body and its cells deteriorate as they age, largely due to changes in cell structure and genetic material.
- Secondary ageing—the results of lifestyle choices such as diet, smoking, declining physical exercise, and drug and alcohol abuse which result in a faster physical deterioration of cells and tissue than would be the case with only primary ageing having an impact.

The psychological effects of ageing are a result of how the human brain is affected by ageing as well as the way the individual thinks and feels about their advancing age. This is an area of considerable research but about which we know the least.

The approach and attitudes to ageing within societies also impact the lives and experiences of older people. Ageist attitudes affect the quality of life of older people and their experiences of life and healthcare. Political influences impact wealth and quality of life in later life. Global shortages of health and social care facilities and workers, for example, can mean that older people often receive inadequate care.

The physical effects of advancing age

Many older people lead healthy and active lives, but there are numerous general effects of ageing that impact both health and quality of life, including:

- Changes in the structure of skin cells, resulting in drier, less elastic skin that is more easily damaged and recovers less well from injury
- Changes in the eye which result in deteriorating sight
- Changes in the ear leading to hearing impairment and loss
- Problems in the vestibular system and perception that affect balance and stability
- Changes in nerves and loss or deterioration of some types of brain cells that result in neurological deterioration, memory loss, and slower cognition

- Reduction in the elasticity of the *lungs* leading to decreased lung capacity and depleted resilience during ill health affecting the ability to increase oxygen levels on demand
- Gradual decrease in elasticity of the *blood vessels* and the *heart* resulting in reduced capacity of the circulatory system with an impact on renal function
- Changes in the *digestive system* that result in diminished taste, loss of appetite, and greater risk of constipation.

Musculoskeletal ageing

An understanding of the ageing of the musculoskeletal system is central to providing effective trauma and orthopaedic care to older people:

- Change in the structure of *bone* as a result of loss of calcium and lower bone density, particularly in cancellous bone, leads to bone fragility (see ➔ Osteoporosis, p. 252) and significantly increases the risk of fragility fractures (see ➔ Fragility fractures, p. 419).
- Loss of *muscle* mass, known as sarcopenia, resulting in declining activity and function along with slower movement and greater risk of falls and poorer outcomes following injury and surgery.
- Changes in the structure of connective tissue, particularly cartilage, that lead to *joint* stiffness and arthritic conditions, affecting flexibility and leading to pain on movement (see ➔ Osteoarthritis, p. 252), affecting function and mobility.

These changes lead to a gradual decline in mobility and stability, resulting in older people becoming less able to move around in their environment and, therefore, less able to interact with the rest of society, leading to social isolation.

Caring for older people in orthopaedic settings

Older people with musculoskeletal disease and injury need carefully planned, age-sensitive, specialized care that takes into account both the orthopaedic condition and the effects of ageing and comorbid health conditions. Care should be provided by practitioners who have received specialist education related to caring for older people. Recovery and re-habilitation (see ➔ Rehabilitation, p. 176) for older people take longer and the principles of ensuring orthopaedic care is tailored to the needs of older people include the following:

Mobilization

The musculoskeletal and neurological effects of ageing mean that older people need more time to regain their mobility after orthopaedic surgery and injury. Setting short-, medium-, and long-term goals and gradually introducing exercise and reintroducing activities that involve movement is key. Older people cannot be expected to remobilize at the same rate as younger adults and need support for much longer periods of time.

Nutrition

Poor nutrition and dehydration result in delayed recovery. Older people often have depleted appetite and thirst, especially when they are incapacitated or unwell, and are the most likely to be under- or malnourished both on admission to hospital and on discharge. Malnutrition is a major cause of complications such as infection and pressure ulcers as well as poor recovery and outcomes. Assessment of nutritional status and carefully planned intervention are needed to prevent this. Long fasting times prior to surgery can lead to or worsen dehydration and malnutrition. Surgery must be planned to ensure that fasting times are minimized and intravenous (IV) fluids are carefully administered. Additional calories and protein are particularly important during recovery from injury and surgery and dietary supplements (high in calories and protein) are an important aspect of maintaining adequate nutrition along with enteral feeding when normal eating is depleted.

Pain

Older people suffer the same pain as younger people following injury or surgery, but they may be reluctant to take regular analgesia because they are anxious about the side effects of medication including becoming constipated or becoming addicted. Communication difficulties due to a stroke or cognitive impairment make pain assessment challenging. Detailed individualized pain assessment and age-appropriate pain management are central to improving the older person's experience of care and enhancing their recovery. An older person's pain tolerance is influenced by many cultural factors, prior experience of pain, and coping mechanisms

Elimination

Older people are more prone to constipation—particularly when they are dehydrated and taking codeine-based analgesics. They are also more prone to frequency of urine, urinary tract infections (UTIs), and incontinence that can lead to delirium, deliberate fluid intake restriction, and greater likelihood of dehydration. Constipation can be avoided by ensuring adequate access to toilet facilities and ensuring that the diet contains sufficient fibre and fluids (see ➔ Nutrition, p. 164). Never assume that urinary incontinence is normal for the individual or an unavoidable aspect of ageing. Some incontinence in orthopaedic patients may be caused by limited mobility due to their musculoskeletal problem (see ➔ Mobilization, p. 170) or can be the result of UTIs.

Senses

Sight and hearing deteriorate with age. Communicating effectively with older people means speaking clearly and slowly and not shouting. It also involves making eye contact and being sure that you are close enough for the older person to see your face and hear you without raising your voice. Written materials need to be prepared with a regard for potential sight problems.

Comorbidities

Primary and secondary ageing lead to increasing ill health. When planning care, practitioners must consider other multiple medical and health problems such as cardiovascular and respiratory conditions that can complicate orthopaedic care. Polypharmacy, multiple medication use, may have an impact on both physical and psychological health. Regular review of medications is essential in both the primary and secondary care settings along with patient and carer education about medication.

Mental health

Depression is a common feature of later life. Living alone, social isolation in their community, and bereavement can significantly affect mood, and motivation. This in turn affects recovery and rehabilitation. Recognizing older people suffering from depression and referring them to mental health services can be a significant factor in improving their health and recovery.

Cognitive function

Cognitive function can be affected by age, illness, injury, and surgery. Delirium is an acute, fluctuating change in mental status that is manifested as inattention, disorganized thinking, and altered levels of consciousness.[1] Delirium must never be assumed to be normal but regarded as a serious medical condition. Prompt assessment for underlying reasons for any confusion, disorientation, or other change in cognition is essential. Common reasons for acute delirium in older orthopaedic patients are dehydration and infection. Practitioners must understand the difference between delirium and dementia as delirium is almost always treatable with the right interventions following careful assessment. Patients with a diagnosis of dementia can also develop delirium, often manifesting in increased disorientation and confusion.

Frailty

Frailty is an important clinical syndrome seen in older people who have increased vulnerability and decreased resistance to physiological and psychological stressors that result in functional impairment and risk of health deterioration and death following illness, injury, or surgery.[2] Recognizing frailty through comprehensive multidisciplinary assessment enables the clinical team to predict and prevent adverse outcomes such as falls, infections, and functional impairment.

Dementia

Dementia is one of the most significant challenges facing health and social care services and society in general. Older people with dementia frequently need orthopaedic and trauma care, especially following injury as falls and dementia are closely linked. Rather than a single condition, dementia is a group of conditions associated with a decline in memory or other cognitive skills that can reduce a person's ability to perform everyday activities. Alzheimer's disease, Lewy body dementia, and vascular dementia are different conditions but have some similarities in care needs. Care needs are complicated by features that can include:
• Memory impairment
• Impaired abstract thinking and judgement
• Speech impairment
• Disorders of mood
• Hallucinations and delusional ideas
• Personality and behavioural changes.

These problems have a devastating effect on individuals and their families and complicate musculoskeletal injury or surgery. A high standard of individualized care and support is needed that includes providing a secure, comfortable environment with sensitive dementia-friendly communication and an understanding of the needs of the person with dementia and their family. It is vital to include the patient's family and usual care providers to inform an understanding of their usual patterns of behaviour and how best to care for them. Families understand the person better than anyone and can advise how best to communicate and manage problems that arise. Both hospital and community settings need to be specifically designed to consider the needs of people with dementia and all staff should be specially trained to ensure they have the knowledge and skills to provide care that is dementia sensitive.

Dignity

Older people can be vulnerable because of declining function and cognition. They are also reluctant to express dissatisfaction with care, making them more likely to tolerate poor standards.

Dignity and respect are fundamental human rights that acknowledge the worth of every human being and the right to be treated as such. Dignity is a major area of concern in providing care, particularly when an older person's vulnerability is increased by healthcare needs and institutional needs are placed above those of individuals. Dignity in care protects and promotes the individual's personhood and is linked with the ethical principles of respect for self and others, autonomy, empowerment, advocacy, and communication. Important aspects include providing high standards of age-sensitive care, involving older people in decisions about their care and communicating with them effectively about that care, as well as assessing their capacity to make decisions. Paying attention to these principles is important in ensuring patients' best interests are served at all times as well as improving and maintaining quality of care for older people and, critically, avoiding care failures such as those highlighted in the 2013 Francis Report.[3]

References

1. Inouye SK, Schlesinger MJ, Lydon TJ (1999). Delirium: a symptom of how hospital care is failing older persons and a window to improve quality of hospital care. *Am J Med* 106:565–73.
2. Marques A, Queiros C (2018). Frailty, sarcopenia and falls. In: Hertz K, Santy-Tomlinson J (eds) *Fragility Fracture Nursing: Holistic Care and Management of the Orthogeriatric Patient*, p. 15–26. Cham: Springer.
3. Francis R (2013). *Report of the Mid Staffordshire NHS Foundation Trust Public Inquiry*. London: The Stationery Office.

Further reading

Hertz K, Santy-Tomlinson J (2014). Fractures in the older person. In: Clarke S, Santy-Tomlinson J (eds) *Orthopaedic and Trauma Nursing*, pp. 236–50. Oxford: Wiley Blackwell.
Hertz K, Santy-Tomlinson J (eds) (2018). *Fragility Fracture Nursing: Holistic Care and Management of the Orthogeriatric Patient*. Cham: Springer. ℘ https://www.springer.com/gb/book/9783319766805

People with a learning disability or cognitive impairments

People with a learning disability or cognitive impairments

It is important to remember that a significant number of people accessing orthopaedic and trauma services may have special needs which makes verbal communication difficult, e.g. people with hearing and/or speech impairment, people with learning/intellectual disability (PWLD), mental health problems, or cognitive disorders such as dementia. Often people with these difficulties and disabilities do not have the same quality of access and treatment within healthcare as those without disability. The evidence for this since the first edition of this handbook has increased and therefore a dedicated topic on supporting PWLD has been added. It is important that nurses in orthopaedic and trauma services work collaboratively with people with learning/intellectual disabilities, their family and carers, specialist learning disability teams, and mental health and dementia services to provide care and treatment that meet their needs. Effective communication is the most important factor in providing sensitive and individualized care. Some of the key considerations for person-centred care are listed here:

- All hospitals in the UK have a legal responsibility to provide reasonable adjustments for PWLD.[1]
- There is a requirement for effective 'flagging systems' to be in place to identify people with learning/intellectual disabilities, cognitive, and/or communication impairments to ensure that these particularly vulnerable people are identified and appropriately cared for.[2]
- High-quality support and implementation of reasonable and achievable adjustments is needed. This requires staff to have specific competencies when caring for people with these difficulties.[3]
- The role of the acute liaison learning disability nurse (in the UK) provides invaluable support and facilitates communication between the PWLD and the staff.[4]
- An individualized and person-centred focus on the quality of the relationship with staff and the PWLD is important and is the same requirement as for a patient without a learning/intellectual disability, communication difficulty, or cognitive impairment.[5]
- Central to this relationship is effective communication.[6]
- Changes to communication methods may be needed and include for example, the provision of easier to read information; use of hospital/communication passports; pictures, photographs, or symbols; signing such as the use of Makaton or British Sign Language; using objects of reference; the Picture Exchange Communication System (PECS) or the use of high-technology alternative and augmentative communication (AAC) devices; and reasonable adjustment to procedures.[7]
- Time must also be allowed for the person to process information and express responses and while some people may be able to understand short and simple sentences, additional time should be allocated to communicate in the most appropriate person-centred way.[7]
- For people with the most complex needs, the carer who knows the person well is often invaluable as communication is most successful with familiar, responsive partners who care about the person they are communicating with.[7]

- Regular assessment and management of pain is vital as this can be overlooked. Reassessment of the pain level is essential as the person's needs may change. Some PWLD may express their pain in a unique or unconventional way and therefore it is of paramount importance to get to know the person, read the hospital passport, and communicate effectively to establish levels of pain and evaluate whether the management of pain has been effective.
- The Disability Distress Assessment Tool known as the 'DISDAT' tool can be used to assess the level of distress. It is intended to help identify distress cues in individuals who have severely limited communication. It is designed to describe an individual's usual cues when they are content, thus enabling distress cues to be identified more clearly.
- Double appointments either at the beginning or the end of a clinic are warranted as the consultation is likely to take longer to allow for the processing of information.
- Constipation can lead to serious health issues and death in PWLD and therefore prevention of constipation is essential; if confirmed, this must be managed effectively.[8] The main management response to constipation in PWLD is laxative use despite limited effectiveness. An improved evidence base is required to support the suggestion that an individualized, integrated bowel management programme may reduce constipation and associated health conditions in PWLD.

References

1. Office for Disability Issues (2010). Equality Act 2010. ℘ https://www.gov.uk/government/publications/equality-act-guidance
2. Drozd M, Clinch C (2016). The experiences of orthopaedic and trauma nurses who have cared for adults with a learning disability. Int J Orthop Trauma Nurs 22:13–23.
3. Royal College of Nursing (2017). The Needs of People with Learning Disabilities: What Pre-Registration Students should Know. London: Royal College of Nursing.
4. MacArthur J, Brown M, McKechanie A, et al. (2015). Making reasonable and achievable adjustments: the contributions of learning disability liaison nurses in 'Getting it right' for people with learning disabilities receiving general hospitals care. J Adv Nurs 71:1552–63.
5. Mansell J (2010). Raising Our Sights: Services for Adults with Profound Intellectual and Multiple Disabilities. London: Department of Health.
6. Bradbury-Jones C, Rattray J, Jones M, et al. (2013). Promoting the health, safety and welfare of adults with learning disabilities in acute care settings: a structured literature review. J Clin Nurs 22:1497–509.
7. Goldbart J, Caton S (2010). Communication and People with the Most Complex Needs: What Works and Why This Is Essential. London: Mencap.
8. Robertson J, Baines S, Emerson E, et al. (2018). Constipation management in people with intellectual disability: a systematic review. J Appl Res Intellect Disabil 31:709–24.

End of life and palliative care

Most patients cared for in orthopaedic settings make a full recovery to health following surgery or injury. However, there are a proportion of patients who will need end of life and/or palliative care because their condition is untreatable or because it may result in unavoidable death due to its severity, complications, or their poor health status. Such patients typically fall into one of the following categories:

• Older, frail, patients who have sustained major fragility fractures
• Patients suffering catastrophic multiple trauma
• Serious postoperative complications such as PE, stroke, and respiratory or cardiac failure
• Individuals being treated for pathological fractures such as those with primary malignant bone tumours and/or those who develop metastatic bone disease.

In acute care settings, practitioners can fail to recognize when curative treatment becomes futile and when palliative and/or end of life care should be considered. This frequently results in a suboptimal death for the patient, distress for their family, and lost opportunities for the patient to decide where they would like to die. Most people who die in hospital would have preferred to die at home but are not afforded the opportunity to make such a decision because staff do not initiate conversations with patients and those close to them, they do not have the skills to do so, or they do not recognize the importance of such actions. In attempts to improve palliative and end of life care, there have been several initiatives that aim to provide guidance relating to how palliative and end of life care should be provided. This guidance is constantly under review and practitioners have a duty to be cognizant with current best practice as well as to understand the distinction between end of life care and palliative care.

End of life care

Death can be expected as well as sudden. When death can be anticipated, e.g. for a frail older person who is unlikely to survive the physiological assault of a major fragility fracture and surgery, end of life care can ensure that the most dignified and least distressing death possible can be achieved through a holistic pathway focusing on the principles of good end of life care that includes:

• Identification of those approaching the end of life and initiating sensitive, open, and honest discussions about preferences for end of life
• Assessing needs and preferences, agreeing a care plan with regular review with the patient/family
• Coordination of care
• Delivery of quality services including symptom control, psychological and spiritual care, and timely referral to specialist palliative care teams
• Management of the last days of life
• Care after death
• Support for patients and families/carers during the illness and after their death.

Palliative care

End of life and palliative care are not synonymous, but palliative care is an important aspect of end of life care. It is a care approach that improves the quality of life of patients and their families experiencing life-threatening or life-limiting illness or injury. Its principles include the prevention and relief of suffering by effective assessment and management of pain and other physical, social, and psychological problems.[1]

Reference

1. Brent L, Santy-Tomlinson J, Hertz K (2018). Family partnerships, palliative care and end of life. In: Hertz K, Santy-Tomlinson J (eds) *Fragility Fracture Nursing: Holistic Care and Management of the Orthogeriatric Patient*, p. 137–45. Cham: Springer. ℘ https://www.springer.com/gb/book/9783319766805

Settings for orthopaedic and trauma nursing

Introduction

Traditionally, orthopaedic and trauma care has been mainly delivered within hospitals. However, there is an increasing drive for healthcare services to be delivered in community and primary care settings. The rationale for this shift away from hospital-based care is based upon evidence that patients' rehabilitation is more realistic in their home environment, hospitals do not provide a good therapeutic milieu, and a policy to reduce the number of in-patient beds as community-based care is more cost-effective. Orthopaedic and trauma services should be integrated across the primary/secondary care interface to provide seamless care. Since the first edition of this handbook, there is an increasing emphasis on minimizing length of hospital stay through either early discharge to HaH schemes or by use of enhanced recovery pathways (see ➔ Models of service delivery: enhanced recovery/fast-track, p. 30) and reducing the number of face-to-face outpatient follow-up appointments through non-face-to-face/telephone clinics (see ➔ p. 31).

Providing orthopaedic and trauma care within the community setting

These changes in service delivery necessitate orthopaedic and trauma nurses to adapt their skills and knowledge to work confidently and competently between hospital, primary care, and community settings to facilitate integrated orthopaedic and trauma services. There are a number of specific differences between working in the community and hospital settings, including:

- Nurses working in the community setting often work alone and without direct supervision
- Practice in the community necessitates higher levels of decision-making and autonomy as access to medical support is limited
- The nurse is a guest in the patient's home and there are specific legal issues around access to private property
- The nurse should have more 1:1 time with the patient with fewer interruptions than in the hospital setting
- Issues around personal safety of the nurse when out in the community and working alone
- Access to clinical investigations such as radiography is not readily available in the community setting.

To acquire the necessary skills and knowledge to work within the community setting the nurse will need to use a blended approach to their learning, which should include:

- Observation and supervised practice with experienced community trained nurses
- Enhancing assessment and decision-making skills through formal education and supervised practice

- A period of preceptorship with an experienced community practitioner/s
- Directed and self-directed study about legal aspects of entry to patients' homes and personal safety.

Conclusion

Increasingly, orthopaedic and trauma care will be delivered in the community and primary care settings. Nurses will be required to work across the interface of primary and secondary care and to provide seamless, integrated patient-focused care.

Models of community-based care

There are two approaches to delivering community-based orthopaedic and trauma services, which are hospital outreach and integration into mainstream community nursing and social services. From the outset when community schemes are being developed, it is important to have the correct skill mix and staff experience to transact expert orthopaedic care in the community setting and to have robust systems of evaluation to ensure patient safety and outcomes are at least comparable to in-patient models.[1]

Hospital at Home

Hospital outreach may be called HaH or the admission prevention/early discharge scheme. This model is staffed by nurses, therapists, and support workers from the hospital-based orthopaedic and trauma team and medical responsibility for the patient is retained by the hospital-based orthopaedic medical consultant. These schemes require both interdisciplinary and transdisciplinary approaches to optimize the patient's experience and avoid duplication of visits. Typically, this type of service facilitates early discharge of patients from the orthopaedic and trauma unit following procedures such as total hip and knee replacement surgery, spinal fusion, and internal fixation of hip fracture. Such schemes provide hospital-level care 7 days a week between the hours of 8 am and 8 pm (with on-call provision for out-of-hours contact) for a clearly defined aspect of the treatment/care pathway and are not a replacement for generic community and social care services. It's important to remember that not all patients are suitable for early discharge to such schemes and patients should be assessed for their suitability preoperatively against specific criteria as listed here:
• Does the patient live with a relative or significant other who is able and willing to provide support during their stay on the scheme?
• Does the patient have any significant comorbid states which increase their risk of postoperative complications, e.g. severe and enduring mental illness, history of stroke, or major heart disease?
• Is the patient's home accessible to the team and within the defined geographical area of the scheme?
• Does the patient's home pose any significant safety risks to the team?
• Does the patient have a telephone?

Such schemes also require clearly defined discharge criteria with systems *in situ* to facilitate referral to generic community and social services if the patient requires ongoing support.

Integration into mainstream community nursing and social services

This model involves the transfer and integration of specific elements of orthopaedic and trauma care provision into mainstream community nursing and social services. Usually medical responsibility for the patient is taken over by their general practitioner (GP) and the service is staffed by nurses and therapists who have expertise and specialist training in community care. Generally, admission and discharge criteria are less clearly defined than hospital outreach schemes and there will be more flexibility around the length of time the patient receives the service. It is important that such schemes liaise closely with specialist orthopaedic and trauma services and that staff are both competent and confident to deliver care to trauma and orthopaedic patients.

Reference

1. Jester R, Titchener K, Doyle-Blunden J, et al. (2015). The development of an evaluation framework for a Hospital at Home service: lessons from the literature. *J Integr Care* 23:336–51.

Models of service delivery: enhanced recovery/fast-track

To facilitate safe and efficient discharge from hospital to home following orthopaedic procedures such as total hip/knee replacement and to minimize hospital length of stay, many countries have adopted fast-track pathways which are also known as enhanced recovery pathways in some countries. Fast-track is a multidisciplinary strategy that begins before surgery and continues after discharge and has become a predictable and safe reality.[1] Fast-track aims to optimize preoperative patient information, multimodal opioid-sparing analgesia, fluid management/nutrition, and rehabilitation. Patients are mobilized ideally within 1–2 hours after surgery. To achieve early and sustained mobilization there is a need for comprehensive preoperative education, optimal pain relief, early oral nutrition and antiemetic prophylaxis, and a proactive interdisciplinary rehabilitation approach.

Fast-track has proven successful in not only significantly reducing postoperative length of stay, but in providing high degrees of safety (morbidity/mortality) and increased patient satisfaction.[2,3] Nurses have a pivotal role to play in supporting patients through fast-track pathways but despite their success there is evidence that patients can experience a number of difficulties following discharge home[4] including:

• Patients struggling with self-medicating for pain relief
• Motivation to continue with rehabilitation and exercises
• Overload of information during the pre-hospital and hospital stages, but feeling uncertain who to contact following discharge.

References

1. Hozack WJ, Matsen-Ko L (2015). Rapid recovery after hip and knee arthroplasty: a process and a destination. *J Arthroplasty* 30:517.
2. Galbraith AS, McGloughlin E, Cashman J (2018). Enhanced recovery protocols in total joint arthroplasty: a review of the literature and their implementation. *Irish J Med Sci* 187:97–109.
3. Kehlet H (2013). Fast-track hip and knee arthroplasty. *Lancet* 381:1600–2.
4. Specht K, Agerskov H, Kjaergaard-Andersen P, et al. (2018). Patients' experiences during the first 12 weeks after discharge in fast-track hip and knee arthroplasty – a qualitative study. *Int J Trauma Orthop Nurs* 31:13–19.

Models of service delivery: virtual clinics

Due to significant increases in the need for outpatient clinics in trauma and orthopaedics, there has been a growing trend in the development of virtual clinics which have become well established over the last decade,[1] particularly for fracture patients and increasingly for follow-up of patients after joint arthroplasty and other elective procedures. These clinics are often delivered by nurses in specialist roles.

Virtual clinics typically involve patients attending X-ray or other radiological investigations, biochemical investigations (written requests sent to the patient's home address), and completion of either paper or electronic versions of patient-reported outcomes measures (PROMs), such as Oxford knee or hip scores, and returned to the clinic ahead of the 'virtual clinic appointment'. The patient is then allocated a virtual clinic appointment usually compromising a telephone consultation and review of the results from the pre-requested investigations and PROMs questionnaires. The telephone consultation will comprise a review of the patient's symptoms and progress and gives feedback to the patient regarding the results of their clinical investigations as well as providing an opportunity for patients to ask questions or seek further advice about their condition/treatment/rehabilitation.

If patients are progressing well and there are no concerns about the results of their clinical investigations, the patient will continue to be reviewed by virtual clinics. However, if either the patient or clinician has any concerns then usually a traditional face-to-face review will be arranged to permit further investigations and physical examination.

Virtual clinics are generally well evaluated by patients[2] who appreciate not having to attend an outpatient clinic and being able to have their clinical investigations at a time of their convenience. Virtual clinics also can dramatically reduce waiting times for outpatient clinics.

Clinicians undertaking virtual clinics must have appropriate training and education to gain competence in undertaking virtual assessment and clinical decision-making without having the patient in front of them.

References

1. Jenkings P, Morton A, Anderson G, et al. (2016). Fracture clinic re-design reduces the cost of outpatient orthopaedic trauma care. *Bone Joint Res* 5:33–6.
2. Gupta S, Jones G, Shah S (2018). Optimising orthopaedic follow-uo care through a virtual clinic. *Int J Trauma Orthop Nurs* 28:37–9.

What is evidence-based care?

Introduction

In contemporary healthcare, ritualistic practice is no longer acceptable. Commissioners and providers of healthcare must demonstrate value for money, effectiveness, and best practice. Despite this, many aspects of orthopaedic and trauma treatment and care are based on individual clinician's preferences and 'doing it the way it's always been done'. All nurses must have the skills to be critical users of research, even if they do not undertake research themselves. Realistically, it's not always possible to underpin all nursing practice with robust research, because there are gaps in the research-based literature and it takes a significant amount of time for findings from research to be published and be available to clinicians.

What constitutes evidence?

There are a number of sources of evidence to underpin nursing practice and a summary of these is provided in Box 1.1.

Using evidence to underpin care

All of the previously described sources of evidence are valuable and can be used to underpin practice. It is often recommended that the gold standard of evidence is empirical research, but we must remember that not all research is of a good standard and the nurse has to decide whether the evidence is robust and relevant for the particular patient based on their preferences and their unique circumstances. For example, randomized controlled trials may indicate that full-length antiembolic stockings are the most effective mechanical means of preventing DVT following lower limb surgery. However, if a patient has a comorbid condition that prohibits their use or finds them so uncomfortable they roll them down then they are not the best option for the patient and may in fact do more harm than good. Therefore, it is essential that the nurse is able to evaluate the use of evidence in the context of the individual needs of patients and be able to critically evaluate research-based literature.

Box 1.1 Types of evidence

Evidence from research—review of research-based literature including systematic reviews and meta-analyses. Protocols and guidelines developed using empirical evidence from research

Evidence based on experiences—reflecting on practice and using non-research publications such as opinion pieces and case studies

Evidence based on theory that is not research based, but based on formal education, symposia, and conference presentations

Evidence gathered from clients and/or their carers about issues of satisfaction/dissatisfaction/complaint and audit data about untoward incidents

How to critically evaluate research

We must not assume that all research published in professional journals is of good quality and that guidelines and protocols developed by healthcare organizations are based on robust evidence. The nurse has a duty to enquire about the source of evidence for all protocols and guidelines, e.g. when, how, and by who were they developed and approved and were the evidence sources robust and up to date. Also, nurses need to be able to critically evaluate a piece of research or a systematic review before deciding if it can be used to underpin practice and seldom should practice or changes to practice or policy be based on a single research study.

Implementing evidence-based care

It is important to remember that there are many sources of help and guidance available to support you in implementing evidence-based care within the orthopaedic and trauma setting, including:
- Research and development departments within NHS Trusts
- Professional organizations such as the Royal College of Nursing—specialist forums
- Access to systematic reviews through the Cochrane Library (% https://www.cochranelibrary.com/) and the National Institute for Health and Care Excellence (NICE; % http://www.nice.org.uk)
- Nursing and health research departments within universities.

Chapter 2

Musculoskeletal anatomy and physiology

Anatomical terminology

It is essential that the orthopaedic practitioner is conversant with the terms used to describe anatomical positions and sites involved in trauma and orthopaedic conditions, injuries, and surgery. The ability to use a common language is central to effective interdisciplinary communication. The practitioner must also be able to translate this language to make it understandable for patients and relatives when discussing their care.

Anatomical position

Anatomical position describes the position of the body when it is in the upright position with the head facing forward, the hands at the side facing forwards, and the feet hip-width apart.

Planes

Understanding of the planes of the body helps practitioners to use accurate terminology to describe the location of the structures of the musculoskeletal system or the direction of movement from a three-dimensional view to guide the diagnosis and planning of treatment and care (see Fig. 2.1):
- *Sagittal plane*—from front to back vertically through the centre of the body
- *Transverse plane*—from left to right horizontally through the centre of the body
- *Coronal plane*—from left to right vertically through the body.

Anatomical terms—describing position

The most common anatomical terms used in orthopaedics and trauma to describe the site of a condition, surgery, or injury are:
- *Midline*—the centre line of the body in the anatomical position
- *Medial*—closest to the midline of the body
- *Lateral*—furthest from the midline of the body
- *Anterior*—the part of the body nearest to the front
- *Posterior* (dorsal)—the part of the body to the rear/back when in the anatomical position
- *Proximal*—the position nearest to the trunk or centre of the body or where a limb joins the body
- *Distal*—the furthest part of a limb away from the trunk or the furthest point away from the body
- *Inferior*—below, under, or less than, away from the head
- *Superior*—above, over, or towards the head
- *Valgus*—deviation away from the midline in the anatomical position
- *Varus*—deviation towards the midline in the anatomical position
- *Epiphyseal*—at the distal and proximal ends of long bones
- *Diaphyseal*—at the shafts of long bones
- *Apophyseal*—a protrusion of bone associated with the insertion of a major tendon.

Many other terms are used to describe the positions of conditions and injuries which relate specifically to a specific area of bone, joint, or soft tissue structure, e.g. intertrochanteric, condylar, talar, etc.

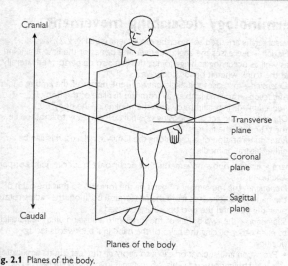

Cranial

Transverse plane

Coronal plane

Sagittal plane

Caudal

Planes of the body

Fig. 2.1 Planes of the body.

Terminology describing movement

Several terms are used to describe movement (see Fig. 2.2):

- *Flexion*—decreases the angle between the bones of the limb at a joint; as well as occurring at hinge joints, this can also be performed laterally at the trunk when it bends sideways
- *Extension*—increases the angle between the bones of the limb at a joint
- *Abduction*—moves a limb away from the midline of the body
- *Adduction*—brings a limb towards the midline of the body
- *Opposition*—the act of opposing one part of the body to another, i.e. the thumb to the fingers
- *Rotation*—rotation of a joint along the longitudinal axis, this can be either lateral or medial.

There are a few body movements that occur only in specific joints or parts of the body:

- *Pronation*—the movement of rotating the forearm so that the palm of the hand faces forwards from the anatomical position; the radius rotates over the ulna and the two bones are crossed
- *Supination*—the two bones of the forearm (radius and ulna) lie parallel to each other placing the palm of the hand in a backwards facing position
  - Pronation and supination can also apply to the feet but its application is less straightforward. This is because it involves the person's gait and how their weight is distributed when they walk, run, or move. Therefore, pronation of the foot means the person's weight is on the inside of the foot when walking and supination of the foot means the weight is on the outside of the foot
- *Plantar flexion*—the toes are pushed down away from the body using the strong flexors on the sole of the foot and contraction of the muscles of the calf
- *Dorsiflexion*—the toes are pushed up towards the body using the strong flexor apparatus of the lower leg
- *Inversion*—movement of the foot and ankle causing the sole to face medially/inwards
- *Eversion*—movement of the foot and ankle causing the sole to face laterally/outwards.

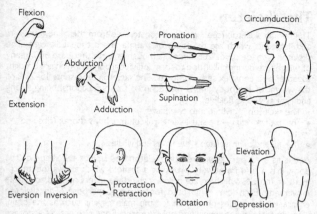

Fig. 2.2 Assessment of musculoskeletal conditions. Reproduced from Castledine and Close, *Oxford Handbook of Adult Nursing*, 2009, with permission from Oxford University Press.

The skeleton

The human skeleton (see Fig. 2.3) is constructed from the bone, cartilage, and ligaments which are the focus of trauma and orthopaedic care. The skeleton is made up of 206 bones (although at birth there are 300, many of which fuse during childhood to form individual bones) which are brought together by a complex series of joints. The skeleton represents 15–20% of the weight of the body and is well adapted for its functions, being strong and light as well as flexible.

The skeleton is divided into two parts:
- *The axial skeleton*—the skull, vertebral column, bony thorax (ribs and sternum)
- *The appendicular skeleton*—the limbs and girdles.

Acting as a support structure, the skeleton determines the shape of the body. It is a rigid framework providing a scaffold which allows the attachment of muscles which create power behind the levers needed to enable movement. Each joint is adapted for a specific purpose. The skeleton encases and provides protection for the main organs such as the brain, lungs, heart, and abdominal and pelvic organs. Bone also acts as a storage receptacle for minerals while the bone marrow contained within its cavities manufactures red and white blood cells (haematopoiesis).

The bones and their structures

There are several different types of bone:

Long bones

Each long bone has a central shaft (diaphysis) and two extremities (epiphysis) and is completely covered with a fibrous membrane (the *periosteum*) except at joint surfaces. Long bones include the femur, tibia, and humerus. The structure of long bones is the same throughout the skeletal system, with each including:
- A *diaphysis*—the shaft of the bone which comprises an outer layer of compact bone with a central canal that contains bone marrow
- The *epiphyses*—expanded areas at each end of the long bone. These have an outer covering of compact bone which is usually thinner than that found at the shaft/diaphysis. The bone tissue within the epiphyses is cancellous/spongy bone which is much less dense than compact bone and helps to keep the bones lighter to facilitate movement
- Long bones also have *epiphyseal cartilages/plates* near each end of the bone which are active in the growth in length of long bones and ossify when growth is completed in early adulthood. These can be seen clearly on radiographs as strips of cartilage which are more opaque than bone because they contain no calcium minerals
- *Periosteum* covers the outer surface of the bone. The periosteum has two layers—the outer *fibrous layer* has a protective function while the inner *osteogenic layer* contains the bone forming and destroying cells responsible for bone growth repair and remodelling (see ➲ Bone physiology, pp. 42–43)
- The inner spongy bone tissue, *bone marrow*, and the canals within them are covered by a more delicate membrane called the endosteum which also contains osteoblasts and osteoclasts which are responsible for the production and absorption of spongy bone.

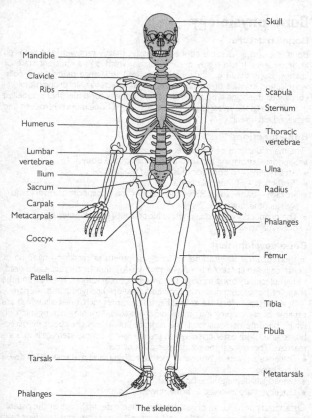

Skull
Mandible
Clavicle
Ribs
Scapula
Sternum
Humerus
Thoracic vertebrae
Lumbar vertebrae
Ilium
Sacrum
Ulna
Radius
Carpals
Metacarpals
Phalanges
Coccyx
Femur
Patella
Tibia
Fibula
Tarsals
Metatarsals
Phalanges

The skeleton

Fig. 2.3 The human skeleton. Shading indicates the axial skeleton and white shows the appendicular skeleton.

Flat bones, short bones, irregular bones, and sesamoid bones

These have no shafts or extremities and vary in size and shape. All have two thin outer layers of compact bone with cancellous bone sandwiched between them containing bone marrow within the trabecular bone, but there is no marrow cavity.

Further reading

(Note: these texts are recommended for further reading throughout this chapter as they provide detailed material about musculoskeletal anatomy and function.)

Soames R, Palastanga N (2019). *Anatomy and Human Movement: Structure and Function*, 7th edn. Philadelphia, PA: Elsevier.

Waugh A, Grant A (eds) (2018). *Ross & Wilson Anatomy and Physiology in Health and Illness*, 13th edn. Philadelphia, PA: Elsevier.

Bone physiology

Bone structure

Bone is a strong, durable connective tissue that is renewed and repaired at tissue level. It is a highly dynamic tissue which is in a constant state of change. Bone tissue is a porous, mineralized substance made up of cells, vessels, and crystals of calcium compounds which vary in proportions according to the bone type and its location. Bone is continuously remodelled in response to the stresses put on it and ~10% of bone mass is removed and replaced each year.

Bone functions

The main functions of bone are:
- Support—providing the solid framework of the body
- Attachment—to bone for muscles and tendons
- Protection—of internal organs
- Storage—bone stores 99% of all calcium and phosphorous reserves as well as other minerals
- The production of red and white blood cells (erythropoiesis)—in the bone marrow.

Bone development

In the fetus, the skeleton begins its development as cartilage, made up of dense collagen fibres. As the skeleton develops after birth, cartilage is gradually replaced by bone through the process of ossification. The size and the shape of bones continue to change and develop throughout the lifespan.

Bone begins in fetal life as undifferentiated mesenchymal cells which are capable of developing into many different cells, including osteogenic cells which become osteoblasts. Bone remodelling is brought about by osteoblasts along with osteoclasts which are derived from the stem cells in bone marrow. There are three main types of bone cell:
- *Osteoblasts* remodel bone and secrete collagen and minerals to lay down new bone
- *Osteoclasts* demineralize bone
- *Osteocytes* are involved in bone remodelling.

Osteoblasts produce an organic matrix called osteoid. Some of the osteoid bone undergoes mineralization (calcium and phosphate ions are deposited on the matrix). Once mineralized, the cells are known as osteocytes.

The osteocytes are accommodated in a space called the lacuna (see Fig. 2.4) and derive their nutrition from tunnels called canaliculi which enclose them. These eventually connect to the blood supply through the Haversian canal system. The outer areas of the bone are covered by periosteum and the inner surfaces by endosteum. The endosteum contains the osteoblasts and osteoclasts that remodel bone tissue. Osteoclasts are found on bone surfaces and function in bone reabsorption.

Types of bone tissue

The human skeleton is made up of two types of bone (see Fig. 2.5):

Cortical bone (compact bone)

Cortical/compact bone is found in ~80% of the skeleton and forms the protective outer shell around all bones. It is very strong bone that has a slow turnover rate and a high resistance to stresses such as torsion and bending. Cortical bone consists of large numbers of Haversian systems (see Fig. 2.4). Each microscopic Haversian system has a central vascular channel surrounded by a tunnel (the Haversian canal). This canal contains capillaries, venules, nerves, and lymphatic vessels. Between each Haversian system are concentric layers of mineralized bone (lamellar). This is a very strong but dynamic structure.

Trabecular bone (spongy/cancellous bone)

Trabecular/cancellous bone is found in 20% of the skeleton. It forms the internal scaffolding which helps bone maintain its shape despite being compressed by great forces. It is rigid but looks like sponge in structure. It is found in most of the axial skeleton (skull, ribs, and spine), the interior of short bones, and the epiphyseal and metaphyseal areas of long bones.

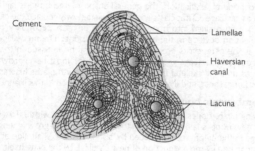

Lamellar bone architecture

Fig. 2.4 Haversian system and macroscopic structure of bone. Reproduced from the *Oxford Handbook of Clinical Specialties*, 8th edition, with permission from Oxford University Press.

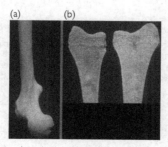

Fig. 2.5 Cross-section through a long bone epiphysis showing a thin outer layer of cortical bone with trabecular bone within and fused epiphyseal plate faintly visible. (a) Cortical and outer shell. (b) Trabecular—spongy/cancellous bone.

Bone growth and development

Bone growth (ossification) begins in the embryo (embryonically). This occurs in two ways:

Intramembranous ossification

Intramembranous ossification is the mechanism by which flat bones develop within membranes. Connective tissue exists where the flat bones will develop which is richly supplied with blood vessels and some of the connective tissue takes on the identity of osteoblasts which lay down bone. The osteoblasts are wrapped within the bone matrix and become osteocytes. Therefore, there are layers of connective tissue with spongy bone in the middle. As more osteoblasts form from the connective tissue they become periosteum and accumulate at the edges of the trabecular bone, laying down further hard matrix and becoming compact bone.

Endochondral ossification

In endochondral ossification, the general shape of the bone is laid down initially as cartilage. Osteoclasts and osteoblasts slowly replace the cartilage which is then ossified into bone. At the time of birth, secondary centres of ossification develop in the epiphyses of the bone. The medullary canal forms as the osteoclasts break down the central bone tissue in the shaft. This process of cartilage growth is responsible for most bone growth and continues until full skeletal maturity when the growth plates fuse and disappear. Long, short, and irregular bones are developed in this manner.

Postembryonic bone growth

Following birth, bones continue to grow in length and width. To grow in width, new bone is laid down under the periosteum. To grow in length the cartilage in the epiphyses is replaced by bone from the shaft side at a rate that is matched by the production of new cartilage by the plate itself. When adulthood is reached, this process stops and hormones cause the cartilage in the epiphyses to become ossified (see Fig. 2.6).

Influences on bone growth

- Nutrition
- Sunlight
- Hormonal secretions
- Physical exercise.

Exposure to sunlight assists bone growth because the skin produces vitamin D. Vitamin D is needed for the absorption of calcium. If vitamin D is not available, calcium is poorly absorbed, the bone is deficient in calcium, and is, therefore, weak.

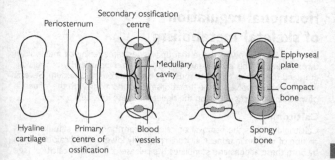

Bone growth

Fig. 2.6 Diagram of long bone development.

Hormonal regulation of bone growth

The hormones that help bone growth and development are (see ➲ Hormone regulation of skeletal metabolism, pp. 46–47):

- Growth hormone—this stimulates activity in the epiphyseal plates and is particularly important during infancy and childhood as it is the main regulator of height
- Testosterone and oestrogens—these influence the physical changes at puberty. They promote closure of the epiphyses and help retain calcium in the bones and do not stimulate osteoblasts but inhibit osteoclasis
- Thyroxin—increases the rate of energy production and protein synthesis
- Parathyroid hormone (PTH)—increases the reabsorption of calcium from the bones to the blood which increases blood calcium levels
- Calcitonin—decreases the reabsorption of calcium from blood, lowering blood calcium levels.

The length and shape of bones does not normally change after complete ossification in early adulthood. However, bone tissue is continuously reabsorbed and replaced throughout life and is remodelled when it is damaged.

Hormonal regulation of skeletal metabolism

Bone is a living, growing tissue that undergoes remodelling by metabolism throughout life. This is necessary both to maintain the integrity of the skeleton and to serve as the storehouse for phosphorous and calcium. Several hormones are involved in the metabolism of bone along with the influence of mechanical forces acting on the skeleton. These include:

Calcitonin

Calcitonin inhibits the removal of calcium from bones and stimulates excretion of calcium in urine. Calcitonin primarily lowers blood calcium levels by both these actions and stimulates the release of PTH and calcitriol (see Fig. 2.7).

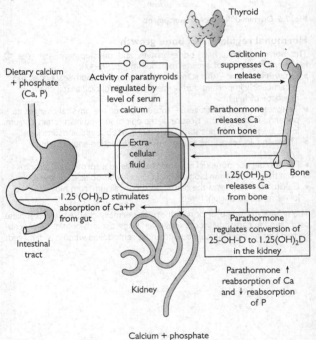

Fig. 2.7 Calcium and phosphate metabolism.

Parathyroid hormone

PTH enhances the release of calcium from bones. Bone reabsorption is the normal depletion of bones by osteoclasts which are stimulated by PTH which binds to the osteoblasts, the cells that create bone. With ageing, PTH production increases and this produces an increase in bone turnover and loss of bone mass, stimulating bone growth; a PTH deficiency in infancy will lead to stunted skeletal development and growth.

Calcitriol (vitamin D)

Calcitriol is a steroid hormone that has an important role in regulating levels of calcium and phosphorus and in the mineralization of bone. It also facilitates intestinal absorption of calcium, phosphate, and magnesium. Calcitriol increases the uptake of dietary calcium in the blood and bone, thereby stimulating osteoblastic activity. Calcitriol is generated in the skin when light energy is absorbed (see Fig. 2.8).

Oestrogens

Oestrogens are multifunctional hormones including one function that involves bone. Calcium is absorbed into bone due to osteoblast action. Oestrogens do not stimulate osteoblasts but inhibit osteoclast activity, protecting bone from excessive bone turnover. They are involved in bone growth, and with testosterone, cause adolescent 'growth spurts'. Once growth spurts have occurred, oestrogen, along with testosterone, will cause ossification of the epiphyseal plates to stop growth.

Growth hormones

Growth hormones stimulate bone growth at the epiphyseal plates. These hormones are particularly important because when there is insufficient, dwarfism will occur and when there is too much, gigantism will result.

This group of hormones control bone remodelling, maintaining the balance between osteoblastic and osteoclastic activities which means that overall bone mass of healthy adults changes very little until normal ageing occurs.

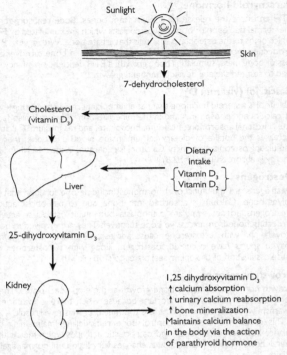

Fig. 2.8 Bone metabolism.

Muscle

Muscles

There are three main types of muscle:

- Smooth muscle—involuntary or non-striated, forms the walls of blood vessels and organs and is controlled by the autonomic nervous system
- Cardiac muscle—specialized for heart pumping activity and also under autonomic control
- Skeletal muscle—voluntary or striated muscle, under the control of both the central and autonomic nervous systems.

Skeletal muscle structure and function

Skeletal muscles contract and relax at varying speeds to bring about movement, providing the power for rapid and controlled movement by acting on the lever system of the bones and joints of the skeleton (see Fig. 2.9).

Skeletal muscles are dense collections of striated muscle fibres. Individual muscle fibres are long, cylindrical structures with multiple nuclei. Their length and width vary depending on the purpose and function of each muscle. The fibres are covered with connective tissue known as endomysium. Bundles of muscle fibres known as fasciculi are bound together by denser connective tissue known as perimysium. In turn, bundles of fasciculi are bound together within a fibrous coating called epimysium. Groups of muscles which function together are bound by coarse sheets of connective tissue known as fascia.

The microscopic contractile units of muscle are thousands of myofibrils contained within each muscle fibre which bring about contraction of the muscle following electrical stimulation in a complex process of sliding filaments within the myofibrils.

Muscles can contract and relax in only one direction; some muscles are longer than others depending on the amount and length of contraction needed to bring about movement. Voluntary control means that most muscles can provide a variety of strengths of contraction depending on the activity required—hence, for example, squeezing with the hand can be controlled to the extent that it can be very gentle to very strong.

Attachment

Every muscle is attached to bone at two points, the origin and the insertion. While in traditional anatomical terminology the origin does not move and the insertion is moved by the muscle contraction, in actuality the insertion can remain static and the origin move (e.g. flexing the trunk forcibly forwards against resistance reverses the origin and the insertion of the iliopsoas muscle). In order to produce movement at the levers created by bones and joints, muscles are attached to bone by tendons which are conglomerates of epimysium and perimysium connective tissue. These attach directly to the periosteum or joint capsule. Bones have numerous ridges, depressions, and roughened areas which often mark the point of attachment of muscles or the tendons associated with them. It is this attachment that enables specific muscles to act upon the levers of the skeletal system by contacting and shortening to bring two parts closer together and relaxing to allow them to move away again. Throughout the body, as one muscle contracts another on the opposite side will relax to bring about reciprocal movement.

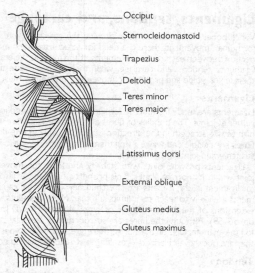

Occiput

Sternocleidomastoid

Trapezius

Deltoid

Teres minor
Teres major

Latissimus dorsi

External oblique

Gluteus medius

Gluteus maximus

Fig. 2.9 Muscle structure: main muscles of the back.

Ligaments, tendons, and cartilage

While bones, joints, and muscles provide the structures and mechanisms for human movement, there is a need for structures which make the connection between each of these elements of the musculoskeletal system; the ligaments, tendons, and cartilage, while they do not create movement in themselves, guide and protect the movement initiated by muscles.

Ligaments

Ligaments are made from *dense regular connective tissue* and join bones together at joints. The bundles of fibres all run in the same direction, offering high tensile strength in the direction of pull but only in one direction. The fibres are flexible and wavy, giving them some elasticity—allowing them to stretch when joints are in motion.

Ligaments provide joints with stability and keep the movement of the joint within its normal planes. This property, however, is also responsible for ligament injury; if joints are stretched beyond normal capacity the ligaments are likely to reach their limits and tear. Many ligaments are thickened extensions of the fibrous capsule of synovial joints (see ➲ Joints 1 and 2, pp. 56–59). Although the fibres are surrounded by fibroblasts, responsible for the manufacture of the fibres, there are few other types of cells and they are poorly vascularized—resulting in structures that do not heal easily.

Tendons

Tendons connect muscle to bone and are also constructed of dense regular connective tissue which provides tensile strength. Tendons contain fewer elastic fibres than ligaments. Where tendons become flattened into sheets connecting muscle to bone or other muscles, they are called *aponeuroses*. Tendons are often surrounded by tendon sheaths, fibrous sacs filled with lubricating fluid designed to protect tendons from friction. Some tendons are protected by larger fibrous sacs known as bursae which act as shock absorbers—e.g. at the knee and elbow.

Cartilage

Cartilage is made from *dense irregular connective tissue* which, although made of fibres similar in structure to ligaments, is laid down in a more irregular fashion, giving it more strength in numerous directions, but less flexibility. Cartilaginous tissue forms sheets within the body which primarily cover the ends of bones at joints ('hyaline' or 'articular' cartilage) and forms the fascial tissue of the muscles and organs. Being tough, but with some flexibility, it provides some protection to more vulnerable structures. Cartilage has no blood or nerve supply and is made up of >70% water, enabling it to recover when compressed and to be nourished by the constituents of tissue fluid such as protein and minerals. Its poor blood supply, however, proves problematic because of its minimal ability to heal.

There are three main types of cartilage:

- *Hyaline (or articular) cartilage*—shiny in appearance, this covers the ends of long bones at joints, joins the ribs to the sternum, and forms the end of the nose as well as the epiphyseal (growth) plates of childhood and early adulthood

- *Elastic cartilage*—is like hyaline cartilage but contains more elastic fibres
- *Fibrocartilage*—may be found at the junction of hyaline cartilage and tendons or ligaments as well as in the intervertebral discs and the menisci (cartilages) of the knee. Its exceptionally fibrous structure allows greater resistance to compression and tension.

Pathology

Ligaments, tendons, and cartilage, like all soft tissues in the body, are prone to injury. Such injuries constitute an important part of orthopaedic practice. It is, therefore, essential that the practitioner has an understanding of the anatomy and physiology of these tissues in order to inform care and treatment (see ➲ Soft tissue injury 1 and 2, pp. 356–359).

Neurovascular supply

The musculoskeletal system is richly supplied with nerves and blood vessels. These supply the nutrients needed for activity such as bone growth and muscle contraction, as well as supporting biofeedback systems. Blood vessels and nerves run side by side in bone through similar pathways.

Blood supply to bone

Bone needs a rich blood supply in order to acquire the nutrients required for bone growth, remodelling, and repair. Each bone is supplied by several major blood vessels depending on its size and position in the body.

Large nutrient arteries enter the diaphyses of bones through holes known as nutrient foramen (see ➋ Fig. 2.6, p. 45); these then divide into the proximal and distal branches and supply the diaphyses and the epiphyses. Large bones have more than one nutrient artery. The ends of long bones also receive a blood supply from metaphyseal and epiphyseal arteries supplying the joint.

Each nutrient artery divides and smaller blood vessels and capillaries enter the central/Haversian canals to supply each individual osteon within the compact bone. Capillaries enter the spongy bone from perforating canals within the compact bone, winding among the trabeculae, supplying the nutrients required for bone cell and bone marrow activity. Hence, when fractured, bones can bleed heavily resulting in significant loss of blood and forming the haematoma which is central to bone healing.

Red marrow is typically found in the centre of long bones and the diploe (central area) of flat bones. This substance, also known as haematopoietic tissue, is responsible for the production of red blood cells. Most of this activity in adults takes place at the ends of long bones and within the centre of flat bones such as the sternum and pelvis. Hence, samples of bone marrow are usually taken from these points.

The nerve supply to bone

Bone is well supplied with myelinated and unmyelinated nerves. This mostly has an autonomic sensory effect, providing feedback as well as being responsible for some of the pain felt when there is bone disease or injury. Nerves within bone run alongside blood vessels and are most prolific in the ends of long bones where they provide autonomic feedback/proprioception from the joints. This gives some of the explanation for pain in conditions such as OA. Again, each osteon receives its own nerve supply through the central canal.

Blood supply to soft tissues

Skeletal muscles provide the power for human movement and require large amounts of energy and other nutrients to accomplish this. For this reason, each muscle fibre has its own supply.

Nerve supply to soft tissues

Autonomic and voluntary nerve supplies enable the control of muscle activity, permitting humans to react quickly to their environment. Each muscle is supplied by at least one motor nerve. The nerve supply to muscle and other soft tissues originates from the spinal cord. The articular cartilage of synovial joints has no nerve supply—meaning, for example, that it cannot be responsible for the pain experienced when it is worn away in OA.

Joints 1

Bones are joined together at joints (or articulations) and act as a fulcrum to facilitate movement in the lever system of the skeleton. Each joint has a specific range of movement and is structured accordingly. Many joints contain a series of soft tissue structures such as ligaments and cartilages which help to provide stability.

Joint classifications

Joints fall into three main classifications:

Fibrous joints

Fibrous joints are the least mobile joint types. Fibrous tissue joins the bones and there is no joint cavity. There are three types of fibrous joints:

- *Sutures* are the remnants of the junctions between the floating bones of the child skull, which have serpiginous interlocking margins, and permit no movement
- *Syndesmoses* are joints in which two bones are connected by a fibrous tissue ligament. Some movement of the joint is possible, but is limited. Examples include the talofibular joint
- *Gomphoses* are joints in which a peg fits into a socket in reference only to the teeth embedded in their sockets.

Cartilaginous joints

Cartilaginous joints also have no cavity and the bones are joined by cartilage. These take two forms:

- *Synchondroses* join two bones with a plate of hyaline cartilage. Their flexibility allows bone growth during childhood and early adulthood, becoming ossified and immobile once growth stops. The epiphyseal (growth) plates at the end of long bones fall under this class as does the first sternocostal joint between the sternum and first rib
- *Symphyses* have pads of fibrocartilage between the two articulating bones. The function of this is shock absorption while allowing limited movement. Two examples are the symphysis pubis and the intervertebral joints between the vertebral bodies of the spine.

Synovial joints

Synovial joints are the most mobile, freely movable, and common and include all the limb joints. The bones are connected at a cavity containing synovial fluid. This arrangement is both strong and flexible and provides lubrication for the joint. There are five main features of a synovial joint

- A *joint cavity* which provides space for movement
- *Synovial fluid* fills the joint cavity; a viscous, glutinous fluid which acts as a lubricant and helps to reduce friction and becomes thinner when it warms up with joint use
- An *articular capsule*—a double layer of fibrous tissue which lines the joint and is continuous with the periosteum
- The *synovial membrane* lines the articular capsule and covers all surfaces which are not already covered by articular cartilage
- *Articular cartilage*—a smooth covering of the bone ends which prevents friction and absorbs shock on compression of the joint.

Many synovial joints are supported by strong ligamentous structures and some have fatty pads known as bursae which cushion bony protuberances such as the trochanters of the upper femur at the hip, the olecranon process at the elbow, and the patella (see Fig. 2.10).

Joints and their surrounding soft tissue structures are well supplied with nerve fibres which help to mediate pain and are responsible for detecting stretching and pressure in and around the joint enabling proprioception.

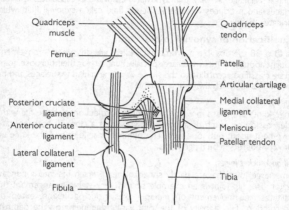

Fig. 2.10 Tendons and ligaments of the knee.

Joints 2

There are several different types of synovial joint. They are classified according to the way in which they move, and the structure of the surfaces involved. Each different type of joint produces specialized movement which reflects its function within the skeleton (see Fig. 2.11). Where the bones meet to form synovial joints, the surfaces are covered with a thin layer of articular cartilage. A very thin synovial membrane encapsulates the joint surfaces and produces a slippery viscous fluid called synovial fluid which lubricates the joint.

Classification of synovial joints

On 🠮 p. 38 the possible movements at joints are described—movements brought about by joints which are specially adapted for their purpose. Joints can be classified according to the shape of the articulating surfaces and the movements of which the joint is capable:

Hinge joints

Hinge joints are those in which a cylindrical projection of bone fits within a depression or notch of another. This enables a close fit that facilitates movement about only one axis. The humeroulnar joint and the knee are both considered to be hinge joints.

Ball and socket joints

Some large joints have a partly spherical head which fits into a concave socket. The hip joint is an example of this very stable arrangement that facilitates free movement on multiple axes including flexion, extension, and rotation. The stability of the joint varies depending on the depth of the socket and the fit of the 'ball' within it. The glenohumeral joint of the shoulder has a shallow socket and is feely movable but, consequently, lacks stability.

Plane joints

The joint surfaces of plane joints are flat, enabling only limited movement where the two surfaces glide against each other in one plane. An example is the intercarpal joints of the hand where little movement is possible because the bones are closely crowded together.

Pivot joints

At the atlantoaxial joint between cervical vertebrae 1 and 2 the odontoid peg of C2 rotates within a fibro-osseous sleeve of C1 around one axis only, demonstrating a pivot joint.

Condyloid joints

Condyloid joints have oval articulating surfaces which are convex on one side of the joint and concave on the other, allowing a close fit. This allows movements around two axes including flexion, extension, abduction, and adduction. The metacarpophalangeal (MCP) joints of the hand are a typical example.

Saddle joints

Shaped like a saddle, with both concave and convex parts of the surfaces, these joints allow greater freedom of movement than condyloid joints. The most often cited example is the carpometacarpal joint (base of the thumb).

Palastanga et al.[1] help to explain complex movements at joints by describing them as 'spin, roll, and slide':

- Spin occurs where one surface spins relative to another around a central axis
- Roll occurs where one surface rolls across the other so that different parts of each surface come into contact with one another at different times
- Slide occurs as one surface slides over the other.

Joint proprioception

Joints, the joint capsule, and ligaments all contain many nerve endings which act as receptors that provide feedback to the autonomic and central nervous systems, enabling a sense of the stretch and position of the joint largely without conscious thought.

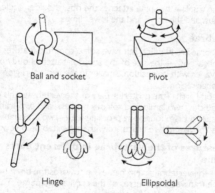

Ball and socket   Pivot

Hinge   Ellipsoidal

Fig. 2.11 Types of joint movement.

Reference

1. Palastanga N, Field D, Soames R (2006). *Anatomy and Human Movement: Structure and Function*, 5th edn, p. 5. Edinburgh: Butterworth Heinemann/Elsevier.

The spine

The vertebral column consists of 24 moveable vertebrae plus the sacrum (five fused vertebrae) and the coccyx (four fused vertebrae). It is strong and flexible, allowing the trunk to remain straight while the back moves and supports the head and the body. When it is viewed from the side the spine presents with four curves: two concave (lordoses) and two convex (kyphoses)—these enhance the strength and mobility of the backbone (see Fig. 2.12).

Functions of the vertebral column

- Vertical posture—the spine is supported and surrounded by muscles and ligaments that enable the spine to support the body in an upright position
- Mobility—the numerous individual bones, and the discs between them, enable movement of the spine
- Protection of the spinal cord—the vertebrae have central cavities that form a channel, providing a strong bony protective covering for the spinal cord
- Axis of the trunk—the spine attaches the ribs, shoulder girdle, and upper limbs, and the pelvis and the lower limbs.

The vertebrae

Not all vertebrae are identical but have some common features:
- The vertebral body—the size of the anterior flattened body of each vertebra varies with its position, smaller in the cervical region and larger in the lumbar region
- The vertebral arch—the posterior part of the vertebrae, this consists of two pedicles, two laminae, a spinous process, and two transverse processes. There are four bony prominences—two articulate with the vertebrae above and two articulate with the vertebrae below.

Special features of the vertebrae in different parts of the spine

- Cervical—the vertebral artery passes up towards the brain through a hole in the transverse processes of the cervical vertebrae. The first two cervical vertebrae are like no other:
  - The atlas—the first cervical vertebrae is a bony ring and two transverse processes; the ring is partly occupied by the odontoid process of the axis held in place by the transverse ligament There are two articulating surfaces on the atlas; these articulate with the skull and allow the nodding movement of the head.
  - The axis—the second cervical vertebrae and has a small body with the upward odontoid process that articulates with the atlas, allowing the head to turn from side to side
- Thoracic vertebrae—the body and transverse processes articulate with the ribs
- Lumbar vertebrae—the largest vertebrae are subjected to the greatest forces
- Sacrum—five vertebrae fused together to form a triangle
- Coccyx—four fused bones forming a smaller triangle and connected to the sacrum.

Intervertebral discs

The vertebrae are separated by intervertebral discs, consisting of an outer rim of fibrocartilage (annulus fibrosus) and the inner, soft, central core (the nucleus pulposus). The thickness of the discs depends on the area of the spine they are in. They absorb shock associated with movement and contribute to the flexibility of the spine.

Ligaments of the spine

Spinal ligaments hold the vertebrae in place and help maintain the position of the intervertebral discs:

- The transverse ligament maintains the position of the odontoid process
- The anterior longitudinal ligament lies in front of the vertebral bodies and extends the whole length of the spine
- The posterior longitudinal ligament extends the length of the vertebral column and lies in the vertebral canal

The spinal cord and vertebral nerves

The spinal cord originates in the brainstem and stretches to the cauda equina. It sits in the channel formed by the central cavities of the vertebrae and is surrounded by the meninges and cerebrospinal fluid (CSF). The spinal cord is one of the nervous tissue links between the brain and the rest of the body; 31 pairs of spinal nerves assist this process, originating in the medulla and exiting the spinal canal via the intervertebral foramina (see Fig. 2.13 and Fig. 2.14).

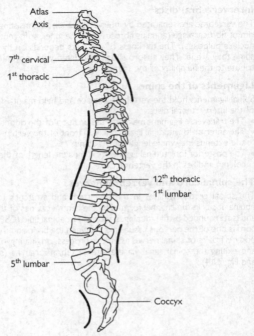

Fig. 2.12 The vertebral column. Reproduced from the *Oxford Handbook of Clinical Specialties*, 8th edn, with permission from Oxford University Press.

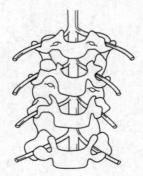

Fig. 2.13 Spinal columns and nerves.

THE SPINE   63

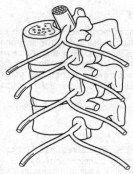

Fig. 2.14 Spinal nerves.

The shoulder

The shoulder is a joint of incredible flexibility. It is central in providing individuals with the ability to manipulate the environment. It connects the upper limb to the axial skeleton where it articulates with the thoracic cage only at the sternoclavicular joint and the scapulothoracic articulation, where the scapula glides directly over the chest wall musculature and is held in place predominantly by muscles, allowing the joint to be freely movable in most directions.

The shoulder (or pectoral) girdle is made up of the clavicle and the scapula.

The scapula

The scapula (shoulder blade) features three distinct areas:
- The broad, flat triangular blade of the scapula
- The posterior longitudinal spine of the scapula which ends in the overhanging prominence, the acromion
- The anteriorly projecting coracoid process.

The scapula articulates with the humerus at the glenohumeral joint and with the clavicle at the acromioclavicular joint. The surface of the scapula is roughened in various places to facilitate the attachment of the series of muscles in which it is 'clothed' and which are responsible for shoulder and upper limb movement. The superior end of the lateral border of the scapula forms a shallow depression, the glenoid fossa, which articulates with the head of humerus to form the glenohumeral joint. This joint is viewed as the main shoulder joint as most movement takes place here.

The clavicle

The clavicles are slender rods with two bends that form the superior border of the chest wall and which articulate with the manubrium of the sternum to form the sternoclavicular joint at one end, and with the acromion to form the acromioclavicular joint at the other.

This acts as a brace for movements, placing stress on the arm and superior chest, making it vulnerable to transferred extreme stress and injury following a fall landing with the body weight on an outstretched hand and arm.

Soft tissue structures

Due to its flexibility, the shoulder is also seen as being a relatively unstable joint. The glenohumeral joint forms only a shallow 'ball-and-socket joint' and can be likened to a golf ball on a golf tee, consequently having minimal bony stability. This is only partly resolved by the muscles, tendons, and ligaments which surround the shoulder and attach it to the thorax, upper spine, and head.

The shallow glenoid cavity is only slightly deepened by a rim of cartilage, this provides little assistance in stabilizing the joint and it is prone to dislocation.

Several ligaments, varying in strength, provide some reinforcement to the anterior aspect of the shoulder, providing support for the arm (see Fig. 2.15). Several muscle tendons cross the shoulder joint, including the *long head of biceps*, and these are central in providing stability of the joint. They act as bands, securing the humeral head in the glenoid cavity. More important still are the rotator cuff tendons—a series of four strong structures which are wrapped around each other and around the glenohumeral joint—the tendons of subscapularis, supraspinatus, infraspinatus, and teres minor. The rotator cuff is frequently injured by a combination of attritional change due to impingement and falling on an abducted arm.

Blood and nerve supply

The rich blood supply to the shoulder is derived from the subclavian and axillary arteries. The blood vessels branch across the scapular region, supplying the large muscles. The nerve supply for the shoulder comes from the major nerve roots derived from C5, C6, and C7.

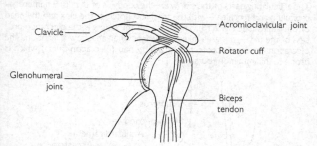

Clavicle

Acromioclavicular joint

Rotator cuff

Glenohumeral joint

Biceps tendon

Fig. 2.15 Shoulder showing rotator cuff.

The elbow

Although the elbow joint is not as flexible as the shoulder or the hand, it has an important role to play in activity. It facilitates flexibility of the upper limb because it allows the arm to bend at the centre. This means that the hand can reach other areas of the body, such as the mouth, to enable feeding, washing, and dressing activities as well as reaching out to undertake activities of daily life. Consequently, when elbow movement is restricted, many activities of daily living can become difficult, particularly if the dominant arm is involved.

The elbow is a synovial hinge joint, which enables flexion and extension (the rotation that facilitates supination and pronation of the lower arm is brought about at the proximal radioulnar joint which is contained within the same joint capsule). There is a relatively lax joint capsule.

Bony structures

The articulating parts of the elbow are the condyles of the distal humerus—capitulum and trochlea—with the trochlear notch of the ulna and the head of the radius (see Fig. 2.16). The 'point' of the elbow is the olecranon process of the ulna—this area takes the weight when an elbow is leant on. The olecranon process is protected by a fatty pad (olecranon bursa) which is prone to inflammation (bursitis).

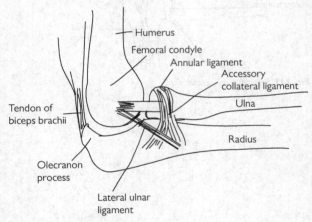

Fig. 2.16 Anatomy of the elbow.

Soft tissues

The soft tissues of the elbow help to provide stability, including strong collateral ligaments (radial/lateral and ulnar/medial) on both sides of the elbow which prevent the joint from rotating. The tendons of the muscles of the upper arm (including biceps, triceps, and brachialis) cross the elbow providing additional stability and strength. Such structures enable a full range of motion, but can 'lock' the elbow in a stable extended position when needed for carrying objects at arm's length and when placing body weight through the arm (e.g. when pushing up from a prone lying position and crawling).

When the arm is fully extended, the bones forming the joint are not fully aligned, resulting in a deviation of the lower arm away from the body when the palm of the hand is facing forwards. This is known as the 'carrying angle' and enables carrying items (such as shopping bags) in a manner that allows them to swing without colliding with the hip or leg. The carrying angle can be disrupted by injury to the elbow. Flexion is performed by the contraction of the anterior muscle brachialis with the contribution of the biceps if the forearm is supinated. Extension is carried out by triceps, which live posterior to the humerus.

Blood and nerve supply

The blood supply to the elbow and lower arm is derived mainly from branches of the brachial artery. The vessels pass close to the distal aspect of the humerus and cross the elbow, offering potential for damage following musculoskeletal injury to this region. The nerve supply is derived from the musculocutaneous, median, radial, and ulnar nerves.

The wrist and hand

The wrist and hand are very flexible, being capable of fine movement. They are formed of 27 small bones (see Fig. 2.17).

The wrist

The wrist is made up of two rows of bones collectively known as the carpal bones The proximal row consists of the scaphoid, lunate, triquetral, and pisiform bones. The distal row consists of the trapezium, trapezoid, capitate, and hamate. There are four articulations among them and the proximal bones articulate with the radius and ulna.

The hand

The hand is made up of five bones, one for each of the fingers, together called the metacarpus. They are long bones and articulate with the carpal bones and the phalanges.

The fingers

These are made up of 14 phalanges, three in each finger and two in the thumb. They articulate with each other and the metacarpals (see Fig. 2.17).

Joints

The hand and wrist consist of a large number of small joints, all of which are synovial. The metacarpophalangeal (MCP) joints are formed by the connections of the phalanges to the metacarpals. The MCP joints work like a hinge to bend and straighten the fingers and thumb. The three phalanges are separated by two interphalangeal (IP) joints. The one closest to the MCP joint is called the proximal IP (PIP) joint, and the one near the end of the finger is the distal IP (DIP) joint. The thumb only has one IP joint between the two phalanges. The IP joints of the digits are also hinges joints for bending and straightening the fingers and thumb.

Ligaments and tendons

The collateral ligaments on either side of each finger and thumb joints prevent abnormal, sideways bending of each joint (see Fig. 2.17).

The PIP joint has the strongest ligament, the volar plate which connects the proximal phalanx to the middle phalanx on the palm side; it tightens as the joint is straightened and keeps the PIP joint from bending back too far.

The extensor tendons of the fingers begin as muscles that arise from the posterior aspect of the forearm bones, they then travel towards the hand, where they eventually connect to the extensor tendons and cross over the back of the wrist joint. As they move up into the fingers, the extensor tendons become the extensor hood. The extensor hood flattens out to cover the top of the fingers and sends out branches on each side that connect to the bones in the middle and end of the finger. When the extensor muscles contract, they tug on the extensor tendons to straighten the fingers.

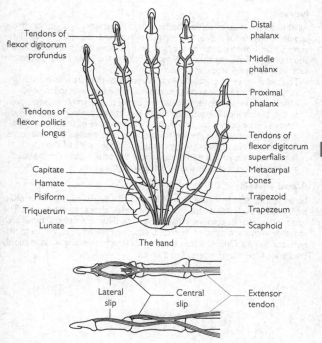

Fig. 2.17 Hand and finger tendon structure.

Muscles

Muscles that control the hand start at the elbow or forearm. The muscles run down the forearm and cross the wrist and hand. They can be broken down into several categories:

- Extrinsic muscles—provide power in flexion and extension of the fingers and the thumb through the long tendons either in the palm or the back of the hand
- Intrinsic muscles—communicate fine movement to the fingers
- Interosseous muscles—allow the fingers to be separated and brought together
- Lumbrical muscles—lie between the fingers and allow for flexion and extension
- Thenar muscle—mobilizes the thumb, helping move the thumb so the pad of the thumb can touch the tips each of each finger on the same hand, this is called opposition
- Hypothenar muscle—mobilizes the little finger.

Nerves

All the nerves that travel to the hand and fingers begin together at the shoulder: the radial nerve, the median nerve, and the ulnar nerve. They carry signals from the brain to the muscles that move the arm, hand, fingers, and thumb. The nerves also carry signals back to the brain about sensations such as touch, pain, and temperature.

- The radial nerve runs along the radial aspect of the forearm, providing sensation to a small area on the dorsum of the first web space only.
- The median nerve travels through the carpal tunnel providing sensation to the thumb, index finger, long finger, and half of the ring finger. It also sends a nerve branch to control the thenar muscles of the thumb. The ring finger innervations are variable between the median and ulna nerve.
- The ulnar nerve supplies feeling to the little finger and half the ring finger. Branches of this nerve also supply the small muscles in the palm and the muscle that pulls the thumb toward the palm.

Blood vessels

Large vessels supply the hand with blood. The largest artery is the radial artery that travels across the front of the wrist, closest to the thumb. The ulnar artery runs next to the ulnar nerve. The ulnar and radial arteries arch together within the palm of the hand, supplying the front of the hand, fingers, and thumb. Other arteries travel across the back of the wrist to supply the back of the hand, fingers, and thumb.

The hip

The hip (coxal) joint is formed from the articulation of the head of the femur and the acetabulum of the innominate bone of the pelvis. It is central in the transfer of weight from the trunk and upper part of the body to the legs placing the joint under considerable stresses throughout life and making it particularly vulnerable to the destructive forces of OA. It is also an important part of the lever system that is responsible for ambulation. As a ball-and-socket joint, the hip is mobile in almost every plane—producing flexion, extension, adduction, abduction, and medial and lateral rotation—enabling the body to twist and turn during weight-bearing movement. This is restricted only by the depth of the acetabulum and the soft tissue structures which surround the joint. The hip is very different from the shoulder joint because it has bony structures which provide stability.

Bony structures of the hip

The almost spherical head of the femur sits within the deep socket of the acetabulum at the junction of the three major parts of the innominate bone. Both are smooth and covered in a thick layer of articular cartilage. The acetabulum is further deepened by a ring of fibrocartilage known as the acetabular labrum. The synovial capsule completely surrounds the joint and includes the, much narrower, neck of the femur from which the rest of the femur angulates away. See Fig. 2.18.

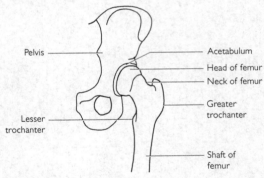

Pelvis

Acetabulum

Head of femur

Neck of femur

Greater trochanter

Lesser trochanter

Shaft of femur

Fig. 2.18 Hip joint.

Soft tissue structures of the hip

The joint is traversed by a series of strong, but relatively short, muscles which link the pelvis to the upper femur and bring about the full range of movement at the joint, often under weight-bearing conditions. Specific muscles bring about specific actions:

- The hip joint is extended by the large mass of gluteal and hamstring muscles on the posterior side of the joint.
- On the anterior and lateral side of the joint the gluteal muscles and the tensor fascia lata provide the abduction movement.
- On the medial side of the joint, the adductor muscles provide adduction.
- The muscles flexing the joint are iliopsoas and pectineus, sartorius, and rectus femoris.
- The hip is medially rotated by some of the gluteals, psoas major, and iliacus.
- Lateral rotation is brought about by gluteus maximus, piriformis, and the obturator and gemellus groups of muscles.

The hip joint is supported by several strong ligaments, most of which are outside the hip joint. A small, weak ligament (ligamentum teres or ligamentum capitis) is attached to a small depression on the crest of the head of the femur, the fovea capitis, but does not provide much additional stability to the joint.

Nerve and blood supplies to the hip

The main nerve supply to the hip joint is the femoral nerves and obturator nerves which are formed from the lumbar plexus. Many of these nerves supply the upper leg down to the knee, so problems in the hip, such as OA, can sometimes manifest as referred pain in the knee.

The blood supply to the hip is derived from branches of the femoral artery and an artery within the teres ligament. The head of the femur is supplied by blood vessels which run over the neck of the femur and enter the head through several small foramens around the subcapital region. This blood supply is easily disrupted in femoral neck fractures, directing the surgical decisions made (see ➲ Hip fracture presentation, pp. 438–439) as this can lead to avascular necrosis of the femoral head.

The knee

The knee is the largest and the most complex joint in the body. With little natural stability, the joint is supported by a complex series of ligaments, tendons, and cartilaginous structures. The knee is mainly a hinge joint, allowing flexion and extension, although there is a small degree of rotation possible when there is no weight borne through the joint. During standing and ambulation, the knee joints carry the full weight of the body and are placed under considerable stress, particularly to excessive rotational movements. Consequently, the soft tissue structures are easily damaged in high-energy and contact sports injuries (see ➲ Soft tissue injury 1 and 2, pp. 356–359).

The bony structures of the knee

The knee joint is comprised of three joints: (1) the *lateral* and (2) *medial femorotibial joints* at the articulation of the condyles of the femur and the tibial condyles (which are separated by the intercondylar eminence—making these appear as two separate joints); and (3) the patella glides over the distal femur during flexion and extension of the knee, forming the *femoropatellar joint*. The condyles of the femur are wheel-like structures, which facilitates their movement during flexion and extension across the much flatter tibial condyles (which are sometimes known as the tibial plateaux). All the articulating surfaces are covered in a layer of articular cartilage. The tibiofemoral joints are contained within one large synovial capsule.

The patella is a small, almost triangular, sesamoid bone suspended in the tendon of the quadriceps. This provides protection to the anterior aspect of the knee, particularly during kneeling, and produces additional leverage from the quadriceps femoris muscle. The articular surface is convex to facilitate the gliding movement.

The soft tissue structures of the knee

There is no stability provided by the bony structures in the knee joint. This is compensated for by several complex ligaments, cartilages, and tendons. See ➲ Fig. 2.10, p. 57.

Two short *cruciate* ligaments cross each other in the centre of the knee. The anterior cruciate ligament (so called because its inferior attachment is anterior) is attached to the medial surface of the lateral femoral condyles, and inferiorly and posteriorly to the anterior tibial spine. The posterior cruciate ligament (so called because its inferior attachment is posterior) attaches to the medial femoral condyle and then tracks anteriorly, attaching to the posterior intercondylar spine of the tibia. These two closely associated ligaments are central to the stability of the knee but are under considerable pressure during rotational movements which occur during weight bearing, resulting in injuries such as complete tears of the ligaments.

Sitting on top of the lateral and medical tibial condyles are two cartilages which help to give additional depth and shock-absorbing properties to the shallow articular surfaces: the medial and lateral menisci or semilunar cartilages. The menisci are attached only to the outer aspects of the joint surface, making them vulnerable to being torn away.

These structures are bathed in synovial fluid which inhibits soft tssue healing, so when injured, healing is impaired.

Outside the joint capsule, on each side of the knee, are the lateral and medial collateral ligaments which laterally attach the lateral and medial femoral condyles to a roughened area inferior to the medial tibial condyles and the fibular head to prevent rotation.

The nerve and blood supply to the knee

The blood supply to the knee is delivered from branches of the femoral artery and the popliteal artery. The popliteal artery crosses the back of the knee and must be considered carefully when bandaging, applying splints, and casting in this area.

The nerve supply to the knee is formed from branches of the femoral nerve, the obturator nerve, and the tibial and the common peroneal nerve. The peroneal nerve winds around the head of the fibula and is prone to injury because of its superficial position here.

The ankle and foot

The ankles and feet allow the body, through their flexibility to balance, to be stable; they carry the body weight, act as shock absorbers, and allow us to stand erect and move around with ease. There are 28 bones in each foot and ankle which add to the suppleness and help to allow adaptation of the foot to a variety of different surfaces (see Fig. 2.19).

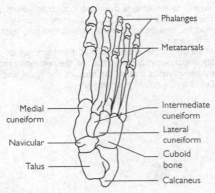

Fig. 2.19 Foot and ankle bones.

The ankle

The ankle consists of one bone—the talus—that articulates with the tibia and fibula.

The hindfoot and midfoot

The hindfoot and midfoot are complex joint structures and consist of:
- The calcaneus—forming the heel of the foot and bearing the most force when walking is taking place
- The navicular—a boat-shaped bone
- The cuboid—articulates with the 4th and 5th metatarsals, forming the 4th and 5th tarsometatarsal joints as well as with the calcaneus forming the calcaneocuboid joint. The calcaneocuboid joint helps with foot stability
- Three cuneiform bones—articulating with each other and the metatarsal bones.

Metatarsal bones of the foot

There are five metatarsals which form the dorsum of the foot and articulate with the tarsal bones and the phalanges. The distal head of the first metatarsal is enlarged, forming the ball of the foot.

Phalanges

There are 14 phalanges arranged very like the fingers, with three in each toe except for the big toe (hallux), which has two.

Arches of the foot

The foot arches are formed by the bones, ligaments, and tendons of the foot and are essential for both movement and weight bearing. The foot has distinct arches—two 'longitudinal' arches (one on each side) and one transverse arch running across the midfoot:

- The medial longitudinal arch—the most prominent foot arch, runs from front to back along the inside of the foot and absorbs most of the shock of impact during walking, jumping, or running
- The lateral longitudinal arch—runs parallel to the medial longitudinal arch along the outer edge of the foot
- The transverse arch—runs across the midfoot from outside to inside, providing support and flexibility to the foot.

The arches of the foot are maintained both by the shapes of the bones and by the ligaments. Muscles and tendons also play an important role in supporting the arches.

Foot and toe movement

Toe movements take place at the joints; the joints are capable of motion in two directions: plantarflexion or dorsiflexion as well as abduction and adduction of the toes.

The foot as a whole has two movements: inversion and eversion.

Muscles, ligaments, and tendons

The tendons and ligaments are vital and give feet their flexibility, allow for movement, and absorb impact (see Fig. 2.20).

- The Achilles tendon—connected to the calcaneum and allows movement to rise up onto the toes and flex the heel
- Tendons surrounding the toes—allow the toes to bend and stretch.

Many of the muscles of the feet work in partnership with those of the lower leg, allowing walking, running, or remaining static. The muscles of the foot are classed as either intrinsic or extrinsic:

- Intrinsic muscles have both attachments within the foot and control the movement of the toes. Several of these muscles also help the ligaments with supporting the arch of the foot
- Extrinsic muscles originate from anywhere in the lower leg, their long tendons cross the ankle joint and insert onto one of the bones of the foot.

Nerves

The nerves permit sensation and send messages to other parts of the body. There are many nerves within the foot, some help us feel the surface we are walking on, others tell the muscles when to contract and relax.

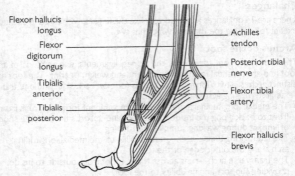

Fig. 2.20 Tendons of the foot and ankle. Reproduced from the *Oxford Handbook of Clinical Specialties*, 8th edn, with permission from Oxford University Press.

Assessment of the musculoskeletal system

Principles of assessment

Introduction

It is important to adopt a structured, timely, and systematic approach when assessing the patient to avoid missing vital information and minimizing repetition. Assessment should be interprofessional and a collaborative shared assessment document is preferable to uniprofessional documentation to avoid replicating questions or investigations and examination. Although the focus of this chapter is assessment of the orthopaedic or trauma patient, it is important to remember the assessment should be holistic and comprehensive and that most patients will have comorbid conditions as well as their presenting musculoskeletal problem. The specific format of the assessment will depend on the presentation of the patient, e.g. acute trauma, initial presentation to orthopaedic services, or ongoing or follow-up episodes. However, regardless of presentation, there are a number of key principles to assessment that should be adopted:

- Always introduce yourself to the patient and explain what the assessment is going to involve.
- Ensure the patient is as comfortable as possible and there is privacy during the assessment and their dignity is respected at all times (specifically in relation to asking sensitive questions and requiring patients to remove clothing for physical examination).
- Check if the patient has any special needs such as communication or learning difficulties and use appropriate aids and support to ensure the patient is able to understand what is being asked (see ➔ People with a learning disability or cognitive impairments, p. 22).
- Be mindful not to overtire older or frail patients with prolonged questioning and examination—patients may need a break and the assessment may need to be undertaken in several smaller episodes.
- Always record all of your findings both positive and negative, e.g. the patient reports no previous or current respiratory problems.

Methods of obtaining information during the assessment process

There are a number of methods of collecting information about the patient during the assessment process including:
- Observation—what we see, hear, and smell
- History taking—see ➔ History taking 1 and 2, pp. 82–85
- Physical examination—inspection for joint swelling, muscle wasting, bruising, scarring indicating previous surgery or trauma
- Use of patient-reported outcome measures (PROMs) and disease-specific and general measures of health
- Clinical investigations.

This list is presented in the order in which the assessment should usually be conducted.

Patients presenting with acute trauma or emergency situations

When a patient presents with acute major trauma such as suspected head injury, spinal injury, or multiple fractures the guiding principle is the rapid identification of life-threatening or life-changing injuries using the structured (C)ABCDE approach[1,2]:

- (Catastrophic haemorrhage)
- Airway with spinal protection
- Breathing
- Circulation
- Disability (neurological)
- Exposure and Environment.

See ➔ Advanced Trauma Life Support (ATLS®), p. 328 for further detail on this approach.[1,2]

General structure of patient assessment

The first stage of assessment is general *observation* of the patient. Observation includes what we see, hear, and smell, and includes:

- General appearance—do they look well groomed or unkempt, significantly under- or overweight for their height?
- Does their body language indicate they are in pain either at rest or when mobilizing?
- Does their gait indicate any lower limb dysfunction/injury, use of any walking aids, splints, or other orthotic appliances?
- Does their skin tone indicate any obvious pallor, flushing, or jaundice?

The nurse should then proceed onto taking a history using the systematic approach detailed on ➔ History taking 1 and 2, pp. 82–85. Dependent on information elicited during the history, the nurse should then decide what type of *physical examination* needs to be conducted taking into consideration that often pain may be referred. Physical examination includes techniques such as palpation, auscultation, and measuring leg length and range of joint movement (see ➔ Principles of physical assessment of the hip, pp. 98–99). Range of movement should be measured using a goniometer. When using a goniometer ensure the movement is free of any muscle contraction and three measurements should be taken of the same movement and a mean value recorded. It is important during observation and physical examination to compare both limbs and to consider that joints and limbs can be grossly distorted by trauma or disease and so identification of key landmarks is essential.

Once physical examination is completed the patient should be made comfortable before proceeding to administer any generic or disease specific indices or PROMs that are relevant to the patient's condition. Finally, based on findings from the history and examination, decisions are made regarding what clinical investigations are necessary to complete the information-gathering process, e.g. X-rays, blood tests, etc.

References

1. NICE (2016). Major trauma: assessment and initial management. NICE guideline [NG39]. ℬ https://www.nice.org.uk/guidance/ng39
2. Parker M, Magnusson C (2016). Assessment of trauma. *Int J Orthop Trauma Nurs* 21:21–30.

Further reading

Flynn S, Pugh H, Jester R (2015). Clinical assessment in trauma and orthopaedic nursing. *Int J Orthop Trauma Nurs* 19:162–9.

History taking 1

Taking an accurate and comprehensive history is the most important step towards completing a holistic assessment of the orthopaedic or trauma patient. The nature of presentation of the patient will determine the time scale and depth of history that is needed. Patients presenting in the emergency department (ED) will need a rapid assessment focusing on airway, breathing, and circulation and often details of the presenting problem will be taken from the ambulance crew and/or accompanying friends or relatives if the patient is unable to communicate themselves. However, patients presenting as elective orthopaedic cases to primary care settings, outpatients, or the inpatient unit will enable the nurse to take a more comprehensive history. Patients are not always accurate historians and the nurse should verify data from accessory sources such as the patient's medical notes, referral letter, and next of kin. Communication difficulties either due to speech or cognition problems require the nurse to access support mechanisms such as interpreters, use of sign boards, and non-verbal communication (see ➲ p. 166). It is important to avoid using medical jargon.

Structure of the history

- Chief complaint
- History of chief complaint
- Recapitulation
- Family history
- Past medical history
- Medications
- Alcohol and smoking habits
- Social and occupational history
- Allergies
- Review of all body systems—head-to-toe approach
- Patient's questions and health promotion opportunities.

Application of the history framework

The nurse should check the patient's identity, introduce themselves, ensure the patient is comfortable, and that the environment facilitates privacy before the history-taking process begins. The patient's medical notes and referral letter should have been read before the consultation begins. Open-ended questions should be posed during the interview and the nurse should avoid asking leading questions to fit the patient into a diagnostic category.

Chief complaint

To elicit the chief complaint ask the patient why they have sought the help of orthopaedic services. Typically, this will be because the patient has pain in a particular joint/s or limb/s. If we take pain as a worked example, the history of the chief complaint will require the following questions:

- Where is the pain and is it localized or diffuse?
- What alleviates or exacerbates the pain?
- When did they first notice the pain and was it associated with a particular trauma or event?

- Is the pain constant or intermittent? Are there any particular times of the day or night that the pain worsens?
- Are there any associated symptoms (e.g. swelling, paraesthesia, locking or giving way)?
- What type of pain is it (e.g. burning, stabbing, dull ache, etc.)?
- What is the severity of the pain? Using a valid and appropriate pain assessment scale.
- What impact does the pain have on their quality of life and functional ability?

Once these questions have been explored, it is important to recapitulate your summary of the patient's condition as they have described it so far. This provides an opportunity to clarify any misunderstanding or to add anything the patient feels is important.

Past medical history

Ask the patient to think about any significant past medical problems, such as surgery and admissions to hospital. Patients may require some prompting as they are often anxious and forget important past illnesses. This is why it is important to have read through the patient's notes before the consultation so you can ask direct questions as prompts, e.g. 'I noticed you were seeing the heart specialist—why was that?' Use of acronyms such as 'MITJTHREADS' (myocardial Infarction, Thromboembolism, Jaundice, Tuberculosis, Hypertension, Rheumatic fever, Epilepsy, Asthma, Diabetes, Stroke) can help you structure your questioning.[1]

Family history

Ask the patient if they know of any illnesses that run in their family, e.g. RA, diabetes, cancer, or heart disease. Often a genogram is the most succinct method of recording the family history. Remind patients this relates to blood relations such as parents, grandparents, and siblings.

Medications

Whenever possible, patients should bring their medications with them to the consultation or at least an up-to-date prescription print-out. It is important to ascertain what medications patients are taking including prescription, over-the-counter, complementary therapies, and recreational drug use. Also, this part of the history gives an opportunity to cross-verify information in the past medical history and elicit the patient's concordance and understanding of the medications they are taking. Drugs such as aspirin and warfarin may need to be stopped prior to orthopaedic surgery.

Alcohol and smoking history

Both alcohol and smoking have an adverse impact on osteoblastic activity and can lead to a reduction in bone density. Smoking history should be recorded as packs per day × number of years. Alcohol consumption should be units per week. The deleterious effects of smoking and excessive alcohol consumption should be addressed with the patient at the end of the assessment process.

History taking 2

Application of the history framework (continued)

Social and occupational history

It is important to elicit the patient's home situation in terms of support from family/friends, social services, and voluntary organizations, along with questions about the layout of their home in terms of access to the property, availability of grab rails, stair lifts, and where the bathroom is situated. Patients may still be in paid or voluntary employment or be the family carer for a dependent relative; this needs to be taken into consideration in terms of discharge planning following surgery or arranging respite care for the dependent relative. Exposure to hazardous substances due to occupation or hobbies should be explored.

Allergies

Eliciting allergies is important for patient safety. Specific questions about allergy to antibiotics, latex, and adhesive dressings should be asked. If the patient declares an allergy, the nurse needs to probe about the nature and the severity of the reaction and these need to be clearly documented in the patient's notes and identified with an allergy sticker.

Review of body systems

Many orthopaedic and trauma patients are older people and are likely to have comorbid conditions. Typically, older patients may suffer with hypertension, atrial fibrillation, and type 2 diabetes as well as their chief complaint of joint/limb pain. Thus, it is important to ask specific questions pertaining to each of the body systems as detailed in Table 3.1.

Table 3.1 Review of body systems

Body system	Example cues
Integumentary	Presence of skin lesions, sores, unhealed wounds, abrasions, rashes, fungal infections of nails
Mental health	Depression and anxiety
Neurological	Fits, faints, headaches, muscle weakness/wasting/altered sensation
	Problems with coordination and/or balance, memory, swallowing difficulties, hearing or sight problems
Respiratory	Shortness of breath, wheezing, bronchitis, asthma, chest infection
Cardiovascular	Chest pain, circulatory problems including leg ulcers, varicose veins
Musculoskeletal	Joint pain, swelling, locking or giving way, limited range of movement, fractures, muscle, tendon, ligament injury
Gastrointestinal	Gastric bleeding, ulcers, stomach pain, oesophageal reflux, abnormal bowel habits
Genitourinary	Frequency and urgency of micturition, nocturia, hesitancy, incontinence, urine infection

In addition to the review of systems detailed in Table 3.1, it is important to ask about the patient's general health status, e.g. weight changes, general well-being, sleep, fatigue, etc. When recording the history, remember to record negative as well as positive responses, e.g. 'Patient reports no neurological symptoms'.

Patient's questions and health promotion opportunities
The final stage of the history-taking process allows patients an opportunity to ask questions and to use the findings from your history to engage the patient in positive health promotion such as advice on smoking cessation, weight reduction, and medication review by their GP or local pharmacist.

Conclusion

A systematic approach to history taking is needed to avoid duplications/ omissions and to conduct the process in a timely manner. Always remember to introduce yourself to patients prior to history taking and gain their consent to proceed. Following history taking, the assessment should continue by conducting a focused examination of the parts of the body pertinent to the chief complaint and any other problems reported through the review of systems. Examination requires knowledge of normal anatomy and physiology and the following skills:
• Observation and inspection
• Palpation
• Auscultation
• Percussion
• Measurement of active and passive range of movement of joints
• Gait analysis.

Reference

1. Fishman J, Cullen L, Gressman A (2014). *History Taking in Medicine and Surgery*, 3rd ed. Oxford: PasTest, University of Oxford.

Further reading

Flynn S, Pugh H, Jester R (2015). Clinical assessment in trauma and orthopaedic nursing. *Int J Orthop Trauma Nurs* 19:162–9.

Principles of physical assessment of the shoulder

The shoulder is a complex area to examine due to its multiple structures, articulations, and extensive range of movements. Occasionally, patients presenting with shoulder pain may have a problem with their cervical spine and therefore it is often necessary to carry out an examination of the cervical spine (see ➋ Principles of assessment of the bony spine, pp. 96–97) to rule out referred pain. Both shoulder girdles and upper limbs should be assessed. The patient will need to be undressed to the waist for the assessment, so privacy and dignity are important issues for the nurse to address.

Assessment of the shoulder complex should include:

History taking

Elicit the chief complaint which is likely to be shoulder pain and/or restricted movement. Shoulder pain can be localized or more diffuse around the shoulder and/or radiating down the arm as pain travels down the nerve pathways. Also patients can present with shoulder pain due to injury or disease to other parts of the body such as the neck, gall bladder, or heart.[1] Apply the questions template presented on ➋ History taking 1 and 2, pp. 82–85 to elicit the nature/details of pain and injury. Also ascertain if specific functional activities are difficult and/or painful such as brushing the front and back of their hair, undoing a bra, or taking something out of their back trouser pocket. Ascertain the patient's activities related to their occupation/sporting and leisure activities. Sports such as tennis, swimming, and golf may precipitate shoulder pain/injury. Injury such as falls onto an outstretched hand or an elbow or generalized reporting of cervical spine and shoulder pain can provide useful clues to the possible cause of the chief complaint.

Observation

Observe anterior/posterior and lateral aspects to ascertain any abnormality in bone and soft tissue outline e.g. muscle wasting of the deltoids, biceps, triceps, trapezius, or subluxation or dislocation of the glenohumeral joint. Also perform general observation of the patient to elicit non-verbal signs of discomfort, pain, or supporting the limb in a protective stance. Listen for sounds of crepitus when conducting active/passive range of movement.

Inspection

Inspect for signs of swelling, redness, inflammation, bruising, and scars from previous surgery or trauma.

Palpation

This should include eliciting signs and symptoms of tenderness, muscle spasm, abnormal bumps or indentations, swelling, abnormal or loss of sensation to touch, and evidence of altered temperature of the joints (increased warmth).

Movement

Active movements should be carried out prior to passive range of movement. It is only necessary to carry out a passive range of movement if the patient has been unable to carry out the full range of active movements. The assessment should be structured so that the most painful movements reported by the patient during the history are left until last, to avoid 'carry over' pain to the next movement. For example, patients with suspected impingement syndrome will typically report difficulty with abduction between 60° and 120°. Range of active movement should include:

- Circumduction (200°)
- Elevation through abduction (180°)
- Elevation through forward flexion (160–180°)
- External/lateral rotation (90°)
- Internal/medial rotation (60–90°)
- Adduction (50–75°)
- Horizontal adduction/abduction (cross-flexion/cross extension 130°)
- Extension (50–60°)
- Elevation through the plane of the scapula (170–180°).

Special physical examination tests

There are many specific tests that may be used to aid diagnosis of joint instability, impingement, labral tears, scapular instability, muscle or tendon injury.

Examples include:

- Scarf test—for acromioclavicular joint pain
- Subscapularis testing using Gerber's lift-off test
- Impingement testing using Neer's sign.

Disease-specific measures of shoulder pain/dysfunction

There are a number of specific clinician- or patient-reported measures that can be used during assessment of the shoulder including:

- Rotator Cuff-Quality of Life (RC-QoL) and the Western Ontario Rotator Cuff (WORC) Index, both used in suspected rotator cuff injury
- Oxford shoulder score—patient self-report measure
- Rowe Score for Instability—clinician administered for joint instability
- DASH (disabilities of arm, shoulder, and hand) score—patient self-report measure.

Clinical investigations

X-rays have a limited role in detecting shoulder problems as they do not show problems with soft tissue (muscles, tendons, cartilage) which are frequently the cause of shoulder pain. However, they are necessary to detect bony injury such as fracture, dislocation, or subluxation and detecting osteoarthritic changes such as reduced joint space and osteophytes. Ultrasound scanning is very useful to detect thickening of soft tissue, damage to tendons and muscles, and the presence of fluid within the joint. Magnetic resonance imaging (MRI) is also very useful in detecting rotator cuff and other soft tissue injury.

Reference and further reading

1. Kenyon P, Flynn S, Marlow W (2018). Assessment of the adult patient presenting with shoulder pain. *Int J Orthop Trauma Nurs* 28:40–5.

Principles of physical assessment of the elbow

Elbow injury and disease is most commonly associated with either occupational or sporting injury, e.g. tennis elbow, with patients presenting with pain on the lateral side of their elbow and difficulty in holding objects at arm's length due to repetitive strain through activities such as sweeping, painting, or playing tennis.[1] Primary and secondary OA are relatively common in the elbow and frequently present as locking of the joint caused by loose bodies. RA also often affects one or both elbows presenting as painful and tender joints, fixed flexion deformity, synovitis, and loss of function of the lower arm. It is very common for patients presenting with loss of function of the lower arm to have both shoulder and/or elbow pathology and therefore it is important to examine both joints. Difficulty with pronation/supination can be related to elbow, wrist, or the ulna and radius.

Assessment of the elbow should include:

History taking

Elicit the chief complaint and the history of its onset which may be:
- Pain over lateral and/or medial, anterior, and posterior aspects of the elbow at rest or when carrying out specific movements such as gripping, wrist flexion, or pronation
- Numbness and tingling below the level of the elbow
- Tenderness and swelling of the joint
- Locking and/or instability of the joint.

Observation/inspection

The patient needs to undress from the waist up to permit observation of the upper arm/shoulders. Specifically look for and note:[1]
- Patients holding their elbow/s in a semi-flexed position due to swelling
- Joint effusion
- Bursitis or rheumatoid nodules
- Muscle wasting above or below the joint
- Tenderness and/or heat over the joint
- Locking or fixed flexion deformities
- Swelling of the olecranon bursa.

Vascular assessment

Check the radial and ulnar pulses and note any skin discoloration or altered skin temperature of the lower forearm.

Sensory assessment

The median, radial, and ulnar nerves are related to various anatomical structures within the elbow joint and its musculature. Check for altered or loss of sensation in the medial/lateral and anterior/posterior aspects of the lower arm. Ulnar nerve palsy generally has a gradual onset following injury to the elbow.

Movement

The range of active extension and flexion should be measured where possible using a goniometer, although a quick visual check of range of active flexion can be assessed by asking the patient to touch both shoulders. The normal range of extension/flexion is 0–145°, but some patients, particularly women, may be able to hyperextend the elbow by as much as 15°. Supination and pronation are assessed by asking the patient to keep their elbows flexed and close to their sides and then turn the palms upward (supination) and then downward (pronation). The normal range for supination is 80° and 75° pronation.

Disease-specific measures of the elbow

Tinel's sign is used to indicate cubital tunnel syndrome (compression of the ulnar nerve). This test involves the examiner tapping the patient's ulnar nerve near to the cubital tunnel several times and the sign is considered positive if the tapping induces symptoms of tingling and paraesthesia. Clinician-completed scores include the Mayo elbow score and patient-completed measures include the Oxford elbow score and the DASH score, which comes in both full and abbreviated versions.

Clinical investigations

X-rays of the elbow are appropriate to diagnose fractures and dislocations and changes to joints due to RA or OA. Nerve conduction studies are still sometimes used to test the amplitude and velocity of nerve conduction, specifically in diagnosing cubital tunnel syndrome. Blood tests such as a full blood count (FBC) may be indicated if infection of the joint is suspected, or inflammatory markers if RA is suspected.

Reference

1. Magee D (2014). *Orthopaedic Physical Assessment*, 6th edn (Musculoskeletal Rehabilitation). St. Louis, MO: Saunders Elsevier.

Further reading

🔊 http://www.orthopaedicscores.com

Principles of assessment of the wrist

The wrist and hand are usually assessed together as nerve, muscle, and ligament problems often affect both the wrist and the hand (see ➔ Principles of physical assessment of the hand, pp. 92–93). The wrist comprises the radiocarpal joint and the radioulnar joint. The most common complaint to affect the wrist is Colles' fracture and a significant number of patients are left with residual pain and deformity following this injury. Other conditions affecting the wrist include RA which is common, less commonly OA, compression problems of the ulnar (ulnar nerve syndrome) and median nerves (carpal tunnel syndrome), and de Quervain's syndrome. Ganglia on the back of the wrist are also common.

Assessment of the wrist should include:

History taking

Elicit the chief complaint and the history of its onset which may be:
- Pain/swelling/deformity/loss of function following a fall onto an outstretched hand—indicating probable Colles' fracture
- Pain over radial styloid process particularly during gripping movement—indicating probable de Quervain's syndrome
- Swelling, pain, local heat, and stiffness of the wrist joint—indicates probable RA
- Altered sensation/tingling of the hand and fingers—may indicate carpal or ulnar tunnel syndrome.

Observation/inspection

This should include the front, both sides, and dorsal aspects. Observe for localized swellings which may be ganglia, deformities, e.g. radial deviation and swelling over the radiocarpal joint. Listen for crepitus on movement of the wrist. Note any scarring indicating previous trauma or surgery.

Vascular assessment

Check the radial pulse and capillary refill of the finger nails. Note any skin discoloration or altered skin temperature of the hand and fingers. The radial pulse may be difficult to locate due to swelling/tenderness around the wrist.

Sensory assessment

Check for altered sensation in the wrist, hand, and digits. Palpate over the median and ulnar nerve to check for tenderness and induction of paraesthesia of parts of the hand and fingers. Phalen's test and Tinel's test (also known as the median nerve percussion test) are often performed to test for carpal tunnel syndrome.

Movement

If the wrist is very painful and swollen and fracture is suspected, measuring range of movement should be delayed until a X-ray is completed. Measure the degree of dorsiflexion (normal range 75°), palma flexion (normal range 75°), radial deviation (normal range 20°), ulnar deviation (normal range 35°), pronation (normal range 75°), and supination (normal range 80°) ensuring the patient's elbows are kept firmly at their sides.

Clinical investigations

X-rays of the wrist and carpal bones are appropriate to diagnose fractures and dislocations and changes to joints due to RA or OA. Nerve conduction studies are still sometimes used to test the amplitude and velocity of nerve conduction, specifically in diagnosing carpal or ulnar tunnel syndromes. Blood tests, such as a FBC, may be indicated if infection of the joint is suspected or inflammatory markers if RA is suspected.

Disease-specific measures of the hand

The most commonly used measure is the DASH score which is available in both full and abbreviated versions and the Mayo wrist score (see ℘ http:www.orthopaedic.scores.com for further details).

Further reading

Hattam P, Smeatham A (2010). *Special Tests in Musculoskeletal Examination: An Evidence-Based Guide for Clinicians.* Edinburgh: Churchill Livingstone/Elsevier.

Principles of physical assessment of the hand

Hand injury and disease is very common and patients can present across many different setting, e.g. the ED, primary care, or in rheumatology or orthopaedic secondary care. The hand is a complex area to assess due to its complicated nerve supply and because often patients presenting with a hand problem can be experiencing referred signs and symptoms from the cervical spine, shoulder, or elbow. It is important to assess and compare both hands and to include the structures above the hands to rule out referred pain or other symptoms such as altered sensation.

Assessment of the hand should include:

History taking

Elicit the chief complaint and the history of its onset which may be a chronic onset of joint pain (unilateral or bilateral), altered sensation and strength in one or more digits, or acute pain and loss of function following injury. If the patient presents with acute injury, establish the mechanism of injury, e.g. scaphoid fracture usually results from a fall onto an outstretched hand. It is important to establish if the patient is left or right handed. Establish if there is any past history of injury, disease, or surgery to the hand and taking an occupational history is very important as often hand problems can be a result of repetitive strain, e.g. keyboard use or musician. Check for diseases such as diabetes which are associated with neuropathy and specifically carpal tunnel syndrome, and use of warfarin therapy which may lead to excessive bleeding into the joints of the hand.

Observation

Check for any bracelets or rings that may cause constriction and remove as swelling is likely to occur. Observe and compare both hands for position and symmetry when in the resting position, note any flexion or extension deformities of the digits. Also observe for muscle wasting particularly over the thenar eminence which may be indicative of carpal tunnel compression.

Inspection

For signs of swelling, redness, inflammation, bruising, and scars from previous surgery or trauma.

Palpation

This should include eliciting signs and symptoms of tenderness, muscle spasm, abnormal bumps or indentations, swelling, abnormal or loss of sensation to touch, and evidence of altered temperature of the joints (increased warmth).

Vascular assessment

Check the radial and ulnar pulses and check capillary refill in each digit.

Sensory assessment

The hand is supplied by three nerves: radial, ulnar, and median. It is important to assess sensation on the dorsal and palmar aspects of all three nerve distributions to ascertain loss or diminished sensation. Phalen's test, the 'prayer' test, and Tinel's test are commonly performed to investigate carpal tunnel syndrome.[1]

Movement

Active movements should be carried out prior to passive range of movement. It is only necessary to carry out a passive range of movement if the patient has been unable to carry out the full range of active movements. The assessment should be structured so that the most painful movements reported by the patient during the history are left until last to avoid 'carry over' pain to the next movement. Range of active movement should include grip strength, flexion and extension of the fingers/thumb, opposition, and abduction and adduction of each digit.

Disease-specific measures of the hand

The most commonly used measure is the DASH score which comes in both full and abbreviated versions.

Clinical investigations

X-rays of the hand are appropriate to diagnose fractures and dislocations and changes to joints due to RA or OA. Nerve conduction studies are still sometimes used to test the amplitude and velocity of nerve conduction, specifically in diagnosing carpal tunnel syndrome.

Reference

1. Hattam P, Smeatham A (2010). *Special Tests in Musculoskeletal Examination: An Evidence-Based Guide for Clinicians.* Edinburgh: Churchill Livingstone/Elsevier.

Principles of physical assessment of the spinal cord

A spinal cord injury (SCI) is potentially a life-threatening situation depending on the level of the lesion and may impact all body systems including respiratory and cardiac function. The nurse may encounter the patient with a suspected or confirmed SCI in the ED, critical care unit, SCI unit, or during the rehabilitation stage either in the inpatient or community setting. As stated on ➔ Spinal cord injury, p. 400 it is extremely important for patients to be transferred to specialist SCI units as soon as possible once they have been stabilized. The priorities for assessment will vary through the clinical journey from initial pre-hospital assessment through to long-term rehabilitation; however, throughout all stages of assessment it is very important to give psychological support to the patient and their family.

At the site of injury

The patient with a suspected SCI may be unconscious and therefore unable to provide a history of their injuries and so any witnesses at the scene should be questioned about the mechanism of injury as this will help to identify the potential severity and region of SCI. The basic principle is that the higher the suspected level of the SCI, the greater the risk of respiratory and cardiovascular complications. It is essential that cervical spine control and stability is achieved by a competent practitioner ASAP using manual in-line cervical immobilization followed by securing the cervical spine position with cervical collar, sandbags, head board, and tape.[1] Assessment should be framed by a primary and secondary survey.[2]

- The primary survey of any trauma patient including those with suspected SCI comprises: cessation of life-threatening exsanguinating haemorrhage followed by airway control, within-line cervical spine immobilization, assessment of breathing, circulation, disability, and exposure—this is referred to as the cAcBCDE approach to assessment.[1] See pp. 80–81 and 328–329 for further details.
- Once the primary survey (following securing of the cervical spine) is complete then move onto the secondary survey which comprises head-to-toe and front to back inspection checking for deformity, contusions, penetrations, asymmetry, and abrasions.[2]

Diagnostic tests

SCI will be confirmed based on:
- Clinical signs and symptoms—neurological assessment of motor and sensory function
- Plain X-rays—lateral and anteroposterior (AP) views of the cervical spine
- Computed tomography (CT)
- MRI
- Dynamic fluoroscopy.

Ongoing assessment of the patient

Once a confirmed diagnosis of SCI has been made, which will include the level of the injury, then ongoing assessment is required to ensure prompt detection of complications and to evaluate the patient's emotional/psychological status when dealing with this life-changing event. The main potential complications are:

Spinal shock

This can occur immediately following the injury and up to 6 weeks after. Depending on the level of the lesion, spinal shock can impact autonomic reflexes controlling blood pressure (BP), heart rate, and body temperature (above T6), diaphragm (C3–5), intercostals (T1–7), and accessory muscles of respiration (C1–8). Therefore, ongoing assessment of vital signs, urinary output, and bowel function are very important.

Deep vein thrombosis

DVT can occur in 60–100% of SCI patients. Assessment for signs are essential including calf swelling, warmth in the calf region, discoloration of the skin (redness, pallor) around the distribution of the tibial, popliteal, and femoral veins, and unexplained low-grade pyrexia. SCI patients will not be able to report calf pain or respond to a Homan's sign test. Investigations for suspected DVT include D-dimer blood test, ultrasound Doppler testing, ultrasonography, and contrast venography.

Autonomic dysreflexia

This is a potentially life-threatening complication that occurs as a response to a noxious stimulus below the level of the lesion, e.g. distended bladder or constipation. Assessment includes observation for signs and symptoms such as severe headache, nausea, anxiety, blotching of the skin across the chest, sweating above the level of the lesion. Monitoring of vital signs to detect increase in BP, bradycardia, and temperature to detect possible noxious stimulus, e.g. urinary infection.

Pressure sores

SCI patients are extremely vulnerable to pressure ulcers and careful assessment of the integrity of the skin is essential for early detection of redness or pressure.

Psychological well-being

Ongoing assessment of the SCI patient's mental health is essential as frequently they can experience depression and anxiety. General assessment of the patient's emotional well-being is integral to the role of the nurse and use of valid and reliable assessment tools such as the Hospital Anxiety and Depression Scale (HADS).[3]

References

1. Parker M, Magnusson C (2016). Assessment of trauma. *Int J Orthop Trauma Nurs* 21:21–30.
2. NICE (2016). Major trauma: assessment and initial management. NICE guideline [NG39]. 🔗 https://www.nice.org.uk/guidance/ng39
3. Zigmond A, Snaith R (1983). The Hospital Anxiety and Depression Scale. *Acta Psychiatr Scand* 67:361–70.

Principles of assessment of the bony spine

Back pain is extremely common and if it becomes chronic and unrelieved can lead to significant psychological and social issues for the patient and their family. It is therefore important to include assessment of patients' stress, coping and depression status, social circumstances, as well physical examination. Back pain may be localized to the back, but often radiates into the buttocks, legs, and feet due to radicular nerve pain. Back pain may also be indicative of problems not associated with the bony spine, such as lower intestine, genitourinary, or renal problems and these should be excluded during the assessment process. The areas of the spine included in the assessment (cervical, thoracic, lumbar, sacral) will depend on the patient's presentation and history. Causes of back pain include sprains and strains, OA, spondylosis, spinal stenosis, ankylosing spondylitis, osteoporotic fractures, and less commonly tumours/spinal metastases and infection. Patients presenting with back pain may actually have pathology in their sacroiliac or hip joints and these may need to be included in the examination.

Assessment of the spine should include:

History taking

Detailed history of what specific movements, activities, and positions bring on or exacerbate the pain, e.g. sitting or standing for long periods, occupational activity, coughing or sneezing, or bowel movements. Also determine what alleviates the pain. Elicit if there is a history of trauma: does the patient report twisting their spine or report any locking? It is important to elicit if there are any neurological symptoms such as sciatica, erectile dysfunction, or loss of bladder or bowel sensation which if reported require urgent investigation. Also ascertain if there is any associated muscle weakness or wasting.

Observation/inspection

The patient will need to undress to their underwear, so maintaining their privacy and dignity is important. The symmetry of the spine should be observed and any abnormal curvature such as lordosis, scoliosis, or kyphosis noted. Observe for limb-length inequality when standing and gait pattern should be noted. Check for protrusions, redness, swelling, and any scars which indicate previous surgery or trauma.

Palpation and percussion

The spine should be palpated with the patient in the sitting and standing positions and any tenderness, heat, misalignment, and protrusions noted. The spine should also be gently percussed with the patient bending forward from the root of the neck to the sacrum noting any pain.

Sensory assessment

The specific assessment of motor and sensory function will depend on the level of the presenting spinal problem and if the patient reports any altered sensation or motor function during the history. For example, patients presenting with lumbar/sacral pain who report sciatica will need to have the sensation and motor function of their lower limbs assessed.

Movement

The amount of flexion/extension, lateral bend, and rotation of the spine should be measured. If a prolapsed intervertebral disc is suspected then the patient's ability to straight leg raise should be included in the assessment.

Clinical investigations

NICE guidelines for management of non-specific low back pain with or without sciatica[1] recommend not to offer X-ray of the lumbar spine for the management of non-specific low back pain and only to consider imaging such as MRI when a diagnosis of spinal malignancy, infection, fracture, cauda equina syndrome, or ankylosing spondylitis or another inflammatory disorder is suspected or if the results are likely to change management plans. If ankylosing spondylitis is suspected, blood tests for inflammatory markers should be taken (C-reactive protein (CRP), erythrocyte sedimentation rate (ESR), plasma viscosity (PV), and human leucocyte antigen (HLA)-B27 antigen); see ➲ Ankylosing spondylitis, p. 236 for further details.

Psychological and social assessment

The nurse has an important role in assessing the psychological status of patients who have chronic back pain. Patients may suffer with depression and anxiety about what the future holds for them as they may be unable to continue with their usual employment and social activities. Observe the patient's general appearance and facial expressions, e.g. do they look unkempt, have low mood, or are withdrawn? There are a number of valid and reliable indices to assess depression and anxiety including the Beck Depression Inventory (BDI) and HADS. The nurse should also ascertain how the patient's back pain is impacting their social and occupational activities.

Disease-specific measures of back pain

There are a number of assessment indices specifically designed for assessing back pain including the Oswestry low back pain score (full and modified versions) and the Back Pain Index; see ☏ http://www.orthopaedicscores. com for further detail.

Reference

1. NICE (2016). Low back pain and sciatica in over 16s: assessment and management. NICE guideline [NG59]. ☏ https://www.nice.org.uk/guidance/ng59/

Principles of physical assessment of the hip

The hip is one of the largest and most stable joints within the body and receives considerable load bearing. This force on the hip joint will vary depending on activities being taken; ranging from 0.3 × body weight to 4.5+ × body weight when running.[1] All weight-bearing joints of the lower limbs, pelvis, and lower spine are adversely affected by excessive body weight and obesity is known to be a contributory factor to degenerative processes of the hip joint. Often patients presenting with hip pain may have a problem with either their lumbar spine or sacroiliac joints and therefore it is often necessary to carry out an examination of these (see ➲ Principles of assessment of the bony spine, pp. 96–97) to rule out referred pain. Both hips and lower limbs should be assessed. The patient will need to be partially undressed from the waist down to conduct the assessment, so maintaining privacy and dignity is important.

Assessment of the hip should include:

History taking

Elicit the chief complaint, which is likely to be hip and/or groin pain. Less frequently patients may report restricted movement, and this is more prevalent when there is a history of trauma rather than gradual-onset pathology. Apply the questions template presented on ➲ History taking pp. 82–83 to elicit the nature/details of pain and injury.

Observation

The patient's gait should be observed from the anterior and posterior aspects. Typically, if the patient has inequality of leg length due to stable hip fracture, subluxation/dislocation, or diminished joint space due to OA they will have a waddling walking pattern. Hip flexion contracture can result in increased lumbar lordosis and this can be observed from the posterior view. Also, general observation of the patient is required to elicit non-verbal signs of discomfort or pain particularly, when walking or rising from a chair. Observe if the patient is using a walking aid and if they are using it correctly. Also inspect their shoes as they will indicate any abnormal gait patterns and weight distribution. Listen for sounds of crepitus when conducting active/passive range of movement. If the patient is unable to weight bear or mobilize, observe the position of the hip/lower limbs with the patient lying down, e.g. external rotation and shortening of the limb may indicate displaced hip fracture/dislocation or subluxation.

Inspection

For signs of swelling, redness, inflammation, bruising, and scars from previous surgery or trauma.

Palpation

This should include eliciting signs and symptoms of tenderness, muscle spasm, abnormal bumps or indentations, swelling, abnormal or loss of sensation to touch, and evidence of altered temperature of the joint (increased warmth). Tenderness over the greater trochanter usually indicates trochanteric bursitis.

Movement

Active movements should be carried out prior to passive range of movement. It is only necessary to carry out a passive range of movement if the patient has been unable to carry out the full range of active movements. The assessment should be structured so that the most painful movements reported by the patient during the history are left until last to avoid 'carry over' pain to the next movement.[1] Examination will require the patient to lie in the supine or prone position, so it is important to ascertain if the patient has any respiratory problems before asking a patient to lie flat in either of these positions. Range of active movement should include:

- Flexion (110–120°)
- Abduction (30–50°)
- Adduction (30°)
- Extension (10–15°)
- Lateral rotation (40–60°)
- Medial rotation (30–40°).

Special physical examination tests

There are many specific tests that may be used to aid diagnosis including Trendelenburg's sign (stability of the hip and strength of the hip abductors) and measurement for true or functional leg-length inequality. True inequality of leg length can be due to reduction of the joint space due to OA or hip fracture. The measurement should be taken from the anterior superior iliac spine to the medial or lateral malleolus. The patient's pelvis must be flat and square to the couch otherwise the measurement obtained could be inaccurate and a false apparent shortening recorded. Thomas's test is performed to test for fixed flexion deformity at the hip.

Disease-specific measures of hip pain/dysfunction

There are a number of specific clinician- or patient-reported measures that can be used during assessment of the hip including:

- Harris Hip Score
- WOMAC
- Oxford hip score
- Mayo hip score.

Clinical investigations

X-rays have an important role in diagnosing problems with the hip. Anterior/posterior views with the patient lying supine will show fractures/dislocation of the hip and signs of OA such as diminished joint space, osteophytes, and migration of the femoral head.

Reference

1. Magee DJ (2006). *Orthopaedic Physical Assessment*, 4th edn. St. Louis, MO: Saunders/Elsevier.

Principles of physical assessment of the knee

The knee is the largest joint within the body and relies on its associated ligaments and muscles for stability. It receives considerable load bearing—specifically at the patellar. Often patients presenting with knee pain may have a problem with their hip, lumbar spine, or ankle joints and therefore it is often necessary to carry out an examination of these to rule out referred pain. Both knees and lower limbs should be assessed. The patient will need to be partially undressed from the waist down to conduct the assessment so privacy and dignity are important issues. The patient will also be required to change from sitting to standing, to lying supine, lateral, and prone through the examination. Ligament injury is very common in the knee so it is very important that these are assessed within the examination. With an acute injury the knee may be very swollen and painful and examining the knee may be very difficult and so the most useful aid to diagnosis in patients presenting with acute knee injury is the patient history.[1] Assessment of the knee should include:

History taking

Elicit the chief complaint which may range from knee/hip pain to low back pain. If the patient presents with an acute knee injury it is important to elicit full details of the mechanisms of the injury. Ascertain if there is a history of the knee giving way, locking, or swelling. Apply the questions template presented on ➔ History taking p. 82 to elicit the nature/details of pain and injury. It is particularly important when examining the knee to identify the location of pain and/or stiffness as well as the type of activities that exacerbate the symptoms due to the complexity of structures within and surrounding the knee.

Observation

The patient's gait should be observed from the anterior, posterior, and lateral aspects. From the anterior aspect it is important to observe for alignment of the knees with the hips and ankles; any varus or valgum deformity should be noted. From the posterior and lateral views the patient should be asked to extend their knees fully and any flexion deformity noted. Also general observation of the patient is needed to elicit non-verbal signs of discomfort or pain particularly when walking or rising from a chair. Observe if the patient is using a walking aid and if they are using it correctly. Is the patient able to fully weight bear and is there evidence of a stiff knee gait because the patient experiences pain on flexion? Also inspect their shoes as they will indicate any abnormal gait patterns and weight distribution. Listen for sounds of crepitus when conducting active/passive range of movement.

Inspection

Inspect for signs of swelling, redness, inflammation, bruising, scars from previous surgery or trauma. Observe the alignment of the patella with the patient lying supine and note any deviation.

Palpation

This should include eliciting signs and symptoms of tenderness, muscle spasm, abnormal bumps or indentations, swelling, abnormal or loss of sensation to touch, and evidence of altered temperature of the joints (increased warmth). It is important to palpate the margins of the patella and to move it both laterally and medially. Muscle wasting of the quadriceps and hamstrings should also be felt for. When a knee is extremely swollen and painful, examination may be of limited value and should be carried out carefully to avoid causing further discomfort.

Nerve and circulatory assessment

Examination should include testing of motor and sensory functions of the nerves of the lower limb. The patellar and medial hamstrings reflexes should be tested. Also observe for altered colour/temperature of the lower limbs and check for popliteal and pedal pulses if vascular damage is a possibility.

Movement

Active movements should be carried out prior to passive range of movement. It is only necessary to carry out a passive range of movement if the patient has been unable to carry out the full range of active movements. The assessment should be structured so that the most painful movements reported by the patient during the history are left until last to avoid 'carry over' pain to the next movement.[1] Examination will require the patient to sit and then lie down, so it is important to ascertain if the patient has any respiratory problems before asking them to lie flat. Range of active movement should include flexion (0–135°); extension (0–15°)—note most people achieve 0° only; lateral rotation (40–60°); and medial rotation (30–40°).

Special physical examination tests

There are many specific tests that may be used to aid diagnosis including:
- Lachman test and anterior drawer test—for anterior cruciate ligament injury
- Posterior drawer sign—for posterior cruciate ligament injury
- Slocum test—anterior/lateral instability
- McMurray test—tears of the meniscus
- Bulge test—assesses effusion in the joint.

Disease-specific measures of knee pain/dysfunction

There are a number of specific clinician or patient-reported measures that can be used during assessment of the knee including WOMAC index, Oxford knee score, and Knee Society Score (KSS).

Clinical investigations

X-rays have an important role in diagnosing problems with the knee. Anterior/posterior and lateral views with the patient lying supine or weight bearing will show fractures, malalignment, and signs of OA such as diminished joint space and osteophytes. MRI scanning is needed for detection of soft tissue problems (ligament ruptures/tears and tears of the menisci).

Reference and further reading

1. Pincher B (2017). Assessment of the adult patient presenting with knee pain: a review article. *Int J Orthop Trauma Nurs* 25:29–35.

Principles of physical examination of the ankle

The ankle and foot are usually assessed together as patients often present with symptoms associated with both. Soft tissue and bony injury of the ankle are very common. The ankle joint is under considerable stress as a major load-bearing joint during ambulation and it is dependent on its bony structure and surrounding ligaments for stability. Degenerative OA is uncommon but usually occurs secondary to previous injury of the joint.

The ankle is largely a hinge joint made up of the articulation between the distal articular surface of the tibia and the upper articular surface of talus. Most injuries occur as a result of excessive inversion or eversion of the ankle and foot, putting the joint under extreme pressure. The practitioner assessing the ankle needs a good understanding of the anatomy and function of the ankle joint.

When injury or other conditions are suspected, examination of the ankle should involve the following:

- *Pain assessment.* The patient should be asked to point to the area that is most painful. This is an important first clue about which part of the ankle is involved.
- *Sensation/circulation.* This should be checked distal to any site of pain, injury, or immobility in order to ensure that neurovascular structures are intact. It is important to check these on both the top of the foot and the base of the foot.
- *Inspection.* The ankle should be inspected for swelling, bruising, and deformities of shape or posture. The amount and spread of swelling must be considered. Both ankles should be inspected so that any asymmetry can be noted.
- *Palpation.* The ankle should be assessed for tenderness over bony points such as the malleoli or over ligaments. This should begin at the area of least pain working towards the site of the most pain.
- *Movement.* Function of the joint should be assessed for the ability to fully perform plantar flexion, dorsiflexion, eversion, and inversion. This will give important clues to the potential structures involved. This should be done actively initially and passively if the patient is unable to undertake active movement. Again, comparisons should be made against both ankles. Any restricted movement and sites of pain should be noted as these indicate sites of both bony and soft tissue injury.
- *Ability to bear weight.* Weight bearing should be assessed as either partial or fully weight bearing. Some patients with ankle problems may be able to weight bear on the toe or ball of the foot but not fully onto the whole foot. The practitioner should observe how the patient arrives for the examination. Patients should always be asked to try to weight bear, even if they say they cannot.
- *Specific movement tests* are available for the ankle which enable the practitioner to assess the condition of specific structures. These include specific tests that identify ligament and tendon damage and possible bony injury within specific areas of the joint, including tests to assess ligament stress and instability. Ankle sprains can be assessed by ligament stress tests including anterior talofibular ligament, calcaneofibular ligament, calcaneocuboid ligament, and medial collateral ligament.[1]

Ottawa ankle rules

Differentiating between ligament injury and fracture has long been a challenge. In 1992, Stiell et al. published a set of rules designed to help the practitioner assessing the patient with an ankle injury exclude fractures.[2]

According to these rules, a series of ankle radiographs are required only if there is:
- Pain on palpation of the bone in the malleolar region and any of the following:
  - Bone tenderness at the tip or posterior edge of the tibia
  - Bone tenderness along the posterior edge of the fibula
  - An inability to bear weight on the ankle for 4 steps both immediately and when asked to do so on examination.

These rules have been shown to be very effective in differentiating between soft tissue and bony injury[3] with a very low rate of false negatives.

References

1. Hattam P, Smeatham A (2010). *Special Tests in Musculoskeletal Examination: An Evidence-Based Guide for Clinicians*. Edinburgh: Churchill Livingstone/Elsevier.
2. Stiell IG, Greenberg GH, McKnight RD, et al. (1992). A study to develop clinical decision rules for the use of radiography in acute ankle injuries. *Ann Emerg Med* 21:384–90.
3. Jenkin M, Sitler M, Kelly J (2010). Clinical usefulness of the Ottawa ankle rules for detecting fractures of the ankle and midfoot. *J Athl Train* 45:5.

Principles of physical assessment of the foot

The foot can be affected by a number of conditions including RA, OA (typically hallux rigidus of the metatarsophalangeal (MTP) joint of the great toe), gout, plantar fasciitis, or injured due to trauma or stress such as March fracture/s. The foot/feet should be observed and compared at rest, weight bearing, and walking to assess gait pattern. The patient's shoes should also be inspected to detect abnormal wear and tear patterns indicating abnormal weight bearing and gait patterns. It is also usual to examine the ankle joint as well as the foot due to the interplay of bony articulations, ligamenture, and muscle insertions and origins.

Assessment of the foot should include:

History taking

Elicit the chief complaint and the history of its onset which may be:

- Pain at the heel within first few steps or after prolonged periods of walking which would indicate possible plantar fasciitis
- Pain and/or numbness and tingling in the plantar surface of the foot which would indicate possible tarsal tunnel syndrome or sciatica radiating from a lower back problem
- Tenderness and/or swelling of the tarsometatarsal/MTP/IP joints indicative of RA
- Pain and deformity of the great toe indicative of hallux rigidus and hallux valgus and bunion
- Pain, swelling, and bruising over the calcaneum following a fall from a height is indicative of a calcaneal fracture (patients who present after falling from a height and presenting with injury/pain to the calcaneum should have a full spinal assessment)
- Pain and swelling over the metatarsal (MT) bones with or without inability to weight bear following direct trauma (someone stepping on your foot) indicates probable MT fracture.

Observation/inspection

This should include the heel, dorsum of the foot, each toe and toe nail, and the sole of each foot. Observe for deformity such as flat foot, hallux valgus, hammer toe, eversion or inversion; note calluses indicating uneven weight bearing, tissue thickening of the plantar fascia, and any ganglion. Note any discoloration, scarring, or fungal infections of the nails.

Vascular assessment

Check the pedal pulses (dorsalis pedis artery and the anterior and posterior tibial arteries) and capillary refill of the toe nails. Note any skin discoloration or altered skin temperature of the foot and toes. Pedal pulses can be difficult to locate and use of a Doppler may be needed.

Sensory assessment

The sural, tibial, medial, and lateral plantar, saphenous, deep, and superficial fibular nerves provide the motor and sensory supply to the foot. Check for altered or loss of sensation over the dorsum, heel, sole, and each digit. Note that diabetic neuropathy often presents in the foot.

Movement

Measure the degree of supination of the foot using a goniometer (normal range is 35°) and pronation (normal range 20°). The degree of flexion and extension of each MT and IP joint of each toe should also be measured.

Clinical investigations

X-rays of the foot are appropriate to diagnose fractures and dislocations and changes to joints due to RA or OA. Nerve conduction studies are still sometimes used to test the amplitude and velocity of nerve conduction, specifically in diagnosing tarsal tunnel syndrome. Blood tests such as a FBC may be indicated if infection of the joint is suspected or inflammatory markers if RA is suspected.

Investigations

Introduction

As part of the assessment process most orthopaedic and trauma patients are likely to require clinical investigations to aid diagnostic decision-making. It is important to remember that investigations can be both expensive and uncomfortable for the patient and so they should only be requested when their results will aid decision-making about the treatment plan. Principles of radiography, MRI, CT scans and ultrasound are presented on ➲ Other types of diagnostic imaging, pp. 110–111. Other investigations are outlined here:

Dual-energy X-ray absorptiometry (DXA)

This is a scan to test the density of the bones and is used to diagnose osteoporosis. The results of the scan will enable the clinical team to assess the risk of pathological fractures and make decisions about prescribing medications such as calcium, vitamin D, bisphosphonates, and hormone replacement therapy (see ➲ Osteoporosis, pp. 252–253). A DXA scan usually takes about 15 minutes and the patient will be required to lie down (fully clothed) while all of the skeleton is X-rayed using very small doses of radiation (equivalent to spending a day out in the sun). The role of the nurse is to explain to the patient what the DXA scan will involve to alleviate anxiety, and to provide information about when they will receive information about the results.

Haematological investigations

The FBC examines three groups of cells: erythrocytes (red cells), leucocytes (white cells), and platelets. A venous blood sample of ~2.5 mL will be required to undertake the laboratory examination. A FBC will be needed preoperatively to detect anaemia, raised white cell count, or platelet dysfunction and should be checked postoperatively to ensure the haemoglobin level is within normal range (10–12 g/dL). A raised white cell count may indicate the presence of infection and will require further investigation to elicit the source of the infection. Low white cell counts may be present in patients with lupus erythematosus and as a side effect of disease-modifying antirheumatic drugs (DMARDs). Blood tests for inflammation are requested to assist in diagnostic decision making when conditions such as RA and ankylosing spondylitis are suspected. The three commonest blood tests for detecting inflammation are:

• CRP
• ESR
• PV.

However, it is important to remember that raised CRP and ESR may also be indicative of infection and/or inflammation so are only to be interpreted in the context of other information such as findings from the physical examination and history. Patients with suspected or confirmed rheumatological conditions will require specific blood tests such as rheumatoid factor (RF), sheep cell agglutination (Rose Waaler test), and the latex agglutination test to assess their rheumatic disease activity[1] (see ➲ p. 231 for further details).

Patients may also require biochemical investigations using a venous blood sample including renal and hepatic function, electrolyte levels and serum glucose preoperatively, postoperatively, and if there is a deterioration in their condition.

The nurse's role in haematological investigations is to explain to the patient what tests are being requested and why and when the results will be available. It is important when carrying out venepuncture to acquire venous blood samples to follow clinical procedure guidelines to minimize risk to the patient and oneself from needle stick injuries. Patients need to have the results of their haematological investigations explained to them in a timely and appropriate manner to ensure their understanding.

Urinalysis

This should be carried out as part of the assessment process to test for:
- Glucose—indicative of diabetes or reduced kidney absorption
- Bilirubin—indicative of hepatic or biliary disease
- Blood—indicative of infection, stones, or trauma
- Protein—indicative of infection or renal disease
- Leucocytes—indicative of infection.

Specific gravity—raised measurement can indicate dehydration and a low value can indicate renal disease or diabetes insipidus. If a urinary tract infection (UTI) is suspected, a midstream urine (MSU) specimen should be obtained and sent to the laboratory. The nurse should ensure that the patient has privacy when asked for a urine specimen and explain the importance of the correct procedure for collecting a midstream specimen to avoid contamination of the specimen.

Further reading

Adebajo A, Dunkley L (eds) (2018). ABC of Rheumatology, 5th edn. Oxford: Wiley Blackwell.

Radiographic imaging

Radiographic imaging (X-ray) is the most important and common form of diagnostic imaging used in orthopaedics and trauma. Radiographic images are created by short bursts of radiation which pass through the body and interact with photographic film or a fluorescent screen. The extent to which the image is blackened depends on the number of X-rays reaching the image which, in turn, depends on the densities of the tissue. X-rays pass easily through soft tissue but are less able to pass through bone which is denser. Radiographs provide images of bony structures, the density of bones, the relationships between bones, their continuity and contour, and the shape of spaces within joints. They are used in all cases of suspected fracture and are commonly used in the diagnosis of musculoskeletal conditions such as OA. For example:

- Radiographs of osteoarthritic joints show narrowing of joint spaces, extra bony growths, and cysts within the subchondral bone
- Radiographs of fractures show a loss of continuity in the structure of bones and any displacement that has occurred.

Health and safety

The amount of radiation used to produce radiographic images is very small and the health risks are very low. Repeated exposure to radiation for both patients and staff, however, can result in cell damage. Guidelines for protection and monitoring such as The Ionising Radiation (Medical Exposure) Regulations (2017)[1] should be followed to minimize risk to patients and staff.

The role of the nurse

Having radiographic procedures or examinations can be painful for the patient with musculoskeletal problems due to movement and positioning on the X-ray table. It is essential that the nurse provides adequate analgesia at an appropriate interval prior to the procedure. For severely injured patients, it may be necessary for pain relief to be provided with Entonox® during the procedure if this is safe and available.

When present at imaging procedures, the role of the nurse is primarily to consider the well-being of the patient but also to assist the radiographer in achieving a good image. The nurse should provide emotional support to patients and assist them to achieve and maintain correct positioning. Some radiographic imaging procedures are difficult and may be painful for patients. For example, the patient may be asked to bear weight on an arthritic ankle or assistance might be required to help patients to depress the shoulders when trying to visualize the 7th cervical vertebrae in cervical spine images.

Radiographs are useful in patient education as they often provide very clear images of musculoskeletal problems. They are used to show patients what bones and joints look like as part of an explanation of their musculoskeletal problem. For this reason, nurses need a sound knowledge of skeletal anatomy and how musculoskeletal conditions appear in radiographic images. Many nurses working at specialist and advanced practice levels request and interpret patient X-rays as part of their roles.

Radiographic image interpretation—principles

Radiographs are often taken from several different angles in order to provide a detailed view of a bone, group of bones, or joint. Increasingly, such images can be viewed on a computer screen, enabling efficient storage, retrieval, and manipulation of the images. Advanced non-medical practitioners working in emergency and orthopaedic settings are now incorporating radiographic interpretation into their practice following relevant training and experience. McRae[2] recommends the following approach to the basics of examining radiographs:

- *Long shot*—a general overview of the radiograph, standing well back, considering the shape, size, and contour of the bones and joints as a whole
- *Medium shot*—noting bone texture, areas of new bone, or bone destruction and deformity
- *Close-up*—tracing methodically around the contours of the bone and noting any abnormalities of the continuity of the outline and structure of the bone.

References

1. Department of Health and Social Care (2018). Guidance to the Ionising Radiation (Medical Exposure) Regulations 2017. London: Department of Health and Social Care.
2. McCrae R (2010). *Clinical Orthopaedic Examination*, 6th edn. Edinburgh: Churchill Livingstone.

Other types of diagnostic imaging

Diagnostic imaging is central to making a diagnosis when musculoskeletal conditions or injury are suspected. Besides radiographs, a number of other diagnostic imaging modalities are available and offer a variety of benefits in diagnosing musculoskeletal problems.

Computed tomography scanning

CT scans are created using radiation beams passing through the tissue from different angles of rotation to provide cross-sectional slice images of a segment of the body. This enables more detailed views of bony structures from many angles as well as greater definition of different types of tissue. In most situations CT scans have now been superseded by MRI. The risks of CT are the same as those for normal radiographs although the scan will take much longer so the dose of radiation may be greater.

Magnetic resonance imaging

MRI is increasingly being used to diagnose musculoskeletal problems. It involves the use of high-strength magnetic fields and electrical pulses which allow the direction and strength of the magnetic field to be varied. This realigns the atoms in tissues, enabling the production of computerized images. It is very useful for providing highly detailed images of both bone and soft tissues. This is particularly helpful in visualizing complex joints and structures such as the knee, shoulder, and spine. MRI images are detailed enough to enable minor tears of ligaments to be seen, assisting in diagnosis and treatment and management planning. Special types of MRI scans called metal artefact resonance scans (MARS) are used to assess metallosis in the hip joint (see ➔ Soft tissue reactions to the wear debris associated with metal-on-metal hip articulations, p. 210 for further reading). No radiation is involved in MRI scans, but the procedure can be quite long depending on the size of area to be scanned and the patient is required to lie completely still. This can be very difficult for some patients—especially if they suffer from anxiety in enclosed spaces. Patients who suffer from claustrophobia may not be able to have an MRI scan. The patient should be warned that there will be a loud noise while the scan is being conducted. Music can be played to help the patient to relax. The patient can also communicate through an intercom with others in the room and instructions can be given and reassurance offered by talking to the patient. When requesting MRI scans any metal within the patient's body must be documented on the request form as metal becomes heated from the MRI scanner.

Ultrasonography

Ultrasound images are created using high-frequency sound waves which 'echo back' in different ways depending on the density of tissues. It is of most value in assessing the presence and amount of fluid in joints and damage to soft tissue structures. It is also useful in assessing pain, inflammation, and infection. The sonographer sends pulses of sound waves through the tissues using a probe. This option is regarded as being risk free as it does not involve the use of radiation. The process is also relatively inexpensive. Ultrasonography can also be used to guide intra-articular injections and is used in the investigation of suspected DVT. Patients who are unable to have MRI scans to detect metallosis may have an ultrasound scan instead.

The role of the nurse

The central role of the nurse in all diagnostic imaging procedures is to ensure that patients are well prepared and informed about the reasons for the procedures and what is likely to happen as well as allaying anxiety about the likely results. The better informed a patient is about what is happening the more they are likely to be able to cooperative with the procedure. Patients should be aware of any risks involved in the imaging process and of any preparations they should make such as wearing appropriate clothing. In the case of MRI, metal jewellery cannot be worn or clothing which contains metal.

Another consideration is that the nurse should ensure that patients have fully understood what they have been told when they are given a diagnosis based on the images produced. It is often helpful for the nurse to be present when results are presented to the patient so that they can answer specific questions later.

Patient-reported outcome measures

Introduction

PROMs are a useful component of clinical assessment because they give patients an opportunity to report their own perceptions of how a musculoskeletal condition or an intervention impacts their quality of life, function, and pain levels.[1] It is good practice to include relevant PROMs within the assessment process. PROMs typically comprise rating scales related to well-being, function, and pain, and contain an inherent component of subjectivity. Self-report measures can be subclassified into generic quality of life/health and disease specific. It is recommended to use both generic and disease specific to optimize the sensitivity and specificity of outcome measurements that are used.

Generic measures of health

Generic measures of health aim to measure the multifaceted nature of health and well-being, so they should be comprehensive and include items relating to social and psychological health as well as physical health. They are useful in assessing health in large diverse populations and across patient groups with different diseases. Examples of commonly used generic measures include:

- Sickness Impact Profile (SIP)
- Nottingham Health Profile
- Short Form 36 Health Survey Questionnaire (SF36)
- Dartmouth COOP Function Charts.

Disease-specific measures

Disease-specific measures are designed specifically to capture the views of patients themselves regarding the impact of a specific disease process or intervention. Bowling[2] suggests disease-specific measures are needed not simply for greater brevity, but to ensure sensitivity to sometimes small, but clinically significant changes in health status and levels of disease severity. There are a significant number of disease-specific PROMs used with orthopaedic and trauma patients. Examples are listed here:

- DASH
- The Arthritis Impact Measurement Scale (AIMS)
- Oxford hip and knee scores
- WOMAC

Establishing the rigor of self-report measures

The examples of generic and disease-specific self-report measures provided earlier have all been through rigorous testing to establish their psychometric properties. Before administering any tool the nurse should ensure the measure is designed and validated for the particular patient group, i.e. orthopaedic and trauma patients. Validation studies should have explored and established the following properties:

- Validity
- Reliability
- Specificity
- Sensitivity
- Practicability.

Practical issues of self-report measures

Many orthopaedic interventions, such as total joint replacement, require long-term surveillance or review systems including the completion of self-report measures for the duration of the patient's life following the procedure. The timing of administration of the measures is usually as follows; baseline prior to procedure then 6 weeks, 6 and 12 months following procedure, and then 3-yearly for the rest of the patient's life. Patients may not always be able to complete the measures accurately without assistance and so the nurse must always offer assistance and support.[1] Patients sometimes report the range of responses afforded them in the scales does not reflect their own particular problems and this can result either in incomplete responses or inaccuracy. Hence there is a move toward patient-developed outcome measures, i.e. the patient assisted by the clinical team develop their own measures of success, e.g. 'Following the surgery, I want to be able to sleep through the night without pain'. The value of this approach is that the outcome measure is highly specific to the patient.

Conclusion

It is strongly recommended that generic self-report measures are supplemented by disease-specific measures and that often patients need assistance to complete these as accurately as possible.

References

1. Jester R, Santy-Tomlinson J, Drozd M (2018). The use of patient reported outcome measure (PROMs) in clinical assessment. *Int J Orthop Trauma Nurs* 29:49–53.
2. Bowling A (2001). *Measuring Disease*, 2nd edn. Buckingham: Open University Press.

Further reading

Jester R, Santy-Tomlinson J, Drozd M (2018). The use of patient reported outcome measure (PROMs) in clinical assessment. *Int J Orthop Trauma Nurs* 29:49–53. ℘ http://www.orthopaedicscores.com

Assessing cognitive function

Introduction

Cognition is an individual's thoughts, knowledge, interpretations, understandings, and ideas. Cognitive processes include perception, memory, and information processing and enable people to problem-solve, plan, and acquire information. There are many types of trauma and disease that can impact patients' cognitive function, such as dementia, stroke, head injury, and alcoholism. Nurses will often meet older patients who appear confused and it is important to ascertain what the cause of the confusion is. It should not be assumed that because a person is older that the cause of their confusion must be dementia. Other causes of confusion include:

- Delirium
- Urea and electrolyte (U&E) imbalance
- Toxicity due to infection
- Abnormal blood sugar levels
- Adverse reaction to medication
- Raised intracranial pressure.

Acute confusion states

Through questioning of family/friends and consulting accessory information, such as the medical notes, the nurse should determine the onset of confusion, e.g. has there been a gradual onset over many months or years or an acute/sudden onset? If the onset is sudden then the nurse should contact the medical team responsible for the patient to organize a full neurological screening. The nurse should complete a baseline assessment of conscious level using the GCS and then begin to collect information to rule out non-neurological causes of the confusion including:

- Blood tests for U&Es, blood sugar, liver function tests (LFTs), CRP, and ESR
- Temperature to determine if there is a pyrexia
- Review medication and discuss any potential adverse reaction with the pharmacist and medical team.
- Urinalysis and MSU if urine infection suspected
- Urine output to determine dehydration or renal impairment.

Once an acute onset of confusion has been ruled out the nurse should complete a baseline assessment of cognitive function using a valid assessment tool. Assessment should take place on admission/initial assessment and re-administered if there is any perceived change in the patient's cognitive status.

Tools to measure cognitive function

There are a number of assessment tools that have been developed and validated to assess cognitive function and the nurse should be sure any tool being used is fit for purpose and has been tested to establish it is:

- Valid
- Reliable
- Specific
- Sensitive
- Practical.

The most commonly used tools in the UK are the Abbreviated Mental Test Score (AMTS) and the Mini Mental State Examination (MMSE). The AMTS comprises ten items as detailed in the box, with each correct item scoring 1 (maximum score being 10). The diagnostic cut-off point varies between authors, but typically <6 indicate cognitive abnormality. The MMSE comprises two parts: verbal and functional. The verbal component affords a maximum score of 21 and the performance section 9 with the total possible score being 30. The cut off point for cognitive dysfunction is <24.

Optimize the environment for administration of the test by starting with friendly informal discussion, a relaxed and private environment, and allowing the patient to set the pace for the test. Avoid administration when the patient has first woken and if in pain or discomfort.

The ten items of the AMTS
- Age
- Time (nearest hour)
- Year
- Name of place
- Recognition of two persons
- Date and month of birth
- Date of First World War
- Queen's name
- Count 20–1 backwards
- 5-minute recall; full street address.

Limitations
Although both the AMTS and MMSE have been extensively tested to validate their psychometric properties, there are limitations in that they are aimed at a specific age and cultural group, i.e. white, older British people. Also, the MMSE does require people to be able to read and have the dexterity to draw a complex shape and this will prove difficult for those with visual problems, those unable to read, or those with deformity of the joints of the hand.

Conclusion
It is important to determine the cause of confusion in older patients and not to assume it is dementia. Tests such as the MMSE and AMTS, although they have their limitations, are a useful initial screening tool to determine cognitive impairment which should lead to referral to specialist dementia services

Further reading
Butler A (2016). Neurological assessment. Int J Orthop Trauma Nurs 22:44–53.

General principles of care

The nature of orthopaedic surgery and the surgical environment

Surgery to bones, muscles, and tendons takes place for two main reasons:

• Planned, non-emergency or 'elective' surgery designed to treat musculoskeletal conditions and correct deformities

• Emergency surgery, usually following traumatic injury to musculoskeletal structures.

Planning for surgery helps to manage some of the risks of surgical procedures and associated anaesthesia. While elective surgery affords the opportunity for planned preparation, it is rarely possible to plan for emergency and trauma surgery, making it more challenging.

Both for children and adults, orthopaedic surgery of any kind usually involves bones, joints, and soft tissues such as tendons and ligaments. In order to reach bones and joints, deep surgical incisions are often needed which require several levels of closure—increasing the risk of haemorrhage, haematoma, and infection deep within the tissues. Much orthopaedic surgery is viewed as routine because it takes place frequently. However, such surgery is often highly invasive, presenting several major risks which the orthopaedic practitioner needs to consider when planning and executing care. These are described in more detail in ➲ Complications and risk management, pp. 190–191.

Orthopaedic surgery can be intricate and necessitates lengthy procedures that increase the risk to patients from remaining under anaesthetic and spending long periods of time on the operating table. This also contributes to their postoperative pain experience. Orthopaedic surgery often involves the implantation of foreign material such as screws, plates, and joint prostheses, usually constructed of metal and/or plastic. These implants have undergone major developments over the last half-century, but they remain foreign bodies within human tissue and, as such, may be prone to adverse tissue reactions including reactions to metal ions leading to metallosis (see ➲ pp. 210–211).

Orthopaedic surgery to the limbs often involves the use of tourniquets to produce a bloodless field within the surgical site. This can increase the risk of haemorrhage and thrombosis in the immediate postoperative period.

Infection

Of paramount importance in orthopaedic surgery is managing the risk of infection. Most surgery involves the exposure of bone to the surgical environment. Osteomyelitis (bone infection) is a serious condition that is difficult to treat, requiring lengthy courses of antibiotics. It can result in necrosis of bone, leading to bone loss and severe deformity so needs to be avoided through good infection prevention measures (see Osteomyelitis, pp. 272–273). Infection prevents bone from healing if it cannot be suppressed and may require the removal of implants, insertion of antibiotic beads and/or bone graft, along with external fixation to try to eradicate it. Antibiotic prophylaxis prior to orthopaedic surgery has been instrumental in preventing both wound infection and osteomyelitis along with special arrangements for orthopaedic operating theatres.

The orthopaedic operating theatre

All practitioners working with orthopaedic patients need to understand the environment in which the surgery took place. Patient safety, including prevention of infection, drives much healthcare practice in operating departments, but particularly in the orthopaedic theatre and especially when implantation is involved. Specialized *laminar ventilation systems* in orthopaedic operating theatres reduce the numbers of potentially infecting organisms in the air and staff may be required to wear specialized clothing for the same reason. Operating rooms also need to be kept at a suitable temperature as patients can lose body heat rapidly during long procedures and this can detrimentally affect their recovery and healing. Staff movement in the operating theatre is kept to a minimum. This can be quite difficult because of the need for access to radiographic imaging equipment and the use of casting equipment during the surgical event.

Minimally invasive surgery

Minimally invasive and arthroscopic surgery in orthopaedics has developed rapidly over the last few decades. This also helps to minimize deep tissue and bone exposure to bacteria. The presence of a small incision does not necessarily mean that the patient will recover more quickly or experience less pain as the internal surgical procedure will be just as extensive (see ➔ Arthroscopy, p. 300).

Further reading

Bowden G, McNally M, Thomas S, et al. (eds) (2010). *Oxford Handbook of Orthopaedics and Trauma.* Oxford: Oxford University Press.

Anaesthesia and the orthopaedic patient

Anaesthesia is the use of a pharmaceutical agent for the prevention of pain sensation; it often also involves the induction of an unconscious state so that the patient is fully insensate, or a selective reduction in sensation to a given body part so that the patient cannot feel pain. Anaesthesia is used throughout healthcare for a variety of procedures including surgery, but may also be used to manage acute and chronic pain.

Types of anaesthesia

There are four main types of anaesthesia:
- *General anaesthesia*—a state of complete unconsciousness and analgesia
- *Spinal anaesthesia*—the patient is conscious and anaesthetic agents are injected into the spinal spaces between the vertebrae, producing numbness and analgesia in the area of the body below the injection
- *Epidural anaesthesia*—a form of regional anaesthesia in which anaesthetic drugs are injected into the epidural space to produce anaesthesia along a specific nerve supplying a specific area of the body. Spinal and epidural anaesthesia can be used in combination
- *Regional anaesthesia*—anaesthetic agents are injected into or near the main nerve supply to the limb or part of the body being operated on, providing analgesia to a large body section such as an entire limb
- *Local anaesthesia*—only the nerves or tissue around the surgical site are injected with anaesthetic agent, providing numbness of the local area only.

Safety

Due to the loss of sensation and/or consciousness when anaesthesia has been administered, the patient is no longer able to exert control over their own safety, identify risk, or communicate effectively so protecting them from the risk of harm created by the surgical environment and procedure is essential.

The main tools for this include the preoperative checklist, monitoring of the patient's condition, and control of the environment. It is essential that the patient's identity, the nature of the surgery, and all safety aspects have been considered and that informed consent to the procedure has been gained before anaesthesia is administered.

The patient must be closely monitored during and after surgery until the anaesthetic agent has worn off and its effects no longer place the patient at risk of injury or health deterioration.

Preparation for anaesthesia

Prior to induction of any anaesthetic, most patients are worried about:
- Fear of what will happen during the surgery and afterwards
- Not being in control of what is happening
- Being able to feel, hear, or see things despite the anaesthesia
- Not being able to ask for help if they need it.

The practitioner should be able to reassure the patient by explaining exactly what will happen to them and by answering any questions. It is vital that the practitioner has a good knowledge of how anaesthesia is administered and the effect it will have. These decisions are made by the anaesthetist or anaesthetic practitioner in conjunction with the care team in the days or weeks prior to surgery and include an assessment of the patient's general health status as well as the type of surgery to be conducted. Many ortho-paedic patients undergo surgery on the day of admission—meaning that information about anaesthesia is essential during preoperative assessment.

Some anaesthetists may prescribe pre-anaesthetic sedatives or other medication designed to reduce anxiety in the period immediately before anaesthesia.

Preparation for anaesthesia and surgery is an important aspect of en-hanced recovery pathways (see ➲ Models of service delivery: enhanced recovery/fast-track, pp. 30–31).

Preoperative fasting

Fasting prior to surgery is essential preparation for surgery Muscle re-laxants affect the swallowing reflex and there is a risk of regurgitation of gastric juices and aspiration because of the patient's inability to respond normally to regurgitation by 'gagging'. The main purposes of fasting are to reduce the gastric contents to prevent regurgitation and to reduce the risk of postoperative nausea and vomiting. Optimum times that patients should avoid food and fluids preoperatively is debated and many patients are still fasted for too long, resulting in malnutrition and dehydration, particularly in elderly and frail orthopaedic patients. Although further research is still required, most guidelines suggest that clear fluids should be allowed up to 2 hours before surgery and a light meal (including milk and formula/breast milk) up to 6 hours before. Patients at risk of dehydration should receive intravenous (IV) fluid replacement, commencing in the preoperative period, and their hydration should be carefully monitored throughout the peri-operative period.

Further reading

Smith A, Kisiel M (2016). *Oxford Handbook of Surgical Nursing*. Oxford: Oxford University Press.
World Health Organization (WHO) (2018). WHO Surgical Safety Checklist. ✄ http://www.who.
    int/patientsafety/topics/safe-surgery/checklist/en/

General anaesthesia

General anaesthesia is a reversible state of unconsciousness induced by medication which provides pain relief, relaxation of muscles, and sedation to enable orthopaedic surgery to take place with minimal stress to the patient. This is usually achieved through a combination of IV administered and inhaled agents.

Preoperative assessment and planning

Consideration of the safety of the patient is central to care before, during, and following general anaesthesia with the aim of ensuring that the patient is not aware of any sensations during the surgery and is in a completely relaxed state. It is this state that renders the patient vulnerable to injury and harm. This requires careful assessment and planning prior to the surgical event.

The general health status of the individual will be assessed by the anaesthetist on the day of, or the day before, surgery so that any risk to the patient's health can be managed during induction, maintenance, and reversal of anaesthesia. The extent of screening and the investigations needed will depend on the general condition and age of the patient as well as the type and length of surgery. The anaesthetic and surgical teams need to fully understand any risks posed by the anaesthetic agents and their effects on the individual patient before making decisions about what type and dose of agents to use. Preoperative investigations may include:

- Chest X-ray
- Electrocardiogram (ECG)
- FBC, haemoglobin, U&E levels
- 'Group, save, and cross-match' of blood; based on the anticipated loss of blood during surgery and possible need for transfusion.

The anaesthetist will also need to consider the impact of joint pathology such as RA and ankylosing spondylitis that lead to reduced cervical spine mobility and the caution required using chin lifts and intubating the patient.

The anaesthetic process

General anaesthesia usually involves three phases:
- Induction—the administration of the anaesthetic drugs
- Maintenance—continuous monitoring of the patient and maintenance of the anaesthetized state
- Reversal—the facilitation of regaining of consciousness and control.

Perioperative monitoring

The unconscious and relaxed state created by general anaesthesia has the potential to compromise the airway. Airway maintenance is, therefore, an important aspect of anaesthetic care and may involve the use of oropharyngeal airways, laryngeal mask airways, or endotracheal tubes. It is important to remember that these can traumatize the airways, leading to pain and discomfort postoperatively.

Respiratory, cardiovascular, and neurological status are monitored carefully throughout the surgical event and immediate postoperative period including the monitoring of oxygen saturation and carbon dioxide levels along with the administration of oxygen. Sedation and muscle relaxation will be maintained during surgery using additional analgesia and muscle relaxants. The effects of these agents, particularly muscle relaxation, may need to be reversed using an anticholinesterase agent when the surgery is complete

Recovery and postoperative monitoring

Once the surgery is complete and the anaesthetic has been reversed, the patient will be transferred to the recovery unit and, when their physical condition and state of consciousness allows, onto a ward or postoperative unit. Patients respond differently to the drugs used in general anaesthesia and some may take longer than others to recover consciousness and muscle control. During the first few hours following general anaesthesia the practitioner must carefully monitor the following aspects of the patient's condition:

- Consciousness levels and orientation, which provide an assessment of the level of sedation which remains and continues to put the patient at risk
- Respiratory function, including the patient's ability to maintain their own airway, may be affected for some hours following general anaesthesia: both respiratory rate and oxygen saturation must be assessed regularly until the patient is fully awake and orientated. Oxygen therapy may be needed for the first few hours
- Cardiovascular function may be compromised by both the anaesthetic and the surgery itself: peripheral tissue perfusion, along with BP recordings and pulse rate, should be monitored closely during the immediate postoperative period
- It is vital that practitioners recognize any abnormalities or deterioration as quickly as possible, using an early warning score (EWS)/National Early Warning Score (NEWS), so that a medical assessment and action can be taken as a matter of urgency.

General anaesthesia has improved considerably but remains a significant factor in perioperative deaths for both elective and emergency patients undergoing orthopaedic surgery. Careful monitoring of patients in all stages of general anaesthesia is central in managing risk.

Regional anaesthesia

While local anaesthesia is confined to local tissue, regional anaesthesia involves the injection of anaesthetic agents into or close to the main nerves (either a plexus of nerves or a single nerve) which supply a whole limb or area of the body. This is also known as a peripheral nerve block. This can enable surgery to take place without the need for general anaesthesia or spinal anaesthesia (although some sedation may be necessary), avoiding the potential complications of general anaesthesia and providing pain relief in the immediate postoperative period. This is particularly useful for minor procedures and day surgery. Femoral nerve blocks are commonly used in lower limb surgery and for chronic pain as well as for managing acute pain in some fractures such as hip fracture. Regional anaesthetic injections are guided by ultrasound imaging and can also be provided continuously for pain relief by regular injections into an indwelling catheter.

Biers block

This is a technique often used in the immediate management of fractures and surgery, usually to the upper extremity, where anaesthesia is required for <1 hour. The blood supply to the limb is exsanguinated using a specially designed bandage or by elevating the limb for 2–3 minutes while using an expressing technique to push blood out of the artery. A tourniquet is then applied to prevent arterial blood entering the vessels. IV local anaesthetic agents are injected slowly via a cannula. Anaesthesia, some muscle relaxation, and a bloodless field are achieved. Normal sensation returns quickly after the tourniquet is released. Risk must be managed by ensuring that the use of the tourniquet is carefully timed, and that protection is provided for the skin under the tourniquet during the procedure. Neurovascular observations must be carried out on the affected limb postoperatively whenever a tourniquet is used.[1]

Preoperative care

Preoperatively, patients should be prepared in the standard manner. Some regional anaesthetic procedures fail, so the patient may be prepared as if for general anaesthesia in case this needs to take place unexpectedly. Patients must be fully informed about what to expect during and after the procedure with careful consideration of consent and capacity.

Postoperative care

A period of postoperative observation is required following regional anaesthesia which includes observation for hypotension, headaches, and dizziness. Regional anaesthesia may also mask the symptoms of other complications such as compartment syndrome, so great attention must be paid to pain levels and neurovascular observations when surgery to a limb has been conducted. The return of sensation and mobility to limbs must be monitored.

Some regional anaesthetic blocks are administered close to the central nervous system. Postoperative monitoring should be conducted in the same way as spinal anaesthesia so that problems can be detected and acted upon quickly (see ➲ Spinal anaesthesia, pp. 126–127).

Pain management

The principles of regional anaesthesia can also be used as pain management interventions either as one-off injections for simple nerve blocks or as regional nerve blocks which affect individual nerve supplies for chronic pain. These interventions are only carried out by specialist practitioners who have been trained to conduct the procedure and are supervised accordingly. Patient information and aftercare must include discussion of the possible side effects of the procedure. The effects can last for several weeks or months.

Reference

1. Murphy S, O'Connor C (2010). So what! if a pneumatic tourniquet is used intraoperatively: a study of neurovascular assessment practices of orthopaedic nurses. *Int J Orthop Trauma Nurs* 14:48–54.

Further reading

Gay J, Parker MJ, Griffiths R, et al. (2017). Peripheral nerve blocks for hip fractures. *Cochrane Database Syst Rev* 5:CD001159.

Spinal anaesthesia

Spinal anaesthesia involves the injection of local anaesthetic and/or analgesia into the subarachnoid space. Numbness and analgesia are produced in the area of the body below the injection site. This is particularly useful for pelvic and lower limb surgery. To administer spinal anaesthesia, a lumbar puncture must be performed along with insertion of a hollow fine-bore spinal needle into the lumbar subarachnoid space, usually at lumbar levels L2–5. Anaesthetic agents mix with the CSF and provide sympathetic nerve blockade.

The advantages of spinal anaesthesia include:

- It has little effect on the respiratory system, making it suitable for patients with respiratory problems and other medical conditions; airway problems in the perioperative period are unlikely because the upper body is not affected
- It is useful in emergency trauma surgery where preoperative preparation can be limited by the time available
- The patient can be awake if they wish, although sedation may be given if preferred
- Recovery is usually rapid and side effects are relatively rare
- Some muscle relaxation is achieved
- Because it is relatively short acting, early mobilization is facilitated, and most activities can resume quickly, including eating and drinking. Nausea and vomiting are uncommon following spinal anaesthesia
- It provides a degree of pain relief in the short-term following surgery which also promotes early mobilization
- There is often a very marked hypotensive effect which can help to reduce bleeding during the surgical procedure.

Patients who are unable to cooperate or have unstable cardiovascular problems are among those for whom this procedure is unsuitable.

Preoperative care

Prior to administration of spinal anaesthesia the patient must be prepared for surgery as usual. Preoperative fasting should be conducted as normal in case spinal anaesthesia proves impossible or difficult and general anaesthetic is required. Patients require additional information about what to expect both in the administration of the anaesthetic and the effects following surgery. Preparation should also include commencement of IV fluids. During surgery, constant monitoring of the cardiovascular system should be conducted—particularly BP and ECG monitoring. Severe hypotension or toxic shock are rare complications, but the patient may require cardiorespiratory resuscitation should either of these occur so resuscitation equipment must be on hand.

Postoperative care

In the first 24 hours postoperatively, the following care should be provided:

- The patent's neurological status below the level of the anaesthesia must be carefully monitored: full sensation and movement should gradually return and any residual deficits should be reported to medical staff immediately
- Frequent assessment and recording of BP and pulse should be conducted
- The site of the lumbar puncture should be closely observed for CSF leak (a rare but dangerous complication), haemorrhage, and infection of the site: persistent headache may be a sign of CSF leak
- Any abnormalities must be reported to medical staff immediately
- Due to the loss of sensation from the bladder and difficulty in passing urine lying down, urinary retention, particularly in men, is a common problem following spinal anaesthesia for orthopaedic surgery.[1] Because of this, urinary catheterization is often needed and this causes an additional risk of infection. See ➔ Urinary tract infections, pp. 204–205 for further information
- Incontinence of urine may also become a temporary problem that is distressing for patients and they should be warned about this preoperatively
- Patients should be encouraged to rest in the recumbent position for the first few hours
- Analgesia and IV fluids should be provided as these will help to prevent headache.

Spinal anaesthesia is now a very common procedure but there remains a need for careful monitoring.

Reference

1. Crew S (2007). A review of the effects of spinal anaesthetic in lower limb orthopaedic surgery on urinary retention. *J Orthop Nurs* 11:104–9.

Further reading

Maher AB (2016). Neurological assessment. *Int J Orthop Trauma Nurs* 22:44–53.

Preoperative assessment

Preoperative preparation has two main functions: to assess the patient's health status to ensure they are fit to undergo surgery and anaesthesia and to prepare the patient for the forthcoming procedure by providing information about the procedure and aftercare/rehabilitation (see ➔ Rehabilitation, pp. 176–177). In accordance with the principles of enhanced recovery (see ➔ Models of service delivery: enhanced recovery/fast-track, pp. 30–31) all patients undergoing surgery, either elective or emergency, require preoperative preparation, although the timing and nature may differ.

Preparation for elective surgery

Elective procedures can be classified as (adapted from NICE guidance[1]):

- Grade 1 (minor)—e.g. excision of ganglion
- Grade 2 (intermediate)—e.g. knee arthroscopy
- Grade 3 (major)—e.g. lumbar discectomy
- Grade 4 (major+)—e.g. total joint replacement (TJR).

The timing and nature of preoperative assessment will depend on the classification of surgery as (listed above) and on the general health status and past medical history of the patient. Anaesthetists and nurses working in preoperative assessment clinics usually use the American Society of Anesthesiologists (ASA) scale[2] to describe a patient's level of fitness to undergo an anaesthetic. The categories of the ASA scale are:

- ASA grade 1—a normal healthy patient without any clinically important comorbidity or clinically significant past/present medical history
- ASA grade 2—a patient with mild systemic disease
- ASA grade 3—a patient with severe systemic disease
- ASA grade 4—a patient with severe systemic disease that is a constant threat to life
- ASA grade 5—a moribund patient who is not expected to survive without the operation
- ASA grade 6—a declared brain-dead patient whose organs are being removed for donor purposes.

For example, a patient undergoing a minor procedure under local/regional anaesthetic who is ASA grade 1 will have minimal preoperative assessment comprising a health screening questionnaire and a set of baseline observations. Patients of ASA grade 3 will usually require assessment and clearance by the appropriate medical physician, e.g. cardiologist, and review by the anaesthetist. Patients with an ASA score of 4 or above would not be suitable for elective orthopaedic surgery.

Typically, preparation for elective procedures such as TJR (grade 4+) will be staged and begin at the time the decision to treat is made in the outpatient department. The first stage will be to administer a health screening tool and take a baseline set of observations. Patients who are categorized as ASA 1 or 2 should then be required to attend a preoperative or anaesthetic review clinic, typically 2–4 weeks prior to the date of their procedure. Some healthcare providers combine this appointment with the information-giving/education component of the preparation, but others separate out these two elements and require the patient and a family member to attend a 'joint class' or 'hip and knee group'.

If health problems are detected at the initial screening process the patient will be referred to their GP or to a specialist to investigate and manage their comorbidity (e.g. uncontrolled hypertension, a leg ulcer, etc.). At this stage, the patient would not be placed on the waiting list for their procedure until the health issues identified have been resolved.

Close liaison and communication between the orthopaedic team and the patient's GP is needed to ensure the patient's health status is optimized prior to their procedure and for appropriate symptom management while they are awaiting surgery. It is important to identify patients unfit for surgery/anaesthetic at the earliest possible point; ideally, the GP should have resolved any underlying unstable comorbidity issues prior to referring the patient to orthopaedic services. Late detection of health problems may lead to postponement of the surgery and to disappointment for the patient and their family and is not cost-effective use of resources.

Preoperative assessment clinics

Preoperative clinics or anaesthetic review clinics are frequently nurse-led services which draw upon the expertise of other practitioners, such as anaesthetists and occupational therapists, who provide specific advice and input. Typically, the review will include:
- Reviewing the patient's home situation and identifying their support needs following discharge
- Referral for any equipment such as raised toilet seat, etc.
- Assessment against criteria for early discharge pathways
- Reviewing the patient's current health status through history taking, examination, and clinical investigations (see → History taking 1 and 2, pp. 82–85 and Investigations, pp. 106–111)
- Making referral to other clinical specialties if comorbidity is identified and expert opinion is required prior to surgery
- Providing information about the procedure and postoperative treatment plan.

References

1. NICE (2016). Routine preoperative tests for elective surgery. NICE guideline [NG45]. ℘ https:// www.nice.org.uk/guidance/ng45
2. ASA (2014). ASA Physical Status Classification System. ℘ https://www.asahq.org/standards-and-guidelines/asa-physical-status-classification-system

Preoperative preparation

NICE issued guidelines to underpin decisions about what clinical investigations should be carried out prior to elective surgery.[1] The evidence-based recommendations are presented by ASA grading of the patient and classification of surgery and are coded as: 1) required; 2) not required; or 3) consider, dependent on the age of the patient and the nature of the comorbidity in ASA grade 2 or 3 patients. For an ASA grade 2 patient (with cardiovascular comorbidity) undergoing a TJR the following investigations may be considered:

- Chest X-ray—consider for all age groups
- ECG—required
- FBC—required
- Renal function tests—required
- Clotting profile—consider for all age groups
- Random glucose—not required
- Blood gases—consider for all age groups
- Urinalysis—required for all age groups.

In addition to the recommended investigations, patients undergoing orthopaedic surgery may need investigations to detect any underlying infection which may lead to infection of the surgical site. Urinalysis should be performed and a urine sample sent for culture and sensitivity. Patients may also require the following baseline assessments:

- Height, weight, and calculation of BMI
- BP, pulse, respiratory rate, and temperature
- Meticillin-resistant *Staphylococcus aureus* (MRSA) screening using nasal, groin, and axillary swabbing according to local policy
- Skin check for signs of infection/ulcers/inflammation, particularly in the area close to the site of surgery
- Oral check for signs of dental decay, gum disease, or loose or broken teeth
- Range of movement of the neck should be assessed in patients with suspected or diagnosed cervical ankylosing spondylitis
- Group and save for potential blood transfusion during or following the procedure.

Patients of North, West, or South African or Afro-Caribbean origin will need to be tested for the presence of the sickle cell gene.

Preparation for emergency surgery

The time scale for preparing patients for emergency orthopaedic surgery is a lot shorter, e.g. patients requiring internal fixation for a hip fracture should be operated on within 24 hours to avoid a deterioration of their general health status. However, they still require preoperative assessment including history taking, examination, and clinical investigations as outlined for elective surgery. Emergency patients are often not as medically stable as elective patients, particularly frail hip fracture patients who may be ASA category 3–5. Working with the anaesthetist and medical team to ensure the patient is stabilized medically as much as possible prior to surgery is essential and may require administration of IV fluids/blood.

Additional aspects of preparation

- *Informed consent*—all patients prior to surgery are required to give informed consent for the procedure. Consent can only be informed if the patient has received information about and understood what the procedure will involve, the risks of the procedure, the potential benefits of the procedure, and consideration of alternative treatment modalities. For patients who are unable to consent due to being too ill or who have cognitive impairment, assent from their next of kin or a medical practitioner (if the procedure is considered to be a matter of extreme urgency) may be required—depending on current local and national guidance and legal requirements.

- *Preoperative fasting*—most elective patients for grade 4 surgery are now admitted on the day of surgery unless they have a significant comorbidity, such as insulin-controlled diabetes. All patients prior to surgery and anaesthesia require a period of preoperative fasting to minimize the risk of asphyxiation due to oesophageal regurgitation. They can drink clear fluids up to 2 hours prior to surgery and food and milk up to 6 hours prior to surgery.[2]

- *Medications*—patients should take their normal medication prior to surgery unless instructed otherwise by the anaesthetist. Some surgeons will ask for anticoagulants such as warfarin and aspirin to be stopped 5 days prior to surgery.

- *Prior to the procedure*—a final safety checklist should be completed between the ward and theatre staff prior to the patient entering the operating suite. Psychological support is essential as most patients feel anxious prior to their surgery.

References

1.. NICE (2016). Routine preoperative tests for elective surgery. NICE guideline [NG45]. ॐ https://www.nice.org.uk/guidance/ng45
2.. Smith I, Kranke P, Murat I, et al. (2011). Perioperative fasting in adults and children: guidelines from the European Society of Anaesthesiology. *Eur J Anaesthesiol* 28:556–69.

Postoperative care

Recovery from surgery to the musculoskeletal system carries a high risk of complications the most severe of which can be fatal. This requires careful monitoring to ensure that any adverse effects from the procedure or the associated anaesthesia are identified and acted upon as soon as possible.

Postoperative monitoring and care

The following aspects of patient monitoring and care must be considered in the immediate period following surgery and should include the use of EWS/NEWS scoring:

- *Level of consciousness*—following recovery from anaesthesia the patient's condition may still be subject to the residual effects of anaesthesia. Consciousness levels should be monitored closely during the first few hours following anaesthetic recovery. Reduced level of consciousness can result in difficulty in maintaining respiratory function.
- *Airway and breathing*—respiratory function can be significantly affected by the substances used in anaesthesia. The patient's airway and respiratory function should be monitored closely until the patient is fully conscious. This includes regular observation for signs of airway obstruction, along with monitoring depth and rate of breathing. To maintain adequate oxygenation, oxygen supplementation may be needed for a few hours following surgery. Once the patient is fully conscious, they should be encouraged to sit up if not contraindicated to facilitate lung expansion.
- *Circulation*—one of the most significant risks is haemorrhage from the surgical site. Observation for bleeding from the wound does not always identify bleeding deep within the site. Tachycardia and hypotension, especially when occurring together, are indicators of bleeding. Pulse and BP should be monitored frequently in the first few hours following surgery and continue to be monitored regularly. Blood loss during orthopaedic surgery is often significant and blood or blood product transfusion may be needed during the immediate postoperative period.
- *Wounds*—drainage from either the wound site itself or any drains that are *in situ*. Any excessive drainage from either should be recorded and reported to medical staff. Excessive drainage of blood indicates possible haemorrhage.
- *Hydration and nutrition*—patients who have undergone orthopaedic procedures often require rehydration because of blood and fluid loss during surgery and following any period of preoperative fasting. Intake and output should be carefully monitored, particularly in the first 24 hours. IV administration of fluids may be needed until the fluid deficit has been resolved and the patient is drinking normally. This is particularly important in frail elderly patients. Confusion may be a sign of delirium which can be caused by dehydration and/or electrolyte imbalance. Postoperative nausea and vomiting is a common feature of recovery and this may exacerbate dehydration. Returning to a balanced diet as soon as possible after surgery will support healing and recovery.

- *Temperature*—due to the procedure and exposure of the patient during surgery, hypothermia can be a significant postoperative problem so body temperature must be monitored. Healing is impaired in tissue that is not at an optimum body temperature as lower temperatures affect perfusion. Patients should be kept warm using blankets and warming devices. Wound infection is a complication of orthopaedic surgery which may not become evident until some days after surgery. Monitoring body temperature from early in the recovery period will also enable a comparison of the temperature over time so that any pyrexia can be quickly identified. Pyrexia may also be a sign of blood transfusion reaction.
- *Limb observation*—surgery to limbs carries risk of damage to the circulation and nerve supply to limbs. During the first postoperative days it is essential that the neurovascular status of the limb is closely monitored (see ➲ Neurovascular compromise, pp. 196–197).
- *Pain*—postoperative pain assessment and management are a central aspect of postoperative care (see ➲ pp. 136–147).
- *Positioning, moving, and handling*—many types of orthopaedic surgery require special consideration of positioning and movement. One of the most important skills of the orthopaedic practitioner is understanding the implications of position for specific types of surgery and being able to assist patients to achieve and maintain correct positioning in the postoperative period. This may include support and elevation of limbs using specialist equipment.

Once the patient has sufficiently recovered from the surgical event and associated anaesthesia, the period of rehabilitation can begin in earnest. Following major orthopaedic surgery any aspects of postoperative monitoring and care will need to continue for several days.

Further reading

Smith A, Kisiel M, Radford M (eds) (2016). *Oxford Handbook of Surgical Nursing*. Oxford: Oxford University Press.

Blood and blood transfusion

Major orthopaedic surgery and trauma can be associated with significant blood loss, requiring blood transfusion either pre-, peri-, or postoperatively. For example, patients can rapidly lose 3–4 L of blood into the abdominal/pelvic cavity following a major pelvic fracture or around 500 mL during and following total knee replacement (TKR). Timely transfusion for major haemorrhage can significantly improve outcomes (see ➜ Haemorrhage, pp. 192–193).

In the past, blood transfusions have been the main method used to manage blood loss from surgery. However, increasing shortages of donated blood, increasing public concern regarding infections acquired from donor blood, and religious beliefs have led to a more prudent approach led by the following principles[1]:

- Transfusion should only be used when the benefits outweigh the risks and there are no appropriate alternatives
- Results of laboratory tests are not the sole deciding factor—transfusion should be based on clinical assessment and evidence-based guidelines
- Transfusion is not the only way to treat anaemia
- Risks, benefits, and alternatives should be discussed with the patient and informed consent gained
- Reason for transfusion should be documented in the clinical record
- Ensuring the right patient gets the right transfusion at every stage of the process is essential: failure to check patient identity can be fatal
- Carful patient monitoring during the transfusion for signs of adverse reaction
- Regular education and training of all staff involved in transfusion.

Blood and blood products

Replacing blood loss due to haemorrhage requires the prescription and administration of blood products in the form of one or more of the following:
Blood components:

- Red cells
- Platelets
- Fresh frozen plasma
- Cryoprecipitate.

Plasma derivatives:

- Albumin
- Coagulation factors
- Immunoglobulins.

Plasma derivatives must be prescribed by a licensed practitioner. Whole blood is now rarely used for transfusion. Autologous transfusion (the transfusion of an individual's own blood) has been shown to be of limited value and is now rarely used.

Pharmacological alternatives

Alternatives to transfusion and have been developed to reduce the amount of blood products used in surgery and traumatic injury. Pharmacological options include:

- Tranexamic acid—a synthetic lysine derivative that inhibits fibrinolysis
- Aprotinin—inhibits many proteolytic enzymes and reduces fibrinolysis
- Tissue sealants—derived from human or animal clotting factors such as fibrinogen: sprayed on surgical fields or raw tissue to promote haemostasis and reduce blood loss. Clinical trials show that they can reduce surgical bleeding and exposure to donor blood, particularly in orthopaedic surgery.

Recognizing and managing risk in blood transfusion

Patients receiving blood transfusion require stringent risk management at all stages of the procedure from cross-matching and prescribing to administration of the blood. Complications due to incompatibility can be serious and life-threatening. All adverse events and reactions related to blood and blood components must be reported to the appropriate authority.

The safe requesting, collection, and administration of blood components form the basis of local transfusion policies. The key principles that underpin every stage of the blood administration process are:

- Positive patient identification
- Good documentation
- Excellent communication.

Reference

1.. Joint United Kingdom (UK) Blood Transfusion and Tissue Transplantation Services Professional Advisory Committee (JPAC) (2014). *Transfusion Handbook*. London: JPAC. ℗ https://www.transfusionguidelines.org/transfusion-handbook

Further reading

Joint United Kingdom (UK) Blood Transfusion and Tissue Transplantation Services Professional Advisory Committee (JPAC) (2014). 4: Safe transfusion – right blood, right patient, right time and right place. In: *Transfusion Handbook*. London: JPAC. ℗ https://www.transfusionguidelines.org/transfusion-handbook/4-safe-transfusion-right-blood-right-patient-right-time-and-right-place

Acute pain

Acute pain has a clearly defined onset, a brief duration (<3 months), and subsides as healing takes place. It is often the chief complaint in traumatic soft tissue injury, fracture, and in the immediate postoperative period. Acute pain is a physiological response to injury and as such provides a protective function and is one of the most common reasons patients will access trauma and orthopaedic services.

Physiological response to acute pain

Acute pain results in several physiological responses including:
• Increased BP
• Increased pulse rate
• Increased respiration rate
• Dilated pupils
• Perspiration
• Nausea and/or vomiting
• Diarrhoea.

These responses are typical of the flight or fight mechanism, the body's response to threat or danger.

Physiology of pain

Both motor and sensory nerve fibres are involved in the transmission and reaction to pain. Pain receptors are densely situated in the dermis, periosteum of bone, and articulating surfaces of joints. Injury or surgery to these structures stimulates the nociceptors and transmission of impulses which are interpreted as pain by the higher brain centres.

Defining pain

Pain is a difficult phenomenon to define due to its subjective nature and the many factors that influence the perception and expression of pain such as:
• Gender
• Ethnicity/culture
• Psychological status
• Past experiences of pain
• Knowledge.

However, a widely accepted definition is 'Pain is what the person experiencing it says it is, existing whenever the person says it does'.[1]

Consequences of acute pain

Acute pain, if unrelieved, can lead to chronic pain and impact on all dimensions of the patient's well-being and function, including:
• Reduced mobility/movement
• Anxiety and stress
• Loss of appetite
• Sleep disturbance
• Inability to concentrate
• Increased risk of pressure ulcers and venous thromboembolism (VTE) due to reduced mobility.

Management of acute pain

Presentation of acute pain requires urgent assessment to determine the cause of the pain. This will involve history taking, examination, and clinical investigations. The practitioner, in collaboration with other members of the MDT, has a duty to assess patients' pain using a valid and reliable method (see ➲ Pain assessment, p. 140) and to provide adequate pain relief in a timely manner (see ➲ Pain management, p. 140 and Pharmacological management of pain, p. 144). If the orthopaedic MDT are finding it difficult to manage a patient's acute pain they should seek specialist support from acute pain services.

Reference

1. McCaffery M (1972). *Nursing Management of the Patient in Pain*. Philadelphia, PA: Lippincott.

Further reading

Brook P, Pickering T, Connell J (eds) (2011). *Oxford Handbook of Pain Management*. Oxford: Oxford University Press.

Chronic pain

Chronic pain is often ill defined and has no clearly identified trajectory. Pain is classified as chronic as opposed to acute when it has been present for >3 months. Chronic pain is a widespread problem that cannot always be resolved by pharmacological and medical interventions. It is estimated that between one-third and one-half of the UK population are affected by chronic pain at some point in their lives,[1] placing tremendous strain on individuals, society, and healthcare resources. This is a common symptom in many orthopaedic conditions such as low back pain, OA, RA, and ankylosing spondylitis. Despite the prevalence of chronic pain, it continues to be sub-optimally managed in many patients, leading to a significant negative impact on their quality of life.

The impact of chronic pain

Chronic pain, if inadequately managed, has physical, social, and psychological consequences and has a significant deleterious impact on patients' quality of life. This can include:

- Anxiety, depression, and/or anger
- Withdrawal from society
- Loss of role function within the family and society
- Social isolation
- Loss of or reduced income
- Muscle wasting
- Reduced mobility/movement
- Altered body image
- Relationship difficulties.

Patients suffering chronic pain can be unfairly labelled as malingerers by the public and sometimes by healthcare professionals. Often there is no clearly identifiable cause of their pain and a poor prognosis. It is important to remember that pain is subjective and what the patient is experiencing, and to adopt supportive and non-judgemental approaches to management of patient with chronic pain.

Supporting patients with chronic pain

Effective management of patients with chronic pain requires a holistic interprofessional approach and working with the patient and their family in partnership. The first stage in management is assessment and diagnostics to elicit the cause of the pain. This will include MRI scans, physical examination, the use of pain diaries, and pain assessment tools, etc. When the cause of the pain is identifiable, such as prolapsed intervertebral disc, then surgical intervention may resolve the problem completely. However, in a significant number of cases the cause cannot be identified and/or cure is not possible. Strategies then need to be adopted to support the patient to effectively manage their pain and cope and adapt to the problem.

Specialist chronic pain management services are becoming more prevalent within orthopaedic centres and bring together the expertise of the MDT. The Royal College of Anaesthetists[2] have provided core standards for pain management services in the UK which should include the use of

Pain Management Programmes (PMPs) based on cognitive behavioural principles. PMPs can be delivered in primary or secondary care settings and are run as individual or group activities which help to normalize the pain experience and provide individuals with strategies for managing their pain. PMPs comprise:

• Patient education on pain physiology, pain psychology, and self-management approaches
• Support and guidance for patients to set goals, plan, and evaluate their progress
• Relaxation, exercise, and self-management techniques
• Challenging negative attitudes and behaviour related to pain and disability.

Other methods of managing chronic pain are outlined in ➲ Pain management, p. 142, Pharmacological management of pain, p. 144, and Patient-controlled analgesia and epidural p. 146.

References

1.. Fayaz A, Croft P, Langford R, et al. (2016). Prevalence of chronic pain in the UK: a systematic review and meta-analysis of population studies. *BMJ Open* 6(6). ℘ http://dx.doi.org/10.1136/bmjopen-2015-010364
2.. Royal College of Anaesthetists (RCA) (2015). *Core Standards for Pain Management Services in the UK*. London: RCA. ℘ https://www.rcoa.ac.uk/system/files/FPM-CSPMS-UK2015.pdf

Further reading

Mackintosh-Franklin C (2014). Pain assessment and management in orthopaedic and trauma care. In: Clarke S, Santy-Tomlinson J (eds) *Orthopaedic and Trauma Nursing*, pp. 120–30. Oxford: Wiley-Blackwell.

Pain assessment

The practitioner has a duty to accurately and regularly assess patients' pain and to ensure that the effectiveness of pain management strategies is evaluated. Inadequate pain management is not acceptable and can have a serious impact on patient well-being and recovery as outlined on ➲ Acute pain, p. 136. Unrelieved pain can affect outcomes following surgery and prolong length of stay. Practitioners frequently underestimate patients' pain but, because of the subjective nature of pain, it is important to use methods of assessment that include the patient as a partner and active participant in the process. The frequency of pain assessment will be dependent on the nature of the pain (i.e. acute or chronic), but assessment should also always be completed following pain management interventions to evaluate their effectiveness.

Methods of pain assessment

Pain should be assessed at rest and during activity as patients frequently report little or no pain when resting, but severe or extreme pain on mobility or performing certain activities or movement. Older adults are least likely to report their pain and are at most risk of having their pain inadequately managed.

Assessment of pain should involve questioning about the nature of the patient's pain, including:
- Onset, duration, and frequency
- Location
- Aggravating and relieving factors
- Intensity
- Description, e.g. stabbing, burning, sharp, dull
- Associated signs and symptoms, e.g. swelling/locking or giving way.

Patients should also be observed for non-verbal signs of pain such as restlessness, agitation, and withdrawal, facial grimacing, and reduced movement/mobility. This is particularly important for patients with cognitive, memory, learning, and communication difficulties.

Patients with chronic pain may benefit from completing a daily pain diary. The use of pain assessment tools is recommended, and it is important that tools used have a robust evidence base and are:
- Valid
- Reliable
- Sensitive
- Specific
- Practical.

Examples of well-tested pain assessment tools include:
- Visual analogue scale (VAS)—the patient is required to make a mark on a 10 cm line to indicate their level of pain, with 0 indicating no pain to 10 being the worst pain imaginable
- Numerical rating scale (NRS)—the patient is asked to verbally rate their pain using numerical values, e.g. 0 indicating no pain, to 10 worst pain imaginable

- Verbal descriptor scale (VDS)—the patient is asked to select a word to quantify their pain from a predefined list, e.g. no pain, mild, moderate, severe, extreme
- Disease-specific PROMs such as the Oxford hip and knee scores, WOMAC; clinical back pain questionnaire include elements of pain assessment.

Assessing pain in patients with special needs

Some patients may not be able to verbally articulate their pain or use pain assessment tools due to communication, cognitive, or learning difficulties. The nurse must assess their pain using physiological indicators as detailed in ➲ Acute pain, p. 136 and/or observe non-verbal signs and behaviour. Several specific tools have been developed for children and people with cognitive or communication problems such as the Wong–Baker Faces pain rating scale which uses six facial expressions ranging from 'no hurt' to 'hurts worst'.

Further reading

Mackintosh-Franklin C (2014). Pain assessment and management in orthopaedic and trauma care. In: Clarke S, Santy-Tomlinson J (eds) *Orthopaedic and Trauma Nursing*, pp. 120–30. Oxford: Wiley-Blackwell.

Pain management

All practitioners have important roles to in the effective management of patients' pain. Management strategies will be dependent on the nature of the pain, e.g.:
• Is the pain acute or chronic? Is the pain localized or multi-site?
• What is the cause of the pain, e.g. postoperative or following trauma?

It is important to adopt an individualized approach to each patient's pain management, drawing upon the expertise of the MDT and seeking further guidance from specialist pain management teams when pain management is complex. Pharmacological approaches to pain management are not the only approach to managing pain and it is widely thought that a variety of approaches are most likely to be successful. This topic, therefore, focuses on non-pharmacological interventions (see ➋ Pharmacological management of pain for pharmacological interventions, p. 144 and Patient-controlled analgesia and epidural, p. 1). Non-pharmacological approaches to pain management include:
• PMPs (see ➋ Chronic pain, pp. 138–139)
• Transcutaneous electrical nerve stimulation (TENS)
• Heat and cold therapies
• Acupuncture
• Other complementary therapies, e.g. massage (see ➋ Complementary and alternative therapies, p. 148).

Other options include positioning, splitting and supporting the affected limb along with other general comfort measures e.g. careful placement of a pillow.

Some of the most common non-pharmacological pain management interventions include:

Transcutaneous electrical nerve stimulation

TENS is often used in the treatment of chronic pain, particularly low back pain. It works in two ways: (1) using high-frequency signals to stimulate beta nerve fibres around the painful area which block pain signals being received by the brain, and (2) using low-frequency current to stimulate the release of endorphins (the body's natural pain killers). An electrical current is delivered through electrodes applied to the skin around the source of the pain. TENS is a safe method of pain relief, with the only known potential side effect being local irritation of the skin where electrodes are applied, although its use is contraindicated in epileptic patients and those with a pacemaker. TENS should not be used in the vicinity of water for safety reasons or electrodes applied to damaged skin. TENS machines allow patients to self-manage their pain and they can experiment with different locations of electrodes and frequency and length of use to suit their own needs.

Use of hot and cold therapies

Ice therapy (also known as cryotherapy) is recommended for the treatment of acute musculoskeletal injury following trauma such as ankle sprain, postoperatively following TKR, or for fatigue injuries such as carpal tunnel syndrome. Ice therapy is not suitable for muscle spasm, e.g. in low back pain. Ice should not be applied directly to the skin but in a plastic or fabric cover and should only be applied to the skin for short periods to avoid ice burn; typically this is the length of time it takes for the area to become numb (around 1–5 minutes). The frequency of application will depend on the depth of the tissue being treated, but usually 2–3 hours between applications is appropriate. Ice therapy should not be used on damaged skin, for patients with diabetes, or those with circulation problems or conditions that affect skin sensation such as neuropathy. When using ice over a surgical wound, use a clean cloth over the wound and put the ice in a plastic bag to avoid the wound getting wet.

Heat therapy such as hot water bottles, deep heat creams, heat pads, wheat bags, and heat lamps are useful in the relief of muscle spasm and with injuries >48 hours old, when inflammation has subsided. Typically heat should be applied for around 20 minutes and then repeated as the area cools or pain reoccurs. Care should be taken to avoid burning the skin and deep heat applications (creams/sprays) should not be used on or near damaged skin or surgical wounds.

Acupuncture

Acupuncture has been used within Chinese medicine for thousands of years and in the last two decades in other countries; it is increasingly being used as either a replacement for, or as an adjunct to, pharmacological management of pain. Acupuncture involves the insertion of fine needles into various points of the body following energy channels or meridians. Only fully trained professionals should carry out the treatment.

Other approaches

Musculoskeletal pain, particularly of the neck, back, and upper limb, account for many lost working days. A report by the Institute for Musculoskeletal Research and Clinical Implementation[1] recommended early assessment and treatment of musculoskeletal pain achieved through partnership between the sufferer, their employer, and musculoskeletal practitioners. Adaptations to the work environment to improve posture and reduce strain are highly effective, e.g. use of wrist supports to minimize strain during computer use, correct height of office chairs, and having workstations at the correct height help to prevent and reduce musculoskeletal pain.

Reference

1. Institute for Musculoskeletal Research and Clinical Implementation (2005). *Improved Early Pain Management for Musculoskeletal Disorders*. The Health and Safety Executive. London: Her Majesty's Stationery Office.

Pharmacological management of pain

Pharmacological pain relief can be administered via the following routes:
- Regional anaesthesia, e.g. femoral nerve block and epidural (see ➔ Postoperative care, p. 132 and Patient-controlled analgesia and epidural, p. 146)
- Orally
- Sublingual
- Topical, e.g. NSAID creams and gels
- Injection—IV, intramuscular (IM), or subcutaneous (SC)
- Intrathecally—into the thecal space of the spine
- Inhalation, e.g. Entonox® for manipulation of closed fractures
- Transdermal—slow-release patches.

Types of analgesia

There are three categories of analgesics:
- Opioid drugs, e.g. morphine and codeine
- Non-opioid drugs, e.g. paracetamol, NSAIDs
- Co-analgesic drugs, e.g. muscle relaxants or antidepressants such as amitriptyline for neuropathic pain.

The analgesic ladder

The analgesic ladder (Fig. 4.1) provides a basic model to decide on the type of analgesia needed. The weakest strength is at the bottom of the ladder, i.e. non-opioids such as paracetamol, rising to a weak opioid such as codeine, and then, at the top of the ladder, strong opioids such as morphine. The analgesic ladder can, for example, be applied to the management of postoperative pain following orthopaedic surgery; the patient returns from surgery with an IV or epidural infusion of morphine which typically stays *in situ* for 24–48 hours, then is removed and the patient commences on oral codeine plus paracetamol, reducing to paracetamol only. Only accurate and ongoing evaluation and assessment of the patient's pain can determine stepping up or down the analgesic ladder.

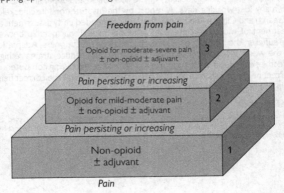

Fig. 4.1 World Health Organization pain ladder.

Clinical decision-making about analgesia

Increasingly, nurses and other practitioners are taking on the role of an independent prescriber following stringent education; deciding on the type, dose, frequency, and route of administration of analgesia under group directives, depending on local policy and procedures. Although evidence-based protocols are often adopted for analgesic regimens following orthopaedic surgery or trauma, it is important to assess each patient individually. This should include the nature and intensity of their pain, any history of allergy to certain types of analgesia and preferred route of administration (consider needle phobia, inability to swallow tablets, etc.). The practitioner must monitor the effect of analgesia through regular re-evaluation of the patient's comfort and pain score. If analgesia is not effective, the prescription should be reviewed as soon as possible to avoid worsening/untreated pain. The patient must also be monitored closely for side effects of analgesia including:

• Respiratory depression
• Constipation
• Nausea and vomiting
• Anaphylaxis
• Skin irritation, itching, rashes.

Patients are often reluctant to take regular analgesia due to fear of addiction, over-reliance, and/or constipation and other side effects. Patient education is essential to ensure that adequate pain relief is achieved and working in partnership with the healthcare team, specialist pain team, and the pharmacist is essential in cases of uncontrolled or complex pain.

Further reading

Mackintosh-Franklin C (2014). Pain assessment and management in orthopaedic and trauma care. In: Clarke S, Santy-Tomlinson J (eds) *Orthopaedic and Trauma Nursing*, pp. 120–30. Oxford: Wiley-Blackwell.

Patient-controlled analgesia and epidural

Postoperative and other acute pain management is often more effective when the sufferer of the pain has control over their own analgesic administration. One option for this is patient-controlled analgesia (PCA). This involves patient self-administration of analgesia using opioids, usually intravenously (or subcutaneously), using an infusion pump and administration device. The patient can press the button on the device when they experience pain to deliver a measured dose of analgesia. 'Lockout' intervals can be programmed into the pump to prevent overdose. This allows rapid uptake of the drug and effect. Such administration can be gradually supplemented and replaced by oral analgesics from the 'pain ladder' (see ➋ Fig. 4.1, p. 144). The aim is for the patient to have no pain or mild pain at rest and mild pain when moving, allowing them to become mobile as early as possible.

Some of the advantages of PCA are:

• Patients are in control of their own pain relief and do not need to wait for someone to administer the analgesia for them, ensuring it is received quickly when it is needed
• The dose can be titrated according to pain levels
• Maintenance of blood levels of analgesia is achieved as small doses are given little and often so that peaks and troughs in concentrations are avoided
• Good pain relief means that patients can move around more easily, helping to prevent the complications of immobility.

Potential problems of PCA include:

• The need for planning, careful patient selection, and patient education, consent, and understanding—this is not always possible after trauma and emergency surgery and for patients with cognitive difficulties
• The patient and the device need constant specialized supervision
• There are several side effects of the drugs that can be unpleasant for the patient including nausea, vomiting, and constipation as well as respiratory problems
• Malfunction of the IV line and/or the pump may lead to inadequate analgesic effect
• Working with patients using PCA requires special training for staff to set up and manage the infusion and pump and the required patient observation
• Bulky pumps and other equipment may restrict patient movement.

As with all opioid analgesia, close monitoring of the patient is vital, particularly as respiratory depression may be a side effect. The patient must be constantly reassessed and pain levels must be carefully monitored through regular pain assessment to ensure that the equipment, drug, and dose are working correctly.

Epidural analgesia

Epidural analgesia involves the administration of pain-relieving medication into the epidural space using an indwelling catheter. This can also be attached to a pump and controlled by the patient. It is particularly successful in the prevention of postoperative and trauma pain, especially involving the lower limb. The aim is for the patient to be pain free or have minimal pain both at rest and on movement. Opioids are the most common drugs used for this purpose, along with local anaesthetic agents.

Monitoring and care must be provided by practitioners who have appropriate knowledge and skills in the management of epidural analgesia and must include:

- Observation for 'total spinal anaesthesia' caused by leakage of local anaesthetic into the intrathecal space; the symptoms of this complication are convulsions, loss of consciousness, apnoea, and hypotension. This is a medical emergency
- Opioids inhibit the parasympathetic nervous system and urinary retention can sometimes be a problem
- The side effects of opioids must be observed for, including respiratory depression, nausea, and vomiting
- The motor system should not be affected by epidural analgesia; muscle weakness and immobility indicate that this has occurred and this is a medical emergency
- Close observation of the catheter site for skin reactions and occlusion or movement of the catheter are required
- All adverse reactions of problems must be reported immediately to medical practitioners.

Further reading

Mackintosh-Franklin C (2014). Pain assessment and management in orthopaedic and trauma care. In: Clarke S, Santy-Tomlinson J (eds) *Orthopaedic and Trauma Nursing*, pp. 120–30. Oxford: Wiley-Blackwell.

Complementary and alternative therapies

Complementary medicine/therapies are those which are seen to complement more traditional healthcare approaches, while the term 'alternative' refers to the use of therapies instead of more traditional practices. What are known in Western cultures as complementary and alternative therapies, have been standard healthcare practices in other cultures for centuries or, even, millennia. Complementary and alternative medicine/therapies (CAMs) are now an increasing facet of healthcare in developed countries. Non-conventional therapies such as these are often used in palliative care and in the hospice setting but are gaining wider acceptance within traditional healthcare and orthopaedic patients are turning to them more often. Because they are contrary to the traditional 'Western' biomedical model, many healthcare practitioners are sceptical about their value. Some of the most common CAMs are listed in Table 4.1.

Table 4.1 Categories of CAMs

Group 1	Group 2	Group 3
Professionally organized alternative therapies:	Complementary therapies:	Alternative disciplines:
Acupuncture	Alexander technique	3a. Long established transitional systems of healthcare:
Chiropractic	Aromatherapy	Ayurvedic medicine
Herbal medicine	Bach and other flower remedies	Anthroposophical medicine
Homeopathy	Massage	Chinese herbal medicine
Osteopathy	Reflexology	Traditional Chinese medicine
	Healing including Reiki	3b. Other alternative disciplines:
	Hypnotherapy	Crystal therapy, dowsing, iridology, kinesiology, radionics
	Shiatsu	

The role of CAMs in orthopaedic care

While there are many different types of therapies, there are several that are commonly considered as having application for orthopaedic practice for their value in facilitating comfort and healing. Those therapies most often used by nurses such as massage, aromatherapy, and reflexology are often viewed as being most useful in this area of practice. Acupuncture and Reiki are being increasingly used by nurses.[1] Relaxation, visualization, and imagery are also used in the management of comfort and pain. Wound pain and wound odour are sometimes treated with essential oils.

In additional to specific physical benefits, many CAMs are thought to have general health benefits and are often used by patients to supplement their own coping strategies. Individual preference and the patients' own health beliefs are significant in the rationale for choosing specific therapies.

Touch is a very simple form of complementary therapy. It is thought that one of the main benefits of CAMs is that they involve one-to-one contact with the practitioner which includes touch and active listening, and these, in themselves, are beneficial. Many patients report physical, psychological, and physical benefits of therapies, although evidence in the orthopaedic setting is limited.

The role of the practitioner and professional issues

While CAMs can be popular with patients and carers, there is often a less positive response from the medical profession. Professions allied to medicine are more likely than doctors to participate in the administration of such therapies, although professional guidelines on this vary and the evidence base is not as well developed or conclusive as that for traditional healthcare.

Consideration of safety and effectiveness as well as desirability to the patient are important aspects of practice. Practitioners should be aware of local and national guidance on providing and administering CAM therapies. Therapies must only be administered by competent practitioners with appropriate qualifications who have undergone training and assessment. CAMs should be used alongside healthcare and medical/surgical interventions where they are most likely to be beneficial. Where complementary and alternative therapies are being used alongside conventional medicine it is important that the patient's medical practitioner is aware of this so that any potential adverse interactions with traditional healthcare interventions, such as drugs, can be avoided.

Reference

1.. Royal College of Nursing (2003). *Complementary Therapies in Nursing, Midwifery and Health Visiting Practice*. London: RCN.

Wound management

An understanding of wound healing and how it occurs enables provision of effective wound care that results in surgical or traumatic wounds that heal without the development of complications such as delayed healing, dehiscence (breakdown), haematoma, or infection.

Wound healing

Wound healing occurs in three phases, each with distinct cellular and tissue activity. Although this does not necessarily occur in the same way in all wounds, there is a general pattern—see Table 4.2.

Table 4.2 Phases of wound healing

Inflammatory	Proliferative	Remodelling
Immediate to 2–5 days	2 days to 3 weeks	3 weeks to 2 years
Haemostasis (clotting):	Granulation:	New collagen fibres form
Vasoconstriction	Fibroblasts lay down	Increase in tensile strength
Platelet aggregation	collagen bed	
Thromboplastin	Defect fills	
makes clot	New capillaries formed	
Inflammation:	Contraction:	
Vasodilatation	Edges pull together	
Phagocytosis	Epithelialization:	
	New epithelial cells migrate	
	across wound	

Types of wound

There are several different types of wound which are common in the orthopaedic setting. These fall into two categories.

Acute wounds

Acute wounds are of sudden onset and normally heal in <6 weeks. This includes surgical wounds and most traumatic wounds. Acute wounds mainly heal by 'primary intention' as the edges are usually closely opposed to each other, thus facilitating the formation of new capillaries and the migration of epithelial cells. Examples of acute wounds that do not readily heal in this way are those where there is tissue loss such as skin tears, degloving injuries, compound fracture wounds, and burns.

Chronic wounds

Chronic wounds are defined as wounds taking >6 weeks to heal. They usually involve significant loss of tissue and/or poor blood supply and include pressure ulcers, leg and foot ulcers, and surgical or traumatic wounds that have dehisced and become cavity wounds. Chronic wounds normally heal by 'secondary intention' from the base of the wound upwards, usually without wound closure although plastic surgery in the form of skin grafting may be undertaken in some cases.

Wound assessment

A thorough and clearly documented assessment of the patient and the wound, including barriers to healing, should be conducted to ensure that the right conditions for effective wound healing are created. This should consider:

- The cause and nature of the wound and the extent of tissue loss or exposure
- The size and location of the wound
- The phase of healing
- The condition of the wound bed and wound edges
- The condition of the surrounding skin and the presence of any exudate
- Any signs of infection such as inflammation, pus, or odour
- The general condition of the patient including nutritional status and underlying medical conditions that may affect healing.

Conditions required for wound healing

- A moist, warm, wound bed is known to facilitate healing; drying out of the wound bed should be avoided
- Good circulation to the wound and surrounding tissue, providing a good supply of oxygen and nutrients.

Barriers to wound healing

Several important factors impede healing:

- The presence of infection (see ❯ Wound infection, pp. 206–207), pus, or slough
- Malnutrition—particularly depletion of protein, calories, vitamin C, and water (see ❯ Nutrition, pp. 164–165)
- Trauma to granulating tissue, e.g. when adhered dressings are removed
- Wounds under physical stress, such as those across the knee or a swollen limb, often heal more slowly.

Principles of wound management

Effective wound management involves the following considerations:

- The patient and their wound site should be kept as warm as possible, particularly during surgery and in the postoperative period.
- Wounds should be disturbed as little as possible and wound care carried out using strict aseptic technique—helping to avoid infection.
- Wound cleansing should only be carried out if wounds are 'dirty' or known to be contaminated.
- Unhealed and open wounds should be covered with a sterile dressing; this dressing should protect the wound from bacteria while maintaining a moist environment where there is exposed unhealed tissue.

Further reading

Donnelly J, Collins A, Santy-Tomlinson J (2014). Wound management, tissue viability and infection. In: Clarke S, Santy-Tomlinson J (eds) *Orthopaedic and Trauma Nursing*, pp. 131–50. Oxford: Wiley-Blackwell.

Surgical wound management

Most orthopaedic surgical wounds have been created in sterile, or at least aseptic, conditions in the operating theatre. The orthopaedic surgical environment is designed to ensure that such wounds are as protected as possible from contamination with microorganisms during the surgery. Consequently, surgical wounds should be expected to heal without complications. It is vital, however, that practitioners know how to intervene when wound problems occur.

Potential surgical wound problems

There are four main complications of surgical wounds:

- *Haemorrhage* is a risk following surgery. In orthopaedic surgery deep tissues are involved. The risk is especially high during the first 24 hours postoperatively, so the wound should be observed closely for any excess wound drainage or bleeding into the dressing. Medical staff must be informed immediately of any continuing blood loss from the wound.
- *Haematoma* may occur deep within the tissues if haemostasis has not been achieved before and during wound closure. A deep haematoma will prevent the deep tissue from healing and may result in breakdown of the wound. Later, the haematoma may liquefy and leak through the dehisced wound. A haematoma can be a major source of infection and drains are used to try to prevent them (see ➔ Wound drainage systems, p. 154).
- *Surgical site infection* (SSI) remains a significant problem in orthopaedic wounds. Deep SSI can lead to infection around implants and prostheses and to osteomyelitis (see ➔ Wound infection, p. 206). Infection around implants means that the implant may need to be removed. The patient should be observed for pyrexia until the wound is sufficiently healed and the sutures or clips have been removed.
- *Dehiscence* of the wound is most often as a result of delayed healing in the presence of infection or poor nutrition. It is also sometimes the result of a deep haematoma. The problem will usually become evident when sutures or clips are removed. The reason for dehiscence needs to be investigated.

Postoperative wound management: general principles

- Immediately following surgery, a protective sterile dressing should cover the wound and be kept in place with a firm adhesive dressing or bandage. The wound should be closely observed for bleeding into the dressing. The initial dressing should be left intact for the first 24 hours to allow the wound to settle and to be kept warm. If there is noticeable bleeding/exudate showing through the dressing it should be changed and the wound closely monitored for excessive discharge.
- Prevention of infection is central to postoperative wound care following orthopaedic surgery. Deep infections of wounds and implants can lead to severe infections and osteomyelitis. Prophylactic antibiotics are often prescribed before, during, and/or after orthopaedic implant surgery. The practitioner must make sure that all antibiotic therapy is administered as prescribed and that the wound is protected by strict aseptic technique.

- When surgical wound dressings are changed this should be done using strict aseptic technique and the wound observed for any signs of the wound problems described previously, such as a gaping suture or clip line, swelling, redness, discharge, or bleeding. The wound should be disturbed as little as possible.
- Any dressing covering the wound should be sterile. Patient allergies to adhesives must be considered when choosing a dressing. It should also help to keep the wound warm and act as a barrier against contamination and irritation from clothing. Cleansing of the wound is only necessary if there is dried exudate, blood, or other wound debris to be removed.
- The dressing may be removed and the wound exposed once there is no exudate. Many patients prefer to keep the wound covered to protect it.
- There is debate about the risks of bathing or showering. It is thought that showering with the wound covered by a dressing and then immediately changing the dressing afterwards is acceptable, but that bathing should be avoided to prevent wound maceration and contamination. The wound should be dried using sterile gauze and a new dressing should be applied immediately.
- Many patients are discharged within a few days of surgery. On discharge, patients need to be given written and verbal instructions on how to care for their wound, how to recognize problems, and how to seek help. Arrangements must be made for the removal of wound closure materials such as sutures or clips.

Wound drainage systems

Orthopaedic surgery takes place deep within the tissues and usually involves bone. Therefore, it is often necessary to ensure that bleeding in the immediate postoperative period is not allowed to collect deep within the wound. During surgery, wound drainage systems can be inserted for use within the first 24–48 hours following surgery. This allows clotting time to stop all bleeding and prevents haematoma from developing at the base of the wound, which may impede healing and act as a focus for infection. There is, however, debate about the value of wound drains and whether they should be used at all—the evidence is inconclusive,[1,2] with some research seeming to show that wound outcomes are not improved by the use of drains and that they increase the risk of infection and the need for blood transfusion.

The care of wound drainage systems

Wound drainage systems provide a portal from the outside environment into the deep tissues and, sometimes, underlying bone. This presents a significant risk of deep wound infection which may lead to osteomyelitis or infection of implant sites so wound drainage systems in orthopaedic surgery should always be closed systems in which there is no open portal that can allow microorganisms to enter the wound. These are made up of a drainage tube with a series of holes at one end and a drainage receptacle which often has suction to assist in removal of fluid from the surgical site (see Fig. 4.2). The care of wound drains involves:

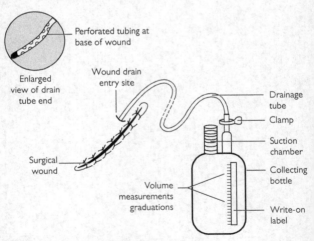

Fig. 4.2 Typical closed suction wound drainage system.

- Close monitoring and recording of amount and type of drainage. Any excessive drainage should be reported to a medical practitioner immediately as this may indicate haemorrhage
- Wound drainage collection receptacles should be emptied, using aseptic technique. This should be done when the receptacle is more than half full and the amount recorded
- All parts of the system should only be handled using aseptic technique and standard precautions for the prevention of cross-infection
- The system should be checked regularly for signs of blockage or displacement; the vacuum on the container should also be checked
- The insertion site of the drain should be covered with a sterile, occlusive dressing at all times and the tubing secured using tape; the tubing may have been sutured into place depending on surgeon preference
- Patients should be informed about what the drain is for and how it works. They should be encouraged to mobilize and not be restricted by or avoid activity because of it.

Removal of wound drainage systems

Wound drains should be removed when drainage has stopped or is minimal (<50 mL in 24 hours). Drains should only ever be left *in situ* for short periods of time—up to 48 hours following surgery. The chances of infection increase the longer the drain is *in situ*. The patient should be carefully prepared for removal of the drain and analgesia given and allowed to take effect before the procedure.

Any sutures securing the drain should be removed. The suction should be removed from the drain before removal and the drain removed using strict aseptic technique and protective sterile gloves. The drain and receptacle should be disposed of carefully following clinical waste procedures.

References

1. Dealey C (2005). *The Care of Wounds: A Guide for Nurses*, 3rd edn. Oxford: Blackwell.
2. Parker MJ, Livingstone V, Clifton VR, et al. (2007). Wound drains in orthopaedic surgery (surgery in joints or limbs). *Cochrane Database Syst Rev* 2007;3:CD001825.

Wound closure

Wound closure aims to keep wound edges close together and minimizes the space between the tissues while healing takes place. It also supports the tissues so that there is minimal tension in the wound. When two wound edges can be closely opposed to each other—as is the case for most surgical wounds—new blood vessels can form, and epithelial cells migrate more easily.

Most orthopaedic surgical and trauma wounds heal by primary intention with edges neatly brought together and held in place to facilitate healing. Closure of the wound immediately, or within 12 hours, is known as *primary closure*. A planned delay (from 1–2 days to several weeks) in wound closure is sometimes required in wounds known to be contaminated, contain foreign material, or occurred >6 hours previously. This allows drainage and close observation of the wound bed. Closure of the wound later is known as *delayed primary closure*. Very deep wounds may not benefit from closure at all and will be left to heal by *secondary intention*. These wounds heal gradually from the base of the wound upwards over much greater time scales.

Traumatic wound closure

Wounds such as those caused by compound fractures and other traumatic wounds, where contamination with dirt/bacteria may cause infection, should not be closed immediately and will be left open initially.

Traumatic wounds should be thoroughly irrigated to ensure there is no dirt or foreign material remaining. Anti-tetanus status of the patient should be ascertained and vaccine given if lack of cover is suspected. Full assessment of the wound should be undertaken before wound closure to make sure there is no foreign material remaining and that underlying structures such as tendons and nerves have not been damaged. Deep and complex wounds, and where there is severe damage to or loss of tissue, may not be closed for some time and may need longer-term specialist wound care, such as vacuum-assisted closure or skin grafting.

Surgical wound closure

In orthopaedic surgery, most wound closure of incisions takes place in the final phase of surgery, often involving suturing of deep tissue such as muscle or fascia and repair of surrounding structures before the skin is closed. Sutures and other closure materials may need to be removed once the wound is sufficiently healed for it to no longer need the additional support usually towards the end of the proliferative phase of healing. The timing of this will depend on several factors which will include the tensile strength of the healed wound, the depth of the wound, the amount of tissue healing required, and the amount of tension the wound is under. Wounds across the knee—particularly those running distally to proximally—often take longer to reach this stage because of the tension on the wound when the knee flexes and extends. Increasingly, dissolvable suture materials are used which do not need removing.

Wound closure materials

There are several different types of wound closure materials available. The main ones are:

- *Sutures*—used to hold together both deep and superficial wound tissue. Deep wound suture materials tend to be absorbable and do not need removal. The main categories of suture material are monofilament (made of a single strand of material) and multifilament (made of several strands of material twisted together). Monofilament materials are more difficult to handle but are thought to be less prone to infection.
- *Clips* or *staples* are commonly used for closure of orthopaedic incisions following suturing of the deeper tissues. They are inserted using specialist equipment in the operating theatre and penetrate only into the upper surface of the wound so are thought to be less prone to infection.
- *Tissue glue* can be used to close superficial traumatic lacerations and is under experimentation in minor surgical wounds.
- *Adhesive strips* are used in minor surgical wounds such as arthroscopic portal wounds or minor traumatic wounds which are under minimal tension and with minimal edge separation. They can also be used with other types of closure to provide additional support and are easily be removed by peeling them gently away from the skin.

Wound closure material removal

- Sutures and clips or staples remain as a foreign body in the skin until they are removed. While the material is present there remains a risk of infection caused by the small wound created by each of the sutures or clips. For this reason, the wound should be kept covered until the wound closure material has been removed.
- Sutures should be removed carefully while ensuring the suture material that has been exposed during wound healing is not pulled back through the suture hole; the holes may remain a focus for infection until healed.
- Removal of clips or staples should be conducted using removal devices specifically manufactured for the purpose.
- Once sutures and/or clips/staples have been removed, the wound should remain covered for a further 24 hours until initial healing of the holes has occurred, and the wound has sealed.

Hygiene and comfort

Comfort and hygiene are basic human needs. Because orthopaedic conditions, injuries, and surgery are often painful and lead to immobility or reduced mobility, hygiene and comfort are difficult for patients to maintain for themselves. This means that a central aspect of care is ensuring that comfort and hygiene are maintained.

Comfort

Patient comfort is a broad concept. It is often defined as a general feeling of well-being brought about by being without pain and having needs for fluid and dietary intake and fulfilment of elimination needs met as well as the maintenance of personal standards of hygiene and dignity.[1] Comfort is also synonymous with being free from pain. In orthopaedic care, comfort enhancement activities not only involve pain assessment and analgesic administration, but also include careful attention to positioning and repositioning in order to achieve a comfortable state that is conducive to recovery, rest, and sleep. Such strategies may be as simple as repositioning a pillow or foam wedge to support a joint more effectively or gently massaging a limb that is suffering from muscle spasm. Attention to such aspects of care is central to the recovery of the orthopaedic patient from injury and surgery as well as in coping with long-term orthopaedic conditions. The skilled orthopaedic practitioner is often able to easily recognize patients who are uncomfortable and in need of assistance to improve their comfort. Such assistance includes the following:

- Ensuring that the environment in which care is provided includes comfortable, supportive surfaces such as beds and chairs with clean linen and covers which do not irritate the skin
- Provision of clothing that is comfortable for the patient to wear and which considers their orthopaedic problem as well as facilitates dignity and personal preferences
- Maintaining an environmental temperature that is comfortable for the patient along with enough fresh air and natural light
- Ensuring the control of noise in the care environment which enables the patient to rest and sleep and not be subjected to sensory overload
- Paying attention to the patient's normal habits regarding positioning. Often patients know best or can feel which position suits their problem. The practitioner can help patients to experiment with different repositioning strategies.

Maintaining personal hygiene

Personal hygiene is an important aspect of an individual's identity and dignity as well as the prevention of skin problems and infection. It may be difficult for orthopaedic patients whose mobility is severely affected to self-care to the level of hygiene that they would normally prefer or need to achieve, and the practitioner is central in helping them to maintain a level of hygiene that ensures their comfort. The interventions which are central to this include the following:

- Assisting patients to achieve clean and dry skin. Particular attention should be paid to skin-fold areas and those which are prone to perspiration and odour such as the axilla, under breasts, perineum, and perianal areas. The level of support needed with washing should be carefully assessed to ensure that the patient is assisted to self-care whenever possible.
- Ensuring that patients have access to adequate toilet facilities either in bed, at the bed- or chair-side or a short distance away.
- Helping patients to avoid excessively dry skin with the judicious use of appropriate cleansing agents and moisturizers/emollients which protect and do not irritate the skin.
- Assisting with washing and dressing and enabling the patient to participate as much as feasible. This should be as close to the standard preferred by the patient as possible and includes hair washing, which can be particularly difficult for someone who is immobile or confined to a bed or chair.
- Ensuring that patients who are unable to access bathroom and toilet facilities can maintain a safe level of hand hygiene before meals and after using the toilet.
- Providing facilities and assistance for adequate mouth, teeth, and denture care which enables the patient to have a clean, fresh, and moist mouth and avoid gum and teeth decay and infection.
- Facilitating the care of the skin and nails of both hands and feet. Feet can be problematic for patients who are unable to mobilize normally and who cannot reach their own feet. Dry, hardened skin can build up and toenails can become long and brittle, restricting mobility and causing pain.

Maintenance of a satisfactory level of comfort and hygiene are central aspects of providing good-quality care to the orthopaedic patient. Such care interventions are often provided by unqualified healthcare assistants. It is essential that the qualified practitioner maintains an oversight of these activities and ensures that those providing such care are appropriately trained and skilled in this fundamental activity.

Reference

1.. Santy J (2001). An investigation of the reality of nursing work with orthopaedic patients. *J Orthop Nurs* 5:22–9.

Moving and handling

Injury and back pain are significant problems for staff working in the ortho-paedic setting. Poor moving and handling practice is often responsible for injuries. Because orthopaedic patients are commonly immobile and need assistance to move, both patients and those caring for them are at risk of injury. In most localities there are a range of local and national health and safety policies, regulations, and guidance which apply to manual handling activities. In order to avoid injury, employers and practitioners must ensure that staff are trained/educated, and that knowledge of safe practice is applied to practice.

Moving and handling activities in the orthopaedic setting

In the orthopaedic setting, common activities of particularly high risk include:
- Moving and handling of patients whose musculoskeletal condition, injury, or surgery restricts their independent movement
- Moving patients from bed to trolley, and vice versa, when admitted and in the perioperative period
- Assisting patients to move who are restricted by casts, traction, and orthoses
- Assisting patients to reposition in bed and move from bed to chair and chair to standing or while walking
- Helping patients to use toilets, commodes, and bathroom facilities
- Assisting patients to move who are in pain, unable to cooperate, or are likely to move in an unpredictable manner or may fall.

Risk assessment

Risk assessment of every patient and every moving and handling situation is an essential step in safe practice. This should include[1]:
- *Task*—that which needs to be done (such as a patient moving from point A to point B)
- *Individual capability*—the skills of the person carrying out the task
- *Load*—that which is to be moved (e.g. the patient or an object) and its properties
- *Environment*—those factors in the environment which affect the task, the load, and the individuals carrying them out.

The need for a task to take place at all and whether it can be conducted using equipment, must be assessed. The identification of risks must be recorded and used to assist decision-making and planning of patient movement and handling. Practitioners must also consider risk and manual handling practice in all aspects of their lives both in the workplace and outside it.

Education and training in moving and handling are essential to all healthcare professionals—attendance at offered training opportunities is the responsibility of the practitioner who must ensure that they attend training and put it into practice in avoiding risk to themselves and others.

Practice

Safe practice is also the responsibility of the individual practitioner. In addition to standard training and education, practitioners need knowledge of the correct methods of assisting patients with musculoskeletal problems and the likely results of movement as well as sound knowledge of current recommended practice. This is also a team responsibility and leadership and change management are important aspects of ensuring compliance to current guidance and policy.

In the spirit of rehabilitation, most orthopaedic patients should be supported in doing as much for themselves as possible, resulting in less risk for both the patient and practitioner. Particularly important is an awareness of movements and positions during positioning and repositioning that place the patient at risk. Examples of this are the movements and positions to be avoided following total/hemiarthroplasty of the hip.

Equipment

An array of equipment is now available to assist in moving and handling tasks. Some of this is in standard daily use in orthopaedic and trauma settings. The practitioner should be trained to use, and be knowledgeable about, the operation and safe working of such equipment and has a duty to use the equipment available when appropriate. Equipment should be freely available at the point of care delivery as well as in good working order. The use of such equipment should be included in patient assessment and documented in a moving and handling plan. Equipment that should be in constant use should be stored near the point of care delivery. Such equipment also includes aids to mobility so that the patient can move themselves as much as possible.

An awareness of the safe working loads of equipment is important, particularly when moving and handling overweight, obese, and morbidly obese patients (often termed 'bariatric') for whom specialist equipment may be needed.

Reference

1.. Smith J (ed) (2011). *The Guide to the Handling of People*, 6th edn. Teddington: Back Care.

Further reading

Talley Holman G, Ellison KJ, Maghsoodloo S, et al. (2010). Nurses' perceptions of how job environment and culture influence patient handling. *J Orthop Nurs* 14:18–29.

Elimination

The elimination of urine (micturition) and of faeces are important physical functions which result in the expulsion of waste from the body in solid and liquid form. The emptying of bowel and bladder are both sensitive issues and these activities are normally conducted in private. Because of immobility and other aspects of care, orthopaedic patients often find that they cannot maintain their normal habits, so helping them to maintain bladder and bowel function is essential.

Because of their immobility, many orthopaedic patients must either use a bed pan, urinal, or commode, or must be assisted to use a toilet. These activities can be embarrassing, and the practitioner must pay attention to maintaining the patient's dignity and privacy. This includes:

• Whenever possible, helping the patient to use a normal toilet behind a closed door
• Providing prompt assistance so that patients do not have to wait
• Ensuring the curtains are fully drawn, patients are covered, and they are not disturbed when using bed pans and commodes at the bedside or a toilet
• Providing all necessary equipment including hand-washing facilities toilet paper, air fresheners, etc.
• Giving patients plenty of time to void their bladder or bowel properly.

Because of immobility, and other factors, bladder and bowel problems are relatively common in the orthopaedic patient and can be the most distressing aspect of their care—see Table 4.3.

Because of the sensitive nature of bladder and bowel function, many patients find discussing these issues difficult and they are unlikely seek early help if they have problems. The practitioner must, therefore, ensure that careful and regular assessment of both bowel and bladder functions are made in a manner which is professional and sensitive, putting the patient at ease.

Bladder care

The bladder is an organ which acts as a holding tank for urine so that it can be emptied at a socially appropriate time. The capacity of the bladder to hold normal amounts of urine and to empty through the urethra can be affected by orthopaedic conditions and injuries, orthopaedic surgery, anaesthesia and blocks, and by immobility. Important aspects of care are as follows:

Table 4.3 Potential bladder and bowel problems in the orthopaedic patient

Bladder problems	Bowel problems
Urinary stasis due to immobility	Constipation
Urinary retention	Incontinence of faeces
Frequency of micturition	Diarrhoea
Urinary incontinence	Haemorrhoids
Urinary tract infection	

- Maintain normal bladder function by ensuring that the patient is adequately hydrated. Ideally, the patient should drink at least 1.5 L of fluid per day—more in warm weather (unless there are health reasons why a patient's fluid intake should be restricted). Being well hydrated means that the bladder will fill with normal amounts of urine and maintain the right concentration of salts and other chemicals.
- Urinary incontinence is distressing, has several causes and is usually a sign of bladder dysfunction. This may be the most distressing problem for any patient and care must begin with an assessment of the causes of the problem. It should never be assumed that the patient was incontinent before admission to hospital, but it should be assumed that there is an underlying cause. Urethral catheterization should be avoided as much as possible and only be used as a last resort as it commonly leads to urinary tract infection (UTI) which may become blood-borne and infect orthopaedic surgical sites and implants.
- UTI is a distressing and dangerous complication for the orthopaedic patient (see ➲ Urinary tract infection, pp. 204–205).
- Urinary retention is also a common problem following surgery (see ➲ Urinary retention, pp. 216–217).

Bowel care

The fact that orthopaedic patients cannot maintain their normal bowel habits can lead to problems with defecation. Bowel habits are very individual, and it is important that an assessment is made of the patient's normal habits so that continuing assessment can ascertain if the patient's norm is not maintained.

Constipation is common in orthopaedic patients and is considered in more detail later—see ➲ Constipation, pp. 214–215.

Patients can also suffer from diarrhoea. It is essential that the cause is identified: there are three main causes in the orthopaedic patient:

1. Infection (usually as a result of food poisoning or other sources of infection such as person-to-person transfer). In all cases stool cultures should be sent to the laboratory. Until the cause of diarrhoea is ascertained, cross-infection must be prevented using standard precautions.
2. When infection has been ruled out, diarrhoea is often due to the administration of antibiotics as they disrupt the normal bowel flora and can lead to *Clostridium difficile* infection.
3. Faecal overflow due to constipation.

Further reading

Burscough S, Smith B (2009). The rehabilitation experience of an elderly female patient following a fractured neck of femur compounded by clostridium difficile infection. *J Orthop Nurs* 13:19–23.
Parker V, Giles M, Graham L, et al. (2017). Avoiding inappropriate urinary catheter us and catheter-associated urinary tract infection (CAUTI): a pre-post control intervention study. *BMC Health Serv Res* 17:314.

Nutrition

Good nutrition is central to good health. Food intake can affect recovery from orthopaedic surgery and trauma and diet can also be responsible for some orthopaedic conditions. Nutrition significantly affects musculoskeletal health. Failure, for example, to eat a diet rich in calcium in the first 20 years of life can be responsible for poor bone health in later life. Obesity throughout the lifespan is deemed to be partially responsible for the development of OA. Improving nutrition in all sectors of society is often a focus of health promotion for both government and non-governmental organizations. In less affluent sectors of society, getting enough to eat is central to health improvement, while in more wealthy societies, improving the quality of what people eat is more important.

Impact of poor nutrition on recovery

Malnutrition is a deficiency of nutrients that influences health. Many individuals eat and drink less than they need and this can result in delayed recovery, increased risk of infection and other postoperative complications, delayed healing, impaired respiratory and cardiovascular functioning, and decreased energy levels and muscle strength.

Nutritional assessment

Orthopaedic patients are at risk of malnutrition if their dietary intake is depleted as a result of their condition, surgery, or other underlying factors that affect appetite and absorption of food. Older patients may be particularly at risk as they may be malnourished on admission. All patients should undergo nutritional screening and assessment which identifies those who need nutritional support.

Patients should be considered at risk if they:
- Have a BMI of <18.5 kg/m^2
- Have recently lost weight unintentionally
- Have a depleted appetite or are unable to feed themselves/find eating difficult.

Appetite is an important aspect of nutrition. Individuals who feel unwell or have suffered trauma or undergone surgery often do not feel like eating. Postoperative nausea and vomiting may affect appetite for a several days.

Good nutrition

A diet rich in all the essential nutrients is not only important in maintaining musculoskeletal health, but supports healing and helps prevent infection and other complications. Although a diet rich in all nutrients is central to maintaining health, the following dietary components need particular consideration:
- *Calories* provide the energy for physical functioning, growth, and recovery. Following injury and orthopaedic surgery, patients need additional calorific intake in order to support healing. Those who do not eat enough calories may begin to derive their energy requirements from the breakdown of lean muscle, resulting in muscle wasting and weakness which can hamper recovery

- *Protein* is an essential component of human tissue and is needed to support healing of both soft tissue and bone
- *Water* is a major component of most human cells, so intake of fluids is central in maintaining cell health and promoting recovery
- *Vitamin C* is required for most metabolic functions and is central to healing and recovery
- *Calcium* is an essential mineral in bone
- *Vitamin D* promotes absorption and use of calcium and phosphate so is essential in maintaining skeletal health
- *Iron* is essential to the production of haemoglobin which transports oxygen needed for general functioning.

Nutritional support

Malnutrition has frequently been reported as a significant problem for hospitalized patients. For orthopaedic patients with depleted dietary intake, three main options for nutritional support are available:
- Extra intake, including special food or drinks
- Diet supplemented by nasogastric tube feeding
- Parenteral nutrition—the provision of nutrients intravenously.

Supporting intake

The following are examples of good practice in ensuring adequate intake:
- Nutritional support is the responsibility of the full MDT
- Ensuring at-risk patients are identified and supported
- The intake of patients identified as at risk is monitored
- Patients who need assistance to eat are given enough help
- Protected mealtimes ensure that patients can focus on eating without unnecessary interruption
- Provision of attractive, appetizing food that considers patient choices
- Additional meals, snacks, and high-calorie drinks are freely available.

Further reading

British Association for Parenteral and Enteral Nutrition (BAPEN) (2012). Standards and guidelines for nutritional support of patients in hospitals. ℘ https://www.bapen.org.uk/resources-and-education/education-and-guidance/clinical-guidance/standards-and-guidelines-for-nutritional-support-of-patients-in-hospitals

Communication

Communication is an important aspect of human behaviour and interaction and is used in every aspect of society to enable individuals to understand each other. It involves the use of verbal and non-verbal messages to convey information between two or more individuals.

Communication in orthopaedic care

In healthcare, communication is used to convey a caring attitude to those receiving care, to help patients and carers to understand what is happening to them, and to facilitate the forming of relationships which facilitate the assessment, planning, delivery, and evaluation of care. By the very nature of their problems and care needs, orthopaedic patients require sensitive and effective communication with all those involved in their care. If communication is ineffective, practitioners cannot understand patients' needs nor receive information about those needs. Failure to communicate effectively results in failure to meet patients' care needs and leads to safety breaches.

Communication is the basis for high-quality care. Practitioners who are skilled communicators build effective interpersonal relationships with patients and others involved in their care. Failures in communication are the most common reason for patients and their families to complain about treatment and care. Skilled practitioners can use their personality and expert communication skills to maximize their therapeutic impact—known as 'therapeutic use of self'. Deliberate use of effective communication and personality on the part of the practitioner can result in patients feeling more confident in those providing care and more in control of their care. This shifts the balance of power in the relationship, so that patients are more likely to act in their own best interests. Patients who feel that practitioners understand their problems are also more likely to be satisfied with their care. Non-verbal communication, and the way in which practitioners use their body language and facial expressions, can make a significant difference to the patient's confidence in them. Most of all, patients want practitioners to be kind to them, listen to them, and demonstrate that they care. Even the careful use of humour can make patients feel more at ease with those caring for them. Orthopaedic practitioners work with patients and families from diverse cultural backgrounds and it is important that cultural norms and language difficulties are considered when communicating.

Communication problems

Assessment of the barriers to communication and ensuring that they are minimized facilitates well-planned and executed care. Orthopaedic patients may experience many problems with communication. Both immobility and physical disability can lead to difficulty in communicating verbally. Body language and position are important aspects of how human beings communicate. An individual who is in a wheelchair or is confined to bed may feel 'talked down to' by practitioners who fail to adapt their body language to the situation. Those who are in pain, recovering from surgery and/or trauma, are frightened, and are less mobile than usual may have difficulty with hearing, speaking, understanding, and writing, leaving them feeling isolated from those around them unless practitioners take steps to overcome these barriers.

Stress, anxiety, and information

It is known that health problems, injury, surgery, treatment, and admission to hospital are very stressful for individuals and provoke intense anxiety. Anxiety levels can be reduced by ensuring that patients, and their families, receive sufficient information that is presented to them in an understandable way. It is important to assess the need and desire for information, and the level of information needed. Some patients have a greater capacity for more complex information than others, while some find the information provided inappropriate for their level of intelligence. Some patients prefer not to share information with members of their family. Some individuals require more repetition and slower delivery of information than others so that they can remember what they have been told; the pace needs to be altered accordingly.

During all healthcare interventions, but especially after injury and before surgery, providing both written and verbal information has a significant impact on the patient's experience of care, recovery and, even, on pain levels. Information and communication are also essential aspects of informed consent prior to procedures and surgery. Backing up verbal information with well-written reading or video material helps patients to remember important aspects of what they have been told. The patient's ability to read and their reading level must be considered and they must be enabled to ask questions and receive appropriate answers.

Further reading

Bach S, Grant A (2015). *Communication and Interpersonal Skills in Nursing*, 3rd edn. London: Sage.

Psychological aspects of care

Psychological health and well-being are important aspects of the care of trauma and orthopaedic patients. Failure to address the psychological support needs of patients can have a negative impact on their physical health, recovery, and concordance with advice and treatment. The link between physical and psychological well-being is well established, but still frequently receives insufficient attention. Psychological distress, if prolonged, will affect physical health, pain tolerance, and the immune system, impacting the body's ability to defend itself against infection. All patients will have psychological needs and the basic principles of psychological support include:

• Treating patients with dignity, kindness, and respect
• Offering information about support available
• Open and honest communication with patients and families
• Listening to patients' anxieties and concerns
• Empowering patients to be active participants in their care
• Providing information at the right time and in an appropriate format.

In addition to these basic principles of emotional care, some patients may have specific psychological care needs, due to:

• Stress and anxiety following trauma or prior to planned surgery
• Altered body image due to musculoskeletal disability or amputation
• Depleted motivation during the rehabilitation phase
• Feeling out of control due to hospitalization or reduced independence.

Stress and anxiety

It is important to recognize when patients are experiencing high levels of stress and/or anxiety. Signs and symptoms may include:

• Inability to concentrate
• Disturbed sleep
• Emotional mood swings
• Altered appetite and digestion
• Increased heart rate and BP
• Lowered immunity.

There are several valid and reliable tools to assess patients' levels of stress/anxiety and depression. The practitioner should engage in therapeutic communication to support the patient and to elicit the cause of their stress and or anxiety. Good information giving may be enough to alleviate their concerns, but referral to specialist mental health or clinical psychology services may be needed if symptoms persist.

Altered body image

Body image is the way individuals perceive that their bodies appear to the external world. There are many conditions and that may alter the way in which an individual views their body image, e.g.:

• RA and OA will disfigure joints, shorten limbs, and necessitate the use of walking aids
• Bone tumours or severe trauma may necessitate amputation of a limb
• Use of external fixators to lengthen limbs or to stabilize fractures
• Scarring from surgery.

Price[1] developed a five-concept model of body image comprising body reality (the body as it really is); body ideal (beliefs about how the body should be); body presentation (how the body is presented to the outside world); and two mitigating personal responses: coping strategies and social support networks. Practitioners need to assess patients' reactions to and coping with a change of body image and offer support through therapeutic communication and, if needed, referral to clinical psychologists and self-help groups.

Motivation

During the rehabilitation phase, high levels of sustained motivation are required by the patient to work towards their goals and the nurse needs to work in partnership with the patient and their family to achieve this. Guthrie and Harvey[2] suggested the following strategies to maximize patient motivation:

- Information, to reduce threat and restore control
- Providing choice and participation in goal setting
- Attention to social and emotional needs
- Discouraging families from being over-protective
- Creating a therapeutic culture of optimism and hope
- Providing positive role models, e.g. patients with a similar injury or disease who have achieved success.

Feeling out of control

Rotter[3] described individuals as considering their locus of control to come from within themselves (internal locus) or believing that they as individuals have little or no control over events (external locus). Through effective communication, empowerment, and advocacy approaches the practitioner can support the patient to have a strong internal locus of control which is important in maximizing independence and concordance with treatment once discharged.

References

1.. Price B (1990). *Body Image: Nursing Concepts and Care*. London: Prentice Hall.
2.. Guthrie S, Harvey A (1994). Motivation and its influence on outcomes in rehabilitation. *Rev Clin Gerontol* 4:235–43.
3.. Rotter JB (1966). Generalised expectancies for internal versus external locus of control of re-inforcement. *Psychol Monogr* 30:1–26.

Mobilization

Mobilization involves the musculoskeletal system (skeleton, muscles, tendons, ligaments, joints) along with the neurological system to initiate, control, and coordinate movement. Pathology in either or both systems can lead to immobility or reduced mobility, but causes of reduced mobility can be multifactorial and include:

- Intolerance to activity, decreased strength and endurance
- Pain and discomfort
- Perceptual/cognitive impairment
- Psychological factors.

There are three essential elements for mobilization: (1) the ability to move, (2) the motivation to move, and (3) the environment to permit and facilitate movement. Practitioners working with orthopaedic and trauma patients will care for patients with impaired mobility due to any of these factors. Patients may have reduced mobility due to a pathological problem, such as a fracture of the lower limbs, soft tissue injury, joint disease, and pain. However, some people may not have a physical barrier to mobilizing but, because of depression, fear of falling, or cognitive impairment, may lack the motivation to mobilize. Others may have the ability to move with or without aids, but are prevented from doing so because of environmental factors such as narrow doorways, preventing access for wheel chair users, or those using a walking frame (see ➔ Disability and enabling environments, pp. 174–175 for further discussion on enabling environments).

Assessment of mobility

Assessment and ongoing monitoring of mobility and movement are essential. Assessment should include:

- Gait assessment
- Assessment of balance and coordination
- Assessment of muscle strength using a recognized scale such as the Medical Research Council[1] scale ranging from 0 (no power) to 5 (normal power)
- Assessment of patients' mental health for issues of depression, anxiety, confusion, or psychosis which may impact their ability and motivation to mobilize
- Assessment of the environment to identify barriers and safety threats
- Assessment of walking aids, e.g. are they appropriate and does the patient know how to use them correctly?
- Walking distance and factors that limit mobility, such as pain, shortness of breath, fear of falling, poor sight, and poor footwear.

Impact of immobility or reduced mobility

Immobility or reduced mobility can have serious implications for patient's health and well-being and can lead to complications including:

- Pressure ulcers
- DVT/VTE
- Reduced independence
- Impact on body image
- Loss of muscle tone and strength
- Elimination problems such as constipation and urinary incontinence.

The practitioner must work collaboratively with other members of the MDT to ensure the patient's plan of care and treatment includes measures to minimize risk of complications. Specific information on prevention and management of pressure ulcers and DVT is provided later—see ➲ Pressure ulcers, pp. 220–221 and Venous thromboembolism, pp. 194–195. A programme of passive and active exercise should be developed with the physiotherapist to restore lost muscle tone and strength and prevent further deterioration. The occupational therapist will be able to provide advice and support regarding aids to assist in maximizing independence. Psychological support for patients having trouble with adapting to altered body image due to a mobility problem is an important aspect of holistic care.

Reference

1.. Medical Research Council (MRC) (2018). Muscle scale. ℘ https://mrc.ukri.org/research/facilities-and-resources-for-researchers/mrc-scales/mrc-muscle-scale/

Aids to mobility

Many orthopaedic and trauma patients will require aids to assist their mobility, either for temporary support while awaiting surgery, following surgery, or trauma, or permanently to enhance their safety and independence. It is important to understand what the various types of mobility aid are, their use, how to ensure the patient is using their mobility aid correctly, and how to measure patients to ensure they have the correct height of walking aid such as a stick or crutches. Mobility aids can assist patients when non-weight-bearing (NWB), partial weight-bearing (PWB), or fully weight-bearing (FWB). Inappropriate or incorrect walking aids or incorrect height and inappropriate use of aids can lead to harm. Axillary crutches, for example, are now rarely used as when they are too long they can cause the patient to exert excessive pressure into the axilla, leading to permanent nerve palsy.

Types of mobility aid

The type of mobility aid will usually be decided by the physiotherapist and will depend on a number of factors including:
- The stability of the patient
- The strength of the patient's upper and lower limbs
- The degree of coordination of the limbs
- The degree of support of weight bearing required (NWB, PWB, FWB).[1]

Types of mobility aid include:
- Wheelchair
- Walking frame
- Metal and wooden walking sticks
- Elbow crutches
- Rollator
- Quadrupod walking stick.

General principles for measuring patients for walking aids

The patient should be measured when standing upright and wearing their shoes. The patient should be able to hold the stick, crutches, or frame with their elbow flexed to a 30° angle and their spine erect with its curves maintained.

General principles for correct use of walking aids

Although it will normally be the physiotherapist who will initially instruct the patient in the use of their walking aid, in the absence of the therapist the orthopaedic practitioner will be required to carry out this role. It is an integral part of the healthcare role to supervise patients when mobilizing with aids and to reinforce correct technique.

Walking frame

When using a walking frame and rising from a sitting position, patients should reach a full standing height using the arms of the chair prior to taking holding of the frame: they should not use the walking frame as leverage for standing as it is not stable and there is a risk of falling. Patients should be instructed to move the frame forward and step into it with the unaffected limb moving forward first.

Two walking sticks or crutches

The principles for use of crutches and two walking sticks for patients who are NWB or PWB are the same, as they both require a three-point gait, i.e. supporting the affected or injured limb with the other limb and the two crutches or sticks. The patient should be instructed to move both sticks/crutches forward around 30 cm at the same time as swinging the injured/affected limb forward to a point level with the sticks/crutches and then stepping forward with the unaffected limb. This is then repeated. When ascending stairs, the crutches/sticks should be held in the hand opposite the wall and step onto the step with the unaffected limb. The crutches/sticks should then be moved with the affected limb onto the step at the same time—and repeat. Descending the stairs should involve holding the crutches/sticks in the hand opposite the wall and then stepping down onto each step with their affected limb and crutches/sticks at the same time, then moving the unaffected limb onto the step.

One stick

Patients should be instructed to use the stick in the opposite hand to the affected limb and to move the stick around 30 cm in front while moving their affected limb at the same time and then bringing the unaffected limb through to complete the gait cycle.

Instructions to patients

Patients should be given both verbal and written instructions on how to use and care for their walking aids once discharged. Hand grips and axillary pads need to be in good condition and the ferrules (rubber bungs to prevent slipping at the end of sticks and crutches) need to be checked regularly for signs of damage and replaced as necessary. Patients should be instructed to report any sensory impairment/swelling/pain or discomfort in the upper limbs due to pressure from using their walking aids.

Reference

1. Lucas B, Davis P (2005). Why restricting movement is important. In: Kneale J, Davis P (eds) *Orthopaedic and Trauma Nursing*, 2nd edn, pp. 105–39. Edinburgh: Churchill Livingstone.

Disability and enabling environments

In 2012, there were over 11 million people with long-term illness, impairment, or disability in the UK. The most common impairments were those that affect mobility, lifting, or carrying. The prevalence of disability rises with age; 6% of children were disabled, compared to 16% of working-age adults and 45% of adults over 65 years.[1] The Equality Act[2] defines a disabled person as someone who:

> ... has a 'physical or mental impairment that has a 'substantial' and 'long-term' negative effect on your ability to do normal daily activities.

Examples of mental impairment include problems associated with memory, concentration, or ability to learn and/or understand. Physical impairments include problems associated with:

- Mobility
- Chronic illness and chronic pain
- Manual dexterity
- Physical coordination
- Continence
- Ability to lift, carry, or otherwise move everyday objects
- Sensory and communication problems with speech, hearing, eyesight.

A significant number of people accessing orthopaedic and trauma services have a disability which may be the principal reason for referral, e.g. patients with chronic low back pain, ankylosing spondylitis, OA or RA affecting multiple joints. Also, patients with musculoskeletal problems may have a disability due to learning difficulties, mental illness, or sensory impairments.

Enabling environments

People with disabilities do not have the same access to healthcare services or receive the same standard of treatment and care as people without a disability. There has been a positive move away from considering that disabled people are the problem and recognition that the problem is the way society fails to support the needs of people with disability. The Equality Act[2] outlined new rights for people with disabilities in relation to:

- Employment
- Education
- Dealing with the police.

In addition, practitioners must consider the impact of healthcare and the healthcare environment on people with disabilities. This should focus on making sure that disability discussed with patients—and not ignored—while enabling the individual to receive care that respects their needs and wishes.

Practitioners working in orthopaedic and trauma settings have a responsibility to support the inclusivity of people with a disability. It is important to ensure that all forms of patient information are appropriate for people with any type of disability, bearing in mind that not all disabilities are visible, and to work with support organizations to gain expert advice on how to achieve this.

References

1.. DPWO/Office for Disability Issue (2014). Disability facts and figures. ℜ https://www.gov.uk/government/publications/disability-facts-and-figures/disability-facts-and-figures
2.. HMSO (2010). Equality Act. ℜ https://www.gov.uk/guidance/equality-act-2010-guidance

Rehabilitation

Most trauma and orthopaedic patients require rehabilitation following either injury or surgery. Rehabilitation is a goal-directed process comprising several stages, and which aims to restore individuals to their maximum potential following disease, surgery, or trauma. Patients and their family/carers should be considered as active partners in the rehabilitation process and not passive recipients. Delaying rehabilitation can be detrimental to patient outcomes, so the process should begin as soon as the patient is medically stable. Care in a rehabilitation context is concerned with maximizing independence and requires a more hands-off approach compared to caring for patients in the critical or acute phases of their journey. Rehabilitation requires the practitioner to motivate and encourage the patient to do as much for themselves as possible with support, rather than doing things for them in preparation for them to return home and adapt to their new circumstances.

The rehabilitation process

The rehabilitation process comprises four stages:
- Comprehensive assessment
- Goal setting (short, medium, and long term)
- A collaborative plan to achieve the goals
- Evaluation of progress toward the goals.

The process should not be linear, but a cyclical process of regular reassessment, review, and adjustment are required.

Comprehensive assessment

It is important to start the rehabilitation process by undertaking a comprehensive assessment of the patient's health status (physical, psychological, and social). Assessment should be systematic and interdisciplinary to avoid repetition of data collection or missing vital information. Integrated care pathways are an ideal way to promote both seamless integration of the acute and rehabilitative phases and interdisciplinary working. The assessment process will help the patient and the MDT to establish a baseline, which subsequent improvement can be measured against. There are various methods of collecting data during the assessment phase, including:
- History taking (see ➍ History taking 1 and 2, pp. 82–85)
- Disease-specific and generic health measures (see ➍ pp. 112–113)
- Observation
- Physical examination
- Clinical investigations
- Functional measurement, e.g. range of movement, gait analysis
- Consultation with other members of the MDT, patient's family, etc.

Goal setting

Goals should always be set *with* the patient, and not *for* them to ensure they are individualized, relevant, and desirable. Goals should be realistic and achievable, but also provide a degree of challenge to the patient who should be supported to set short-, medium-, and long-term goals. Goals should be reviewed regularly, and patients should receive positive feedback about their achievements. Motivation is a key role of the practitioner in the rehabilitation process. Many rehabilitation teams meet at least once weekly with patients and their relatives for goal setting and review.

Collaborative planning

Once goals have been agreed, the practitioner needs to work with the patient and other members of the MDT to plan treatment and actions. It should be identified which member/s of the team have specific expertise to help the patient with each goal and that all members of the team understand their contribution to helping the patient achieve their goals. Treatment and care should be based on best evidence (see ⟴ What is evidence-based care?, pp. 32–33) and tailored to the individual's needs. For example, if the evidence suggests that hydrotherapy is the best method of managing a fixed flexion deformity, but the patient has a fear of water, then alternatives need to be found.

Evaluation of progress

Progress toward patients' goals needs to be reviewed regularly and should involve the patient and their family. Progress should be measured by the same methods used during the assessment process, e.g. patients' self-report measures (disease specific and generic quality of health), direct observation by clinicians, functional assessment, and clinical investigations. Goals should then be re-set or modified at this point.

Rehabilitation settings

There is a significant amount of evidence indicating that rehabilitation outcomes are best achieved in specialist rehabilitation units, rather than on general trauma and orthopaedic settings, and also that rehabilitation is more realistic in the patient's home setting. However, nurses working on acute trauma and orthopaedic units must start the rehabilitation process in collaboration with the MDT as soon as the patient is medically fit and not wait until the patient is transferred to a rehabilitation unit or rehabilitation team in the community.

Further reading

Jester R (2007). *Advancing Practice in Rehabilitation Nursing*. Oxford: Blackwell Publishing.

Social aspects of care

Social aspects of care are those which relate to the individual's place within a community, their interaction with others in society, and those which impact their care needs. Health and social care are interrelated and the practitioner must ensure that the two are not separated, thus ensuring holistic thinking about an individual's needs. To effectively plan, deliver, and evaluate care, orthopaedic practitioners need knowledge and understanding of social factors and the part they play in the development of orthopaedic conditions and trauma as well their impact on recovery and rehabilitation.

Social and living conditions

Where, with whom, and how patients live can have a significant effect on both their musculoskeletal health and the process of recovery from injury or surgery. Social factors such as family, work, leisure, diet, and exercise have an important bearing on musculoskeletal health across the lifespan, but particularly in childhood, early adulthood, and in later life.

Patients who have warm, comfortable homes, adequate financial resources, and the social support of others are much more likely to thrive during their recovery from trauma and orthopaedic surgery. Those who live in cramped, inappropriate accommodation, are isolated, with poor physical and financial resources are more likely to have a less smooth recovery or adapt less well.

A person's living accommodation needs to be considered as early as possible in the care episode so that change and adaptation can be considered, resources sought, and early intervention planned. Where disability is the result of musculoskeletal health problems, adaptation and rehousing may need to be considered and funding sought.

Social deprivation, poverty, and homelessness are increasing features of twenty-first-century society, even in more resource-rich countries. Individuals without a permanent home are discriminated against socially and financially and have limited access to healthcare so are, therefore, more vulnerable when they have orthopaedic care needs.

Age, race, ethnicity, cultural background, religion, ill health, disability, and numerous other aspects of life may also lead to discrimination and social exclusion which often results in a cycle of isolation and poverty. It is well documented that poverty and deprivation lead to ill health.

Education, work, and disability

In most societies, less well-educated individuals tend to suffer more deprivation and ill health, are less likely to seek healthcare and take longer to recover from episodes of ill health. Unemployment is also a feature of life for individuals who have less education and skill. The practitioner must consider patient, family, and carer ability to understand and interact with the world around them depending on their level of education.

Many chronic musculoskeletal conditions can lead to disruption of an individual's education and/or occupation with a significant impact on their role in society and within the family, and often impacting their role identity.

Due to musculoskeletal problems, injury, or surgery, many orthopaedic patients are either temporarily or permanently classed as living with a physical disability. This can result in social discrimination and difficulty in finding or maintaining employment. Lack of, or inability to, work can lead to social isolation and is a contributing factor in poverty.

Social support

Orthopaedic practitioners cannot resolve major social problems in isolation, but are instrumental in helping to identify sources of social support. The availability and quality of such support can have a significant impact on recovery and rehabilitation. This might include, for example, different types of physical, psychological, and financial help. Such support is often provided by families, friends, and informal carers, but for many reasons, orthopaedic patients may be living in loneliness and isolation. This is particularly an issue for those with disability and those who are older and/or whose partners and friends may have died. The migration of families can also mean that people are isolated, and many others may never have had strong family ties. The notion of family is a socially derived concept and its ability to provide support may be affected by many cultural issues. Social isolation and loneliness lead to depression and restrict the individual's ability to cope. Strong family and other forms of social support can have a significant positive impact on recovery and rehabilitation. The orthopaedic practitioner can also be instrumental in coordinating social networks.

Social care professionals, government departments, and voluntary organizations have extensive knowledge of the services available to individuals in need of support following orthopaedic surgery, injury, and disability. It is essential that the orthopaedic practitioner knows what is available and what modes of referral exist so that patients can receive timely and appropriate support.

Further reading

Alan H, Traynor M (2016). *Understanding Sociology in Nursing*. London: Sage.

Discharge planning

Timely and coordinated planning for discharge is essential in avoiding unnecessary use of scarce hospital resources. Prolonged length of stay has financial implications for healthcare organizations and a detrimental impact on the individual's well-being. It is well recognized that prolonged periods in a hospital setting have a deleterious impact on patients' physical, social, and psychological health. Delayed discharge can lead to elective orthopaedic patients not having a bed to be admitted to, often leading to postponement of surgery. Alternatively, trauma patients may be admitted to non-orthopaedic units within the hospital where specialist expertise and knowledge about their care is not available.

Key problems with discharge

Several key problems relating to hospital discharge have been identified[1], including:

- *Occurring too soon*—due to pressure on acute beds when appropriate intermediate or rehabilitation services are not available
- *Delayed*—often due to poor planning; timely referral for support services in the community has not been made or because of indecision by the patient or family members about the discharge destination/plan
- *Dissatisfaction* with the discharge process from the patient and/or family perspective—usually due to suboptimal communication and lack of partnership working between the MDT and the patient/family
- *Discharge to unsafe environment*—this can result in the patient not being able to cope and possible re-admission.

Principles of good discharge planning

There are several basic principles that support successful discharge from hospital including:

- Planning should occur at the earliest opportunity—for elective orthopaedic patients this should begin in the pre-admission phase either at the time of decision to admit and/or in the preoperative assessment clinic
- Assessment of suitable discharge destination, i.e. directly home supported by an outreach team, intermediate care, or rehabilitation service should be addressed as soon as possible and timely referrals made
- Involvement of patients and their families as partners in the discharge planning process
- One identified member of the MDT should coordinate the discharge planning process. Managed care pathway approaches provide structure and process to discharge planning
- The patient and family must receive both verbal and written information on discharge regarding follow-up, specific instructions regarding medications, exercise regimens, and who to contact in the event of post-discharge complications

- Decisions about discharge planning should be clearly documented in shared MDT records to ensure all members of the team are working towards the same discharge goals with the patient
- Discharge planning is a dynamic and ongoing process and initial discharge plans may need modification depending on the patient's progress or changes in health, or social circumstances
- Accurate and timely discharge information sent to the patient's GP and any community nurse/physiotherapy services.

When problems with discharge planning are identified either through patient or family complaint or unplanned re-admission it is important to analyse which factors contributed to the failed discharge so that remedial strategies can be introduced.

Reference

1.. Department of Health (DoH) (2003). *Discharge from Hospital: Pathway Process and Practice.* London: DoH.

Further reading

NICE (2015). Transition between inpatient hospital settings and community or care home settings for adults with social care needs. NICE guideline [NG27]. https://www.nice.org.uk/guidance/ng27

Patient and carer education

An integral part of the practitioner's role is to promote patient and carer understanding of the patient's health needs. There is well-established evidence highlighting the positive benefits of patients and carers being well informed including:

- Reduced anxiety and stress
- Increased concordance with advice and treatment regimens
- Enhanced therapeutic relationships
- Increased satisfaction with healthcare services.

Conversely, inadequate or inappropriate education can have a detrimental impact on both the individual patient and increased cost to the health service. For example, if a patient undergoing a total hip replacement (THR) is not adequately educated about potential risks and prophylactic interventions, this can lead to complications such as hip dislocation or VTE which, not only cause pain and present risk to the patient, but will require additional resources to treat the complication. Practitioners need to work with other members of the MDT to ensure that patient/carer information is presented in the appropriate format and at the right time for the individual. Consideration needs to be given to people with special needs in relation to information giving, e.g.:

- People with a learning disability or cognitive impairment—use picture and communication charts and boards, avoid using complex language and medical jargon
- People with visual, speech, or hearing problems—always sit facing the patient and speak clearly, ensure hearing aids are *in situ* and working, use large text or Braille in written information. Provide access to sign language assistants
- People whose first language is not that of the health professional— access to interpreters and provision of written information in their native language.

When people are anxious and afraid this will also impact significantly on their ability to receive and retain information given to them.

Best practice in providing patient and carer education

It is important to provide information/education in an environment conducive to active listening and learning, e.g. that the process is not rushed, privacy is protected, the patient is comfortable, pain free, and relaxed, and noise and disruption are kept to a minimum. Establish what the patient and/or carer already know so that you can tailor the information to their specific needs. The following principles should be adopted:

- Organize information in a logical manner
- Give information in manageable chunks (avoid information overload)
- Use visual information such as information booklets, online materials and videos, DVDs, and models to supplement verbal methods
- Avoid using medical jargon and abbreviations
- Check patients'/carers' understanding at regular intervals
- Use summarizing and recapping to embed key messages

- Check non-verbal signs for anxiety or confusion
- Always give the patient/carer an opportunity to ask questions and seek clarification.

Patient education literature needs to be evidence based and reviewed and updated regularly. Organizations such as Versus Arthritis (formed following a merger of Arthritis Care and Arthritis Research UK) produce useful patient information booklets which are a useful adjunct to specific information provided by individual healthcare providers.

Further reading

Silverman J, Kurtz S, Draper J (2013). *Skills for Communicating with Patients*, 3rd edn. Boca Raton, FL: CRC Press.

Health promotion

Health is a state that varies widely between individuals. It is about much more than the absence of illness or disease, but is related to general well-being. Determinants of health include physical, psychological, emotional, cultural, and social aspects. The achievement of health and its maintenance are not only a goal of individuals but a societal responsibility.

Bone, joint, and muscle health (collectively, musculoskeletal heath) are an important aspect of the well-being of all individuals across the lifespan. Without an effective musculoskeletal system, general health suffers, and disability may ensue. Bone, joint, and muscle tissue are in constant use throughout life and are constantly growing and being renewed, depending on the prevalent physiological and environmental conditions. In turn, general health and well-being has an impact on musculoskeletal health. The role of the practitioner is to assist patients to achieve optimum musculoskeletal health as well as good general health.

Health and health promotion

Health promotion is often loosely defined as activity designed to improve the health of individuals or communities. Several other concepts are related to the notion of health:

Well-being

An important aspect of life and is seen, along with health, as vital in people achieving their potential.

Lifestyle

Perceived as a particularly important determinant of health. The way in which a person lives their life, and the choices they make, can have a significant impact on health. For example, poor diet, particularly under- and malnutrition and obesity, significantly affect musculoskeletal growth, development, and repair as well as the individual's ability to protect themselves from disease and injury. Obesity is seen as a major threat to health (see ➋ Obesity and the orthopaedic patient, pp. 186–187) as are smoking, alcohol, and drug use—these all impact the musculoskeletal system as well as having well-known effects on other systems.

Fitness

A state in which individuals are able to resist assaults to their health and are less likely to suffer from disease and ill health. For example, regular exercise, particularly that which is weight bearing, helps to maintain muscle strength as well as improve bone density along with benefits to the cardiovascular and respiratory systems.

The health professional

It is important to recognize that individuals need to maintain autonomy and choice in their lifestyles and that there are many reasons why individuals choose unhealthy behaviours. The health professional must remain non-judgemental about the causes of ill health.

Practitioners play an important part in health promotion and are well placed to help patients to make changes. The focus of health promotion for the orthopaedic practitioner is often musculoskeletal health. It is important, however, to remember that such a goal is also linked with the health of other systems such as the cardiovascular and respiratory and each is often interdependent with the other.

Health promotion is about much more than educating the orthopaedic patient to undertake health-promoting activity. It involves an assessment of and the provision of support in changing behaviour. Practitioners can use specific opportunities to achieve goals. For example, accident prevention can be central within the trauma setting, focusing on those particularly at risk of accidental injury. Individuals <25 or >65 years suffer more accidents than other age groups.

Health promotion practice

Once an assessment of health promotion needs has taken place both individual and community health promotion activities require careful planning, execution, and evaluation. Practitioners can support health promotion and behaviour change through advocacy and support by:

- Assessing and understanding individuals' health beliefs and behaviours
- Providing information and education about *health issues*
- Assisting patients to set realistic goals and plan changes and adaptations
- Providing discussion, advice, and support to motivate and assist patients in lifestyle or health behaviour change
- Referring patients to other services such as smoking cessation clinics and drug and alcohol services to help support change.

Rather than a separate entity, health promotion activities should take place as an integral part of daily practice in the orthopaedic setting.

Further reading

Naidoo J, Wills J (2016). *Foundations for Health Promotion*, 4th edn. London: Elsevier.
Whitehead D (1999). Health promotion within an orthopaedic setting: a different perspective. *J Orthop Nurs* 3:2–4.

Obesity and the orthopaedic patient

Obesity is often referred to as a modern epidemic. In many developed countries more than half the population are overweight or obese. Issues such as the constant availability of food which is high in calories and fat and low in other nutrients, and societies in which physical activity is becoming less of a feature of daily life are considered central to the problem. Orthopaedic patients are often less mobile because of their musculoskeletal condition, making obesity more difficult to avoid.

Defining and measuring obesity and overweight

Most definitions of obesity refer to weight gain that severely impacts on the health of the individual. BMI is currently the most widely used method designed to measure overweight and obesity in adults. It is a relatively simple calculation derived from weight in kilograms divided by the square root of the height in metres. For example, an adult who weighs 70 kg and whose height is 1.75 m will have a BMI of 22.9, i.e.:

$$BMI = 70 \text{ kg}/(1.75 \text{ m})^2 = 70/3.0625 = 22.9$$

Ranges of BMI vary but the normal range is generally considered to be 18.5–25. Overweight is considered to be >25 and obese >30. The practitioner should use BMI as one part of a health and nutritional assessment for orthopaedic patients.

The impact of overweight and obesity

Due to the pressure that additional body weight places on joints and its impact on posture, there is a clear link between obesity and musculoskeletal problems such as arthritis and back pain. There is also a much higher risk of other problems such as cardiovascular diseases and cancers, as well as numerous other health conditions. This makes obesity a great concern for the orthopaedic practitioner. Many commissioners of elective orthopaedic procedures, such as TJR, set limits for the BMI of patients before they can be referred for and/or undergo procedures. This varies, but typically ranges from a BMI of 35–40 as the cut-off point. The evidence regarding impact of obesity/morbid obesity and absolute body weight rather than BMI on outcomes following TJR (especially TKR and THR) is inconclusive, but many studies suggest that obese and morbidly obese patients who undergo TKR/THR do not go onto lose weight following the procedure, despite their mobility and function being improved.[1]

The role of the practitioner

The orthopaedic practitioner has an important role in helping patients at any stage in their treatment and care to maintain or achieve a healthy weight. However, there is evidence to suggest that there is a lack of knowledge and inconsistent practice regarding how best to support patients to lose and sustain weight loss prior to and following orthopaedic procedures such as TKR.[2] Simply providing dietary and exercise advice is not necessarily the solution as there are many reasons why individuals choose not to following healthy eating guidelines or exercise regularly. NICE highlight the following considerations[3]:

- Assessing an individual's readiness to make lifestyle changes as well as their existing knowledge of dietary and exercise advice
- Exploring barriers to lifestyle and dietary change
- Providing care that is non-judgemental, whatever the patient's weight
- Tailoring advice to meet age, cultural, and other needs. Working with children and young people needs specific consideration and guidance
- Helping patients to find ways to follow dietary and exercise guidelines for achieving a healthy weight
- Assisting patients to find support mechanisms for lifestyle change both within and without their families
- Supporting motivation by explaining to patients the impact that their weight is having on their health and treatment and what risks might be involved.

Caring for the bariatric orthopaedic patient

Losing weight often proves difficult or impossible for some patients. Providing non-judgemental, safe care to overweight and obese patients is, therefore, essential. 'Bariatric' is the term currently used to refer to healthcare for patients who are overweight or obese. In caring for patients who are obese, practitioners need to consider the following:
- Focusing on assessing and recording the risk to the patient's health during care, treatment, and surgery as part of the assessment and preparation for admission and surgery. These risks must be communicated to all members of the MDT
- Advising patients and their families of any identified risks and ensuring that this is included in discussions about informed consent
- Planning and executing care and treatment that manages identified risk where possible
- Ensuring that equipment such as beds, mattresses, operating tables, and manual handling equipment is available which is recommended for the patient's weight and safe working. Most manual handling equipment is only safe for patients weighing approximately 160 kg, so appropriate equipment must always be available
- Following guidelines for safe manual handling practice for bariatric patients. This may involve seeking expert help and training
- Ensuring that care workers involved in the patient's care following discharge are fully informed of any residual risks.

Reference

1.. Teichtahl A, Quirk E, Harding P, et al. (2015). Weight change following knee and hip joint arthroplasty – a six month prospective study of adults with osteoarthritis. *BMC Musculoskelet Disord* 16:137.

2.. Hill D, Freudmann M, Sergeant J, et al. (2018). Management of symptomatic knee osteoarthritis in obesity: a survey of orthopaedic surgeons' opinions and practice. *Eur J Orthop Surg Traumatol* 28:967–74.

3.. NICE (2014). Obesity: identification, assessment and management. ℘ https://www.nice.org.uk/guidance/cg189

Further reading

Cohen S (1997). Using a health belief module to promote increased well-being in obese patient with chronic low back pain. *J Orthop Nurs* 1:89–93.

Complications

Complications and risk management

Complications are undesirable events in the care of the orthopaedic patient. An important focus of orthopaedic care is their active prevention and management. Being an orthopaedic patient involves a degree of risk to the patient's health beyond the original musculoskeletal problem, injury, or surgery. These risks threaten patient safety and may lead to serious health problems and even death. The most common cause of death in orthopaedic patients, for example, is PE secondary to VTE which are discussed in more detail on ➲ Venous thromboembolism, pp. 194–195.

Complications in the orthopaedic patient are usually related to one or more of three factors (Table 5.1):

- The physiological impact of injury or surgery on bone and soft tissue
- Being immobile or less mobile than previously leading to stasis or sluggishness within organs and blood vessels
- The use of orthopaedic appliances and devices such as traction, fixation devices, casts, and splints.

Some major complications such as VTE may be related to all three causes. The orthopaedic practitioner needs an in-depth knowledge of these complications including their aetiology, pathology, prevention, and how to recognize them, to maintain the patient's health and well-being. This begins with an understanding of the risk factors for the complications most likely to affect patients under different circumstances. These are described in more detail for specific complications in the following sections.

Clinical risk assessment and management

Providing harm-free care is an important aim of modern healthcare. Identification, assessment, and control of risk are fundamental to providing effective care to the orthopaedic patient. The recognition and management

Table 5.1 Main orthopaedic complications according to possible underlying cause

Immobility/reduced mobility	Injury/surgery	Orthopaedic appliances
Venous thromboembolism	Venous thromboembolism	Venous thromboembolism
Chest infection	Neurovascular compromise	Neurovascular compromise
Urinary tract infection	Compartment syndrome	Compartment syndrome
Pressure ulcers	Fat embolism	Plaster/cast/splint sores
Muscle wasting, joint stiffness, and contractures	Haemorrhage	Muscle wasting
Falls	Wound infection	Pin site infection
	Failure of surgical implants	

of risk helps to control some of the uncertainty about hazards and potential complications. Most complications are foreseeable and can be predicted based on evidence, previous experience, and an understanding of risk factors. The occurrence of a foreseeable complication is viewed as a breach in patient safety. The assessment of risk and the instigation of risk management measures can protect the patient from harm related to these risks. There are legal implications when practitioners do not adequately recognize known risks and act accordingly. Failing to act upon risk that might reasonably be anticipated can be deemed negligent, particularly in relation to complications that occur often. While it is not always possible to prevent complications, failure to recognize their symptoms, act accordingly, and document appropriately is poor practice.

Orthopaedic teams must use systematically developed guidelines for practice that include advice about the minimization of the risk of complications. These should be based on the best available evidence so that the practitioner knows that care based on the guidance is likely to be effective. This is the principle on which 'clinical governance', 'patient safety', and 'continuous quality improvement' in healthcare are based and the practitioner has both a legal and professional duty to operate within these principles. The practitioner has a responsibility to:

• Make regular and full assessments of the patient to facilitate identification of those aspects of their condition and care that might result in harm
• Plan and deliver care which reduces or minimizes the risks identified
• Ensure the whole clinical team is aware of the risks identified and the care prescribed
• Continuously monitor the patient and his/her condition for signs of the development of complications
• Document and maintain records about the risks, results of observation, and the measures to be taken to manage the risk
• Evaluate the success of care aimed at preventing and recognizing complications
• Monitor, record, audit, investigate, and learn from clinical incidents where risk management fails to prevent complications.

Knowledge of the risks and signs of complications is essential as the practitioner is required to implement risk management strategies as an independent aspect of practice. The active recognition and management of the risk of complications in the orthopaedic patient is one of the central aspects of care and is of vital importance in ensuring patient safety, recovery, and effectiveness of care.

Further reading

Fisher M, Scott M (2013). *Patient Safety and Managing Risk in Nursing*. London: Sage.

Haemorrhage

Haemorrhage may occur following musculoskeletal trauma such as fracture, perioperatively, or postoperatively following orthopaedic surgery. Haemorrhage can be internal, (a patient with a pelvic fracture can lose between 3 and 4 L of blood into the abdominal cavity) or external, significant and/or prolonged bleeding from the surgical wound. Haemorrhage is life-threatening if it is not detected and treated promptly.

Patients at increased risk of haemorrhage

There are several factors that increase patients' risk of haemorrhage including:

- Patients with low platelet counts—thrombocytopenia
- Patients with prolonged prothrombin time, e.g. haemophilia
- Patients on anticoagulant therapy (e.g. warfarin, heparin, aspirin) or antiplatelet agents (e.g. clopidogrel).

Major elective orthopaedic surgery carries a moderate to high risk of haemorrhage. As part of the preoperative assessment process all anticoagulation therapy should be reviewed by the medical team and withdrawal of medication planned under medical instruction, according to local and national guidelines.

Patients requiring emergency surgery for orthopaedic trauma who are taking anticoagulants or antiplatelets should receive prothrombin complex and vitamin K intravenously to reduce the risk of haemorrhage.

Clinical signs of haemorrhage

Patients presenting with internal haemorrhage may have no obvious sign of external bleeding. For example, a patient with a pelvic fracture may incur damage to the blood supply of major pelvic organs and interruption to the blood supply to the lower limbs. Internal bleeding will manifest as pelvic tenderness, swelling over and near the area of bleeding, and ischaemia to areas distal to the vessel damage with or without obvious bruising to the area. Haemorrhage, if left untreated, will result in hypovolaemic shock, which is commonly described as having four stages:

- Grade 1: <15% loss of blood volume (750 mL)—the patient presents with normal BP, urine output, and respiratory rate, and pulse rate <100 beats per minute
- Grade 2: 15–30% loss of blood volume (750–1500 mL)—the patient presents with normal BP, pulse rate >100 beats per minute and thready, respiratory rate 20–30 breaths per minute, cool skin, reduced urine output
- Grade 3: 30–40% loss of blood volume (1500–2000 mL)—the patient presents with reduced BP, respiratory rate 30–40 breaths per minute, pulse rate >120 beats per minute and thready, urine output significantly reduced to 5–15 mL per hour, anxiety, and confusion
- Grade 4: >40% loss of blood volume (>2000 mL)—the patient presents with very low BP, respiratory rate >40 breaths per minute, urine output <5 mL per hour, pulse rate >140 per minute, confusion, and lethargy.

Prevention and treatment of haemorrhage

Early recognition and treatment of haemorrhage and hypovolaemic shock is essential to prevent serious organ damage and death. This requires regular and careful monitoring of patients following trauma and surgery including their vital signs, fluid intake, and fluid output (including wound drainage). Principles of treatment for hypovolaemic shock are:

- Apply the ABCDE approach to assessment and resuscitation (see → ATLS®, pp. 328–329)
- If the source of haemorrhage is external, then pressure should be applied to the wound using a pressure dressing
- Alert the medical team promptly to changes in the patient's vital signs that indicate hypovolaemic shock
- Secure venous access using a wide-bore cannula as quickly as possible and commence rapid re-expansion of circulating volume
- Take venous blood samples for FBC, clotting screen, group and cross-match
- Insert a urinary catheter to accurately monitor urine output
- Reassure the patient who will be anxious and possibly confused.

Further reading

Tait D, James J, Williams C, et al. (2015). *Acute and Critical Care in Adult Nursing*. London: Sage.

Venous thromboembolism

Venous thromboembolism (VTE) is the collective term for deep vein thrombosis (DVT) and pulmonary embolism (PE) and is the most significant cause of death in orthopaedic patients. DVT is a particular risk following lower limb orthopaedic and spinal surgery. There is very strong evidence that VTE can be prevented through risk assessment and prophylactic measures.

Pathophysiology

VTE usually begins in the deep veins of the calf and is the result of three main factors known as 'Virchow's triad':
1. Trauma to blood vessels due to trauma or surgery
2. Venous stasis due to immobility
3. Hypercoagulability of the blood due to the physiological response to tissue damage and bleeding.

A blood clot (thrombus) forms in a deep vein which may break off and become an embolus, lodging in smaller vessels, most often in the lungs. Pulmonary emboli result in damage to lung tissue and have a high rate of mortality due to respiratory arrest.

Risk assessment

There are a range of factors which indicate that a patient may be at risk of VTE and recognizing these should help to identify those who require preventive measures (Table 5.2).

Table 5.2 Major risk factors for VTE in the orthopaedic patient

• Age—especially >60 years	• Surgery—especially prolonged, especially to the lower limb or spine
• Obesity	• Acute traumatic injury
• Varicose veins	• Anaesthesia—general and spinal
• Previous VTE and other recent thrombotic events (e.g. myocardial infarction)	• Hormone therapy (inc. contraception)
• Prolonged immobility	• Central venous catheter *in situ*
• Casts and splints	• Blood clotting disorders

Prevention

Measures for preventing VTE are based on management of the factors which are considered in Virchow's triad and on increasing blood flow and venous return in the lower limb, falling into two main categories:

Mechanical measures

Mechanical measures of prevention aim to improve blood flow in the lower limbs and aid venous return. These non-pharmacological measures do not add to the risk of bleeding, are relatively inexpensive, and can be implemented by all practitioners. They include:
• Graduated compression (antiembolism) to reduce venous stasis. It is essential that stockings fit correctly, are worn at all times, and are

removed at least daily for skin care and circulatory observations. Calf-length stockings may be more comfortable for some patients

- Intermittent pneumatic compression uses mechanical compression to increase the efficiency of the 'foot pump' which is instrumental in venous return from the lower limb and normally functions when walking
- Early mobilization, active leg exercises which utilize the calf muscle pump, leg elevation, and maintaining hydration are all simple measures which can also help to improve venous return.

Pharmacological methods

When the risk of VTE is very high, as in many orthopaedic patients, pharmacological methods are used in addition to mechanical methods. They include low-molecular-weight heparin (LMWH) or other drugs which reduce blood coagulability. Pharmacological measures often carry increased risk of bleeding.

As more evidence is incorporated into local and national guidance, it is essential that practitioners are aware of the contents of the most up-to-date guidance.

Signs, symptoms, and management

It is essential that the practitioner recognizes the symptoms of DVT. Not all DVTs are symptomatic, but the most common symptoms are leg pain (often in the calf), swelling, and warmth and redness of the skin of the calf. Medical staff must be informed immediately if DVT is suspected.

PE is a medical emergency. The main symptoms are acute shortness of breath, chest pain, tachycardia, and coughing with or without haemoptysis. If a patient has a suspected PE, urgent medical attention should be sought immediately.

DVT must be treated immediately. This involves carefully controlled doses of oral anticoagulants and regular follow-up which includes assessment of blood clotting.

PE may be fatal, and the first indication of its occurrence may be a cardiac arrest. If a PE is suspected, it may be diagnosed by a lung perfusion scan and is treated using anticoagulant therapy.

Further reading

NICE (2018). Venous thromboembolism in the over 16s: reducing the risk of hospital-acquired deep vein thrombosis or pulmonary embolism. NICE guideline [NG89]. ℰ https://www.nice.org.uk/guidance/ng89/

Neurovascular compromise

Bones, muscles, and joints require good local nerve and blood supply in order to function effectively. Compromise of either or both the blood or nerve supply to an area can be caused by compression of, or injury to, nerves, and/or blood vessels, particularly in limbs and their extremities. Depletion or interruption of the blood or nerve supply can lead to serious, irretrievable damage to nerve, muscle, and soft tissue due to ischaemia or direct/indirect nerve damage. This is a significant risk for orthopaedic patients and those at risk usually have:

- Accidental physical injury/damage to nerves or blood vessels during surgery
- Compression or injury of neurovascular structures following blunt or sharp tissue trauma—especially crushing injures of limbs
- Compression of neurovascular structures caused by bleeding or swelling of the surrounding tissues, especially when this is within a fascial compartment (see ➲ Compartment syndrome, p. 198)
- Casts and splints where there is swelling within an encircling device and pressure builds up within the limb and cannot be released.

Monitoring

When neurovascular compromise occurs, damage to tissue worsens as time passes, so it is essential that the practitioner closely monitors patients following limb trauma and surgery to recognize any compromise and ensure it is treated quickly.

Physiological indicators of vascular compromise are caused by lack of oxygen within the muscles and other tissues and resultant ischaemia and necrosis. Indicators of neurological compromise are caused by interruption in the nerve supply to the tissues. Collectively these result in the following main indicators of neurovascular compromise:

- *Pain*—the most important sign of neurovascular compromise, indicating tissue ischaemia. It is often severe and unrelenting. Such pain is often not relieved by even opioid analgesia and must be taken very seriously as an early sign of neurovascular compromise.
- *Sensation*—reduced sensory perception may occur in an area of tissue supplied by the affected nerves. Altered sensory perception (resulting in tingling, pins and needles, or numbness) is also a significant sign.
- *Movement*—inability to move a limb or digit within normal range of motion.
- *Colour*—change in colour of the skin, any blueness or mottling indicating a diminished blood supply.
- *Warmth*—change in skin temperature, particularly coldness of a limb or extremity, when compared to the other limb.
- *Capillary refill*—usually assessed by placing light finger pressure on the skin or nail bed for 5 seconds and then releasing it. This should result in whitening of the area but colour returns within 2 seconds. Any delay in colour return indicates reduced distal perfusion, either due to arterial disease, surgical injury, or a cast, splint, or dressing that is too tight.
- *Pulses*—diminished or absent pulses are a very late sign of vascular compromise.

These observations should be carried out at least hourly in the immediate period following surgery or injury—reducing gradually over a period of days as the patient's condition stabilizes. Patients should be engaged in monitoring their own limb whenever they are able and any observations they make must be taken seriously.

Documentation and action

For patient safety, professional, and legal reasons it is essential that regular neurovascular assessment is clearly documented, preferably using a chart where any change over time can clearly be seen, even if staff caring for the patient change frequently, as this will alert the practitioner to changes in physiological signs. Any suspicion that there is any neurovascular compromise must be reported to medical staff and urgent action taken to resolve the cause. This most often means emergency surgical intervention.

Further reading

Royal College of Nursing and British Orthopaedic Association (2014). *Peripheral Neurovascular Observations for Acute Limb Compartment Syndrome: RCN Consensus Guidance*. London: RCN.

Compartment syndrome

Although uncommon, acute compartment syndrome is an extremely dangerous complication of injury or surgery to the limbs. As it is so dangerous, it is essential that the orthopaedic practitioner can recognize and act on its signs and symptoms.

Aetiology

Both the arm and leg contain fascial compartments where the nerves, blood vessels, and muscles travel to the extremities. These structures are contained in an enclosed space within the muscle and bone structure (compartment) and are surrounded by a membrane (fascia). When injury or surgery to the bone or soft tissues leads to bleeding or swelling, fluid collects within the compartments. Because of the relative inflexibility of the surrounding fascia, fluid from tissue swelling is unable to escape and pressure builds up within the compartment, compressing the nerves and blood vessels within it. This can lead to permanent damage due to poor oxygen supply to the neurovascular and muscular structures leading to death (necrosis) of tissues such as muscle, resulting in long-term disability and other medical problems caused by the release of toxins from necrotic muscle tissue.

Signs and symptoms

Compartment syndrome is recognized by several important signs and symptoms. Some, or all, of the following may occur:

- Pain (the most important and earliest sign)—severe, and out of proportion to the injury sustained or the surgery; the pain is unrelenting and often not relieved by even opioid analgesia
- Swelling and tenseness of the limb
- Loss of sensation, numbness, or tingling distal to the injury or surgery (this is a late sign)
- Pallor or blueness of the foot or hand (a late sign)
- Loss of pulses to the foot or hand (this is a very late sign)
- Loss of movement of any part of the limb distal to the surgery or injury (this is also a late sign).

The earliest and most obvious sign of compartment syndrome is pain. It is increasing, out of proportion to the injury or surgery and does not respond well to analgesia. The pain is often described as deep and throbbing and worsens when the associated muscles are used.

Observations

Particularly in the first 24–48 hours following injury or surgery careful observations must be undertaken and recorded. Observations should take place at least hourly for the first 24 hours. Compartment syndrome usually occurs within the first 6–8 hours but can occur up to 2 days after surgery or injury. If the nurse is concerned about observation results or feels that it has deviated in any way from the normal, assessment should be repeated within the half hour. These observations must include:

- Pain assessment—it is essential that pain assessment is conducted thoroughly. Any complaints of pain from the patient should be taken seriously. It should not be assumed that if the patient is asleep they are not in pain—especially following general anaesthesia and strong analgesia.

- Check for colour, sensation, capillary refill, and movement in the limb distal to the site of injury or surgery. Specifically ask the patient if there is any numbness or tingling. It is also important to differentiate between numbness, loss of sensation or movement that is related to spinal or regional anaesthesia. It is not safe to assume that such loss of sensation or movement is related to anaesthetia or nerve blocks without checking with an anaesthetist or surgeon.
- Check the presence of pulses distal to the site of surgery or injury. Loss of pulses is a very late sign of compartment syndrome.

What happens if compartment syndrome is suspected?

If there is *any* suspicion of compartment syndrome the practitioner should remove or cut through any bandages, splints, or appliances. Supervision by a more experienced practitioner will be required if the nurse/practitioner is not experienced in this procedure. If a cast is involved it is important that this is bivalved properly (see ➜ Cast: removal and bivalving, pp. 374–375).

A senior member of medical staff/orthopaedic surgeon must be contacted immediately and informed of the symptoms. It is essential that the practitioner impresses on the doctor (who is often at the other end of the telephone and cannot see or hear the patient) that compartment syndrome is suspected. The signs and symptoms should be clearly explained. Clinical assessment by an experienced surgeon is essential. Tissue pressure measurement may also be used.

If compartment syndrome is present, decompression is performed by a fasciotomy (linear incision of the fascia over all compartments) in order to release all pressure. The wounds are often left open until all of the swelling has subsided and will be closed at a later date.

Further reading

Ali P, Santy-Tomlinson J, Watson R (2014). Assessment and diagnosis of acute limb compartment syndrome: a literature review. *Int J Orthop Trauma Nurs* 18:180–90.

BOA/BAPRAS/RCN (2016). BOAST 10: diagnosis and management of compartment syndrome. ♪ https://www.boa.ac.uk/wp-content/uploads/2015/01/BOAST-10.pdf

Infection control and prevention

Healthcare-associated infections (HCAIs) are a major problem for the NHS. In England, in 2011, the prevalence of HCAIs was reported as 6.4%, mostly respiratory infections, UTIs (17.2%) and SSIs.[1] Infection control and prevention is an important aspect of care. Spread of infection to bone and/or soft tissue following fracture, internal/external fixation, or joint replacement is a serious complication that can lead to:

- Osteomyelitis (see ● Osteomyelitis, p. 272) and delayed/non- or mal-healing of a fracture/s (see ● Fracture healing problems, pp. 348–349)
- Pain
- Delayed discharge
- Increased cost to the health service
- Revision surgery (see ● Revision joint replacement, pp. 290–291)
- Patient distress and dissatisfaction
- Bacteraemia, septicaemia, sepsis, and death.

Principles for preventing infection

The standard principles of infection prevention are included in national guidelines[2]:

- Hospital hygiene
- Hand decontamination (patients and staff)
- Personal protective clothing
- Safe use and disposal of sharps
- Isolation of patients with some infections
- Aseptic technique.

In the orthopaedic setting, specific measures include:

- Screening of elective patients for MRSA and other infections prior to surgery according to current protocols and guidance
- Preoperative assessment for any existing infections such as skin lesions, infections of toe nails, respiratory and systemic infections, and dental decay which may act as a portal for infection during or following surgery
- Use of dedicated 'clean' orthopaedic operating theatres with laminar airflow systems
- Judicious use of prophylactic IV antibiotics pre-, intra-, and postoperatively for major orthopaedic/trauma procedures.

Early detection and treatment of infection

Early detection and management of local or systemic infection is vital to avoiding spread. Signs and symptoms of infection will depend on the source and location, but include the following:

- Pyrexia
- Redness/heat/swelling/inflammation of wounds and/or soft tissue
- Wound discharge that is odorous/purulent
- General malaise
- Delirium
- Joint inflammation and swelling
- Offensive/cloudy urine

- Discolour (green/yellow/brown) sputum
- Nausea, vomiting, diarrhoea.

If infection is suspected, samples such as wound swabs, urine, stool, and sputum specimens should be sent for laboratory analysis as soon as possible so that appropriate antimicrobials can be prescribed. Laboratory request forms should clearly state the symptoms of suspected infection. Isolation of infected patients and the use of universal precautions are needed to minimize the risk of contamination of other patients.

References

1. NICE (2014). Infection prevention and control. Quality standard [QS61]. ℘ https://www.nice.org.uk/guidance/qs61/chapter/introduction#footnote_2
2. Loveday H, Wilson J, Pratt R, et al. (2014). epic3: National evidence-based guidelines for preventing healthcare-associated infections in NHS Hospitals in England. *J Hosp Infect* 86:S1–70.

Respiratory tract infection

Respiratory tract infection is a common complication of immobility, trauma, and surgery and a significant cause of death in orthopaedic patients.

Infections can be divided into upper respiratory tract infections (URTIs) involving the nose and pharynx (usually viral and the result of the common cold or influenza viruses) and lower respiratory tract infections (LRTIs) which involve the lungs, bronchi, and trachea. A URTI can lead to an LRTI in patients who are frail, ill, undergo major surgery, or suffer significant trauma.

Pneumonia is a potentially life-threatening infection that infects the alveoli, resulting in impaired gaseous exchange respiratory function and X-ray changes. It is a significant cause of death in orthopaedic patients, particularly in older adults. The types of organisms responsible for respiratory tract infection and pneumonia vary but are often hospital acquired in inpatient orthopaedic patients.

Some patients are more vulnerable to infection than others. Predisposing factors for respiratory tract infection include:
- Orthopaedic surgery and trauma and consequent stasis of the respiratory system due to anaesthesia and immobility
- Chest injuries and other conditions resulting in poor chest expansion when breathing
- Anaesthesia—particularly general anaesthesia
- Immobility and pain
- Pre-existing respiratory problems such as asthma and chronic pulmonary disease
- Smoking and associated respiratory disease
- Advanced age, comorbidity, frailty, and poor nutrition
- Hypothermia
- Having a current or recent cold or influenza.

These factors need to be considered when planning and delivering care and need to be considered in preoperative planning.

Postoperative chest infection

Chest infection is a significant cause of perioperative morbidity and mortality. Its prevention in the perioperative period is based on the following strategies:
- Assessment, prior to surgery, of the patient's risk of respiratory tract infection, considering the factors previously listed, so that preventive measures can be instigated
- Encouraging patients to stop or reduce smoking for as long as possible before elective surgery and not to start again postoperatively or abstain for as long as possible
- Close observation of vulnerable patients for signs of chest infection which include:
  - Dyspnoea and increased respiratory rate, with cyanosis in severe cases
  - Pyrexia and tachycardia
  - Productive cough, with green sputum and/or chest pain on coughing
  - General malaise, loss of appetite, and feeling unwell

- Mobilization as early as possible and careful positioning of the patient in an upright position when possible, using pillows for support, to support good chest expansion
- Involvement of the therapist in providing chest physiotherapy
- Effective pain management will enable the patient to achieve good chest expansion when breathing and prevent them from avoiding coughing
- Avoiding and promptly treating dehydration and providing nutritional support.

Management

Treatment of respiratory tract infection requires antibiotic therapy. Sputum microbiology may help in identifying the exact organism, although in practice this is often unhelpful and treatment with antibiotics is determined by the physician based on the likely origins of the infection. Initially, broad-spectrum antibiotics may be prescribed until microbiology results are available. Humidified oxygen may be administered as prescribed to ameliorate the effects of hypoxia.

Monitoring of respiratory function is essential in all patients with actual or suspected respiratory infections which includes rate and depth of respirations and observation for dyspnoea and cyanosis.

Patients should be encouraged and assisted to sit upright so that chest expansion can be maximized, and they should be encouraged to breathe deeply and cough in order to expectorate sputum. Where this is difficult, the patient may require physiotherapy and nebulizer therapy to help loosen sputum and make expectoration easier.

Urinary tract infection

The urinary tract is the most common site of HCAI. UTI is a common complication of orthopaedic surgery and traumatic injury. Bacteriuria, the presence of bacteria in the urine which may be asymptomatic, presents a risk of bacteraemia (the presence of bacteria in the blood). This can lead to remote infection of orthopaedic prosthetic implant sites and wounds. It is important to avoid bacteriuria and UTI in orthopaedic patients as they increase the risk of wound and implant infection.

UTI is caused by the entry of bacteria into the urinary system via the external meatus and urethra. The causative organisms are often bowel or skin flora. Untreated or frequent lower urinary tract (urethra and bladder) infections can lead to upper urinary tract (ureters and kidneys) and renal infections with associated risk of acute kidney injury. Urinary tract infections are the second most common reason for antibiotic prescription in orthopaedic patients.

Diagnosis

A diagnosis of UTI is made based on the symptoms and signs outlined in Table 5.3. The purpose of culture of urine samples is only to identify the bacteria involved and their antibiotic sensitivity. Microbiology cannot diagnose UTI.

Table 5.3 Symptoms and signs of UTI

• Dysuria (pain on urinating)	• Suprapubic pain
• Frequency	• Haematuria
• Cloudy urine	• Back pain
• Odorous urine	• Fever, malaise and/or generally unwell
• Delirium	

Specimen collection

If patients have symptoms of UTI, a urine sample should be sent for microbiology culture and sensitivity to ascertain the causative organism and the antibiotic to which it is sensitive. Urine specimens should be collected into a sterile container aiming to provide a sample that is not contaminated by external surfaces and is from the middle of the stream. Hand decontamination should be conducted and the sample collected while using a gloved hand to part the labia or gently pull back the foreskin. The first part of the urine stream should be wasted into the toilet or pan, then the sample collected, and the remainder of the stream voided into the toilet. The specimen should be labelled and sent to the laboratory. Samples from catheters should be taken using the catheter port and sterile equipment.

Prevention

Prevention of UTI involves taking measures to maintain a healthy urinary system. This includes:
• Avoidance of urinary catheterization wherever possible and removal as soon as possible

- Universal infection prevention precautions when handling catheters and catheter bags
- A daily fluid intake of at least 1.5 L unless contraindicated, consisting mostly of water and avoidance of caffeinated drinks and alcohol
- Maintenance of a high standard of personal hygiene involving daily washing of the perineum and/or penile meatus. Women should wash from the front towards the back to avoid contamination of the urinary system with faecal matter
- Urinating as often as possible and avoidance of bladder stasis by returning to normal physical activity as soon as possible, including normal toileting rather than use of bedpans.

Catheter care

Indwelling catheters are a significant cause of hospital-acquired infections. If catheterization cannot be avoided, it is essential that the catheter is inserted using strict aseptic technique. The principles of effective catheter care include:

- Careful maintenance of a closed drainage system
- Avoidance of unnecessary emptying of the system or changing drainage bags unless necessary or when recommended by manufacturers
- Emptying of the system/bag should be conducted following hand decontamination and wearing clean gloves. A clean container, specifically for each patient should be used and contact between the container, hands, and the drainage tap minimized
- Urine samples must be obtained using aseptic technique from specially designed sampling ports
- Drainage bags should be kept below the level of the bladder to facilitate drainage and prevent reflux. Bags should be hung carefully and not allowed contact with the floor. If bags leak, they must be changed
- Routine personal hygiene including gentle cleansing of the urethral meatus should be carried out with unscented soap and water, preferably during normal bathing or showering
- Catheters should be removed using strict aseptic technique.

Management of infection

Following culture of the urine, infection should be treated with an appropriate course of antibiotics. A further urine sample may be needed once the course of antibiotics is complete. Oral or IV hydration should be maintained so that the urine is not concentrated and flushing of the bladder takes place. Pain relief and standard hygiene measures should also be administered where required.

Further reading

NICE (2015). Urinary tract infection in adults. Quality standard [QS90]. ℘ https://www.nice.org.uk/guidance/qs90

Wound infection

Infection is the most common and feared complication of orthopaedic surgical and traumatic wounds:

- It is painful and distressing for patients, is known to impair the process of wound healing, and is instrumental in delayed recovery and lengthy treatment
- Wound infection following orthopaedic surgery can mean that implants need to be removed and can lead to osteomyelitis (infection of bone)
- Intact skin is the first line of defence against infection: exposure of subcutaneous tissue during surgery or trauma provides a moist, warm, and nutrient-rich environment that is ideal for bacterial growth
- A clean surgical wound, subjected to primary closure with sutures or clips, should only require minimal intervention and should be 'sealed' to bacteria within a few days if healing progresses normally
- Traumatic wounds are a significant worry as they are usually contaminated with bacteria at the time of injury
- Surgical wounds will heal rapidly if the blood supply to the area is maximized, ensuring that oxygen, nutrients, and cells of the immune system can reach the site of the wound quickly and there is little opportunity for microorganisms to colonize the wound.

The *infection continuum* is a conceptual representation of the development of wound infection. It describes how a *sterile* wound, without any bacteria (a rare situation), can become *contaminated* with organisms. If the organisms that have colonized the wound continue to multiply successfully despite the action of the immune system, the numbers of bacteria reach a point known as *critical colonization*. Growth of organisms reaches a level where the immune system can no longer prevent bacteria from damaging tissue and *infection* has taken hold.

Preventing wound infection

There are many factors that increase the risk of wound infection—these fall into two main categories:

- Extrinsic factors—the environment, care workers' practices, surgical technique, contaminated wound drainage systems, and poor wound care technique
- Intrinsic factors that are related to the host defences of the patient—nutritional status, smoking and alcohol consumption, cardiovascular and respiratory problems, and other diseases such as diabetes.

Infection prevention is based on managing these risk factors and includes:

- Good hygiene (such as hand-washing) practice for staff, visitors, and patients
- Maintaining good patient nutrition and hydration
- Minimal disturbance of the wound and protection from contamination with a suitable dressing
- Aseptic management or handling of wounds and wound drains. Wound drainage systems should be removed as early as possible
- As short as possible stay in hospital
- The use of prophylactic antibiotics during the perioperative period is shown to be effective in many types of orthopaedic implant surgery.

Recognizing wound infection

The presence of wound infection leads to an inflammatory response in the tissues resulting in five main signs of infection:
• Pain
• Erythema (redness)
• Oedema/swelling
• Heat
• Purulence (not always present).

As well as these symptoms, other signs include pyrexia, a wound that breaks down (dehiscence) or does not heal normally, or has excessive wound discharge.

   Taking a wound swab for laboratory analysis may not be helpful as this may only identify superficial bacteria or commensal organisms growing on the skin. Most wound infections are caused by a small number of organisms. Wound swabs are most useful in identifying the infecting organism when antibiotic therapy is not successful in resolving the infection.

Managing wound infection

Suspected orthopaedic wound infections must be treated quickly and effectively as soon as they are recognized to prevent spread to other tissue, bone, and implant sites. Any suspected wound infection must be reported to medical staff immediately so that an appropriate systemic antibiotic can be prescribed and administered. The wound must then be monitored for signs of improvement or worsening. Sterile wound dressings should be used along with strict aseptic technique and all standard prevention precautions to prevent cross-infection.

Further reading

Donnelly J, Collins A, Santy-Tomlinson J (2014). Wound management, tissue viability and infection. In: Clarke S, Santy-Tomlinson J (eds) *Orthopaedic and Trauma Nursing: An Evidence-Based Approach to Musculoskeletal Care*, pp 158–67. Oxford: Wiley-Blackwell.

Wound blistering

The practitioner has an important role in ensuring optimal would healing and to minimize the risk of infection (see ⊃ Wound infection, pp. 206–207). Skin blistering can occur lateral to surgical incisions following any orthopaedic surgery, but specifically surgery of the hip and knee. It is reported that skin blistering lateral to the surgical wound occurs in 13% of hip and knee replacement patients.[1] See Fig. 5.1.

Causes of wound blistering

Skin blistering occurs when the epidermis is separated from the dermis because of continued friction to the skin. The deep finger-like projections which hold the epidermis and dermis together weaken due to this friction causing separation of the layers of the skin. There have been few studies to date that have investigated the causes of skin blistering lateral to hip and knee surgical wounds, but the most likely cause is the combination of postoperative oedema surrounding the surgical wound combined with the application of wound dressings which have little elasticity. The lack of elasticity of wound dressings applied under tension to prevent haemorrhage following surgery does not facilitate the increased pressure caused by postsurgical oedema.[1]

Impact of wound blistering

Blistering around the surgical wound has a number of negative consequences, including:

- Discomfort for the patient
- Scarring
- Inhibition of the range of movement due to fear of blisters bursting
- Potential for infection as blisters burst and leave exposed wounds
- Increased cost due to extra wound care and possible increase in length of stay.

Care of the patient with wound blistering

The most important point is to try and reduce the risk of blistering by controlling postsurgical oedema by elevating the lower limbs above the level of the sacrum and the application of wound dressings with capacity for expansion (elastic properties for stretch). If blistering does occur, the nurse should observe the area carefully for signs of infection and ensure the patient's pain and discomfort is assessed using valid pain assessment tools and provide adequate pain relief. The nurse should report blistering to the medical team for consideration for the prescription of prophylactic antibiotics. Patients should be informed preoperatively that skin blistering can occur and patients' anxieties about scarring from wound blisters addressed.

(a)

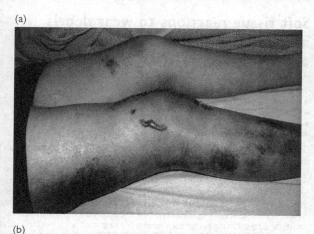

(b)

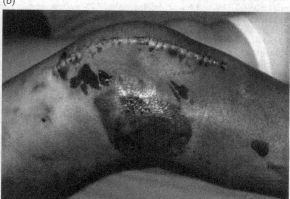

Fig. 5.1 Examples of skin blistering. Reproduced with permission from Jester R, Russell L, Fell S, et al. (2000). A one hospital study of the effect of wound dressings and other related factors on skin blistering following total hip and knee arthroplasty. *J Orthop Nurs* 4(2):71–7.

Reference

1. Jester R, Russell L, Fell S, et al. (2000). A one hospital study of the effect of wound dressings and other related factors on skin blistering following total hip and knee arthroplasty. *J Orthop Nurs* 4:71–7.

Soft tissue reactions to wear debris associated with metal-on-metal hip articulations

The articulating surfaces of hip replacements and hip resurfacing prostheses can be made from several types of materials including:
- Stainless steel
- Chrome/cobalt
- Titanium alloy
- High-density polyethylene (HDP).

Since 2012 there has been a dramatic reduction in the number of metal-on-metal (MoM)[1] replacements and resurfacing procedures carried out due to increasing concerns regarding adverse soft tissue reactions caused by the debris from wearing of metal surfaces and migration of chromium and cobalt ions. This adverse reaction is often referred to as metallosis. The Medicines and Healthcare Products Regulatory Agency (MHRA) have issued several alerts since 2012 regarding the safety of MoM hip replacements and re-surfacing prostheses due to high rates of early revision surgery (19.06–22.21% at 14 years compared to 7.2% average revision rate for all types of prostheses)[1] and necrosis of surrounding soft tissue around the prostheses often leading to formation of fluid-filled cysts sometimes referred to as pseudo-tumours.

Patients who develop metallosis may develop symptoms including:
- Development of hip and or groin pain
- Muscle pain in the thigh
- Development of a limp and/or weakness on the affected side.

However, patients may be asymptomatic, and, for this reason, it is now required that every patient with a MoM prosthesis is monitored annually for the lifetime of the prosthesis. Many of the specialized surveillance clinics are nurse led. The annual surveillance aims to detect adverse reactions as promptly as possible and should include a patient consultation to enquire if they are symptomatic and the following clinical investigations should be carried out:
- X-ray hip, anterior and posterior views and comparison with previous films
- Serum cobalt and chromium ion levels
- Cross-sectional imaging including MRI (specifically metal artefact resonance scanning (MARS)) or ultrasound scan to detect fluid around the joint.

If serum cobalt and chromium levels are raised and there is evidence of adverse reaction on X-ray and/or scan, prompt referral for consideration of revision surgery is required. Patients, understandably, are very anxious about developing metallosis and psychological support is important. If, between annual surveillance clinics, patients become symptomatic, they should know to contact the team to have their monitoring appointment brought forward to avoid delays in investigations and prompt detection.

Reference

1. National Joint Registry for England, Wales, Northern Ireland and The Isle of Man (2018). 15th Annual Report. ℘ https://www.hqip.org.uk/wp-content/uploads/2018/11/NJR-15th-Annual-Report-2018.pdf

Further reading

Elliot S, Langford S (2016). Meeting the demands of on-going metal-on-metal hip surveillance through nurse led services. *Int J Orthop Trauma Nurs* 20:40–4

Fat embolism syndrome

Fat embolism is the presence of fat globules in the lungs and peripheral circulation. Fat embolism syndrome (FES) is a manifestation of fat embolism that presents with several clinical features, including acute respiratory failure. This is a potentially fatal complication that can follow fractures, orthopaedic surgery, and bone trauma. It is relatively uncommon, occurring in 3–4% of patients with fractures of the long bones,[1] but more common following multiple trauma. It is a significant cause of morbidity and mortality and an important cause of adult respiratory distress syndrome following trauma. Apart from long bone fractures, other risk factors include radiotherapy for bone metastasis and surgery to long bones where there has been reaming (drilling or boring) of the medullary canal. FES is an uncommon, but life-threatening, emergency and it is essential that the practitioner can recognize the signs and symptoms so immediate action can be taken.

Aetiology

There are two proposed mechanisms of development:
- Following a fracture, fat from the bone marrow and tissues is released into the circulation. The globules of fat accumulate and become trapped in the small vessels of the lungs, brain, kidneys, or other vital organs. The occlusion of vessels in the lungs causes pulmonary pressure to rise, leading to oedema and haemorrhage in the alveoli which impairs the transport of oxygen and results in hypoxia.
- The metabolic response to the stress of injury alters the physiological emulsion of fat in plasma. Embolic fat globules from circulating blood lipids accumulate, leading to an increase in pulmonary perfusion pressure. Vessels are over-loaded, and the lungs become rigid, increasing the workload of the right side of the heart.

What to look for

FES symptoms usually occur within 72 hours of sustaining a long bone fracture or 12–48 hours following trauma or surgery to a long bone. Observations should mirror those routinely carried out following surgery. The patterns of observations are shown in Table 5.4.

Some or all symptoms may be present, but any of them should alert the practitioner to the possibility of FES. The most important, early, and often neglected observation is an increasing respiratory rate. The severity of symptoms will depend on where the occlusion of the vessel/s occurs and the degree of occlusion. If not treated rapidly the patient may become unconscious and can ultimately die.

What happens if fat embolism is suspected?

If fat embolism is suspected, the practitioner should:
- Inform senior medical practitioner of the symptoms immediately
- Sit the patient upright if their condition allows and reassure them
- Administer high-dose oxygen
- Instigate pulse oximetry
- Establish venous access and arrange for blood gases to be taken to identify hypoxia

Table 5.4 Distinction between normal and abnormal observations in FES

Symptom/sign	Normal	Abnormal
Respirations (breaths/min)	16–20	>20
Pulse (beats/min)	65–85	>85
Temperature (°C)	36.5–37.3	>37.3
Blood pressure (mmHg)	110–130/70–85	Systolic >130; diastolic >85
Mental state	As previously	Confused/disorientated/restless
Signs of cyanosis	None	Blue lips, blue periphery of the limbs
Urine output	50–100 mL/hour	<50 mL/hour, fat globules in the urine
Fluid balance	Normal	Low output compared to input
Haemorrhages	Not normal	Petechial haemorrhages on the upper body

- A chest radiograph may show patchy shadowing of the lungs
- Take a urine sample—this may show fat globules in the urine
- Be prepared to commence resuscitation if required.

The practitioner must clearly inform the medical practitioner that FES is suspected so that there is an awareness of the potential severity of the problem. Mechanical ventilation in a high dependency or intensive care unit may be required. Steroids are sometimes used to help reduce inflammation and oedema. Constant reassurance will help the patient to understand what is going on and lessen anxiety. Anxiety is likely to lead to worsening symptoms.

Prevention of FES

The chances of FES occurring can be reduced by early fracture immobilization. Avoiding intramedullary reaming in the first 24–96 hours may reduce the chances of fat emboli developing. While these measures do have a positive effect on prevalence, the practitioner's focus should always be on prompt recognition, reassurance, and education.

Reference

1. Fukamoto L, Fukamoto K (2018). Fat embolism syndrome. *Nurs Clin North Am* 53:335–47.

Constipation

Constipation is a major cause of discomfort and anxiety. It occurs when there is a failure either of the bowels to propel faeces towards the rectum or when the rectum itself fails to empty. The stool is hard, dry, and difficult to pass. This may result in the patient feeling unwell, suffering abdominal pain and cramps, nausea, and loss of appetite. It may also lead to straining, rectal bleeding, and bowel obstruction.

Causes

The most common reason for constipation is that the faeces have become hard and dry. For the orthopaedic patient, this has multiple causes which can include:

- Reduced mobility caused by orthopaedic conditions and surgery
- Analgesia and other drugs known to cause constipation, such as iron and antidepressants; many of these, especially codeine-based and other opioid drugs, cause bowel action to slow down
- Difficulty in maintaining normal bowel habits due to loss of privacy and dignity and the bowel becomes overfull: patients may choose not to use a toilet, commode, or bedpan due to embarrassment
- Change in diet—many orthopaedic patients lose their appetite following injury or surgery, sometimes simply because they are less active; taking in less food than normal results in a longer gut transit time and increased water reabsorption, making the stool harder
- Insufficient intake of dietary fibre and oral fluids
- Muscular weakness caused by conditions such a spinal injury and ageing of the muscles controlling the bowel
- Occasionally, the cause of constipation can be serious conditions such as bowel obstruction; in older people, particularly following hip fracture, pseudo-obstruction of the colon may occur due to anatomy of the colon muscles.

Assessment

Stools which are dry and hard and straining to pass faeces are the most common symptoms of constipation. The patient is unlikely to tell the practitioner if they have problems so they should ask daily, in a sensitive manner, if patients have had their bowels open and if their stool was normal for them. It is important to base this assessment on an understanding of the patient's normal bowel habits. This will enable problems to be recognized early so that they can be treated before they become severe.

Prevention

Preventing constipation involves considering the causes by:

- Ensuring that a change in bowel habit is recognized as soon as possible
- Facilitating sufficient intake of dietary fibre and oral fluids
- Enabling provision of toilet facilities with as much privacy and as near normal as possible
- Regaining physical mobility as soon as possible.

Management

Treating constipation can involve several measures, the choice of which will vary, depending on the severity of constipation and the patient's preferences. Mild constipation may respond to:

- A gradual increase in dietary fibre and oral fluids, including foods known to be particularly helpful such as citrus fruits, dried stone fruits, and kiwi fruit
- Encouraging patients to defecate when they have the urge to do so and not to rush the activity
- Increased levels of physical activity within the limitations of their ability.

If these measures prove to be unsuccessful or constipation is thought to be more severe, laxative/aperients treatment should be prescribed; these are substances that assist evacuation of the bowel in mild to moderate constipation. They include:

- *Bulking agents*—help to retain water in the stool and promote microbial growth; these must be taken with plenty of oral fluids to assist their action
- *Stool softeners*—contain substances such as glycerol and docusate sodium that make the stool softer and increase its mobility within the bowel

If these measures fail or constipation is severe it may be necessary to use stronger purgatives including:

- *Osmotic agents* to increase the intake of fluid into the bowel through an osmotic effect
- *Stimulant laxatives* which act upon the nerve supply to the bowel wall to increase peristaltic action.

These preparations must be used with caution and patients must be able to drink sufficient fluids to replace that taken up by the bowel.

Enemas

Enemas involve the administration of liquid into the rectum which stimulates the emptying of the bowel. It can sometimes be used to treat severe constipation when other options have been unsuccessful. This procedure is invasive and distressing for the patient and should only be carried out by practitioners who fully understand the procedure and its implications.

Further reading

Bardsley A. (2017). Assessment and treatment options for patients with constipation. *Br J Nurs* 26:312–18.

Dougherty L, Lister S (2015). Elimination. In: *The Royal Marsden Hospital Manual of Clinical Nursing Procedures*, 9th edn, pp. 133–96. Oxford: Wiley-Blackwell.

Urinary retention

Postoperative urinary retention (POUR) is a common complication following major orthopaedic and trauma surgery such as TJR and hip fracture. It is an inability to void the bladder following a surgical procedure. Overall incidence of POUR following any surgical procedure ranges from 4% to 25%.[1] It is associated with pain and discomfort, UTIs, and increased length of stay.

Causes of retention and treatment strategies

The exact aetiology of POUR is not known, but a number of factors have been identified including:

- Postural—difficulty in urinating when lying in bed
- Use of spinal anaesthetic—especially combined spinal–epidural anaesthesia and spinal anaesthetics containing opioids
- Opioid analgesia and other drugs affecting the nervous system such as sedatives
- Prostatic enlargement.

It is important to carefully monitor urine output postoperatively and, even if the patient reports they are passing urine, it may be only a small amount, leaving a large residual volume of urine within the bladder, so the volume should also be recorded.

Signs and symptoms and management

Signs and symptoms of POUR include:

- Suprapubic pain
- Inability to pass urine and/or incomplete emptying of the bladder
- The distended bladder that is palpable and tender when compressed
- Ultrasound bladder scanning is frequently used to determine the amount of urine within the bladder and is a usual adjunct in assessing potential POUR
- Acute postoperative delirium can be caused by POUR, so may be an additional sign.

In most cases, retention is resolved by assisting the patient to get out of bed and use the toilet, bottle, or commode if their condition and postoperative instruction allow. However, for patients whose retention does not resolve when they are ambulant (or because the patient's circumstances prohibit mobilization), insertion of a urinary catheter will be needed, either as a one-off to empty the bladder or it may need to be left *in situ*. Insertion of a urinary catheter places the patient at risk of urinary tract infection, bacteraemia, and deep joint sepsis (see Urinary tract infection, pp. 204–205). The initial insertion of the catheter and removal should be carried out following local and national guidelines.

In men, any prostate enlargement should be explored as part of the pre-operative assessment. Typically, the signs and symptoms of prostatic enlargement include:

- Frequency and urgency of micturition
- Nocturia
- Poor flow of urine and dribbling
- Hesitancy
- Degrees of retention of urine.

In some orthopaedic centres the International Prostate Symptom Score is administered preoperatively, and treatment may be indicated before the patient undergoes orthopaedic surgery.

Reference

1. Zelmanovich A, Fromer D (2018). Urinary retention after orthopedic surgery: Identification of risk factors and management. *J Clin Exp Orthop* 4. ⅒ http://orthopedics.imedpub.com/urinary-retention-after-orthopedic-surgery-identification-of-risk-factors-and-management.php?aid=22148

Further reading

Durat A, Choquet O, Bringuier S, et al. (2015). Diagnosis of postoperative urinary retention using a simplified ultrasound bladder measurement. *Anaesth Analg* 120:1033–8.

Postoperative delirium

Delirium is the acute and sudden onset of fluctuating altered consciousness with changes in perception, cognitive function, and behaviour. Nurses sometimes refer to this an 'acute confusional' state in which the patient is suddenly agitated or aggressive or their demeanour changes. The condition is frightening and dangerous, leading to worse outcomes following surgery.[1]

Causes of acute delirium

Prevention of delirium is based on recognizing and managing known risk factors. Causes of delirium can be physiological, psychological, or environmental, or a combination. Potential causes include:

- Dementia and other cognitive impairment—recognizing delirium superimposed on dementia is difficult
- Dehydration and malnutrition
- Hypovolaemic shock
- Hypoxia and respiratory depression
- Polypharmacy and reaction to drug therapy, particularly opiates and tranquillizers
- Infection with or without pyrexia
- Urinary retention
- Hypoglycaemia or hyperglycaemia
- Constipation
- Drug or alcohol withdrawal
- Pain—untreated or overuse of analgesics
- Depression and/or anxiety
- Sleep deprivation
- Unfamiliar environment, sensory impairment, and loss of sensory cues.

Assessment

A baseline cognitive assessment should always be conducted on admission using a valid and reliable screening tool. Delirium may manifest itself in several ways including agitation, disruptive behaviour, or uncharacteristic drowsiness and appearing withdrawn, depending on whether the delirium is hyperactive or hypoactive. It is the last group whose change in cognitive state is often missed. It is important to listen to family members when they report this is 'not the usual' for the patient.

The 4AT is a simple tool for assessing for delirium (see ℜ https://www.the4at.com/) involving questions about alertness, memory, attention, and acute changes in cognition. This should be used for initial assessment and daily screening.

Management of delirium

Interventions will depend on the probable cause, e.g. dehydration will require fluid replacement and ongoing monitoring of fluid balance and electrolyte levels. Irrespective of the cause, the MDT need to provide a protective environment and to manage risk of injury to the patient or others. Close and frequent monitoring should be conducted in a calm, quiet environment alongside psychological support. Involvement of and reassurance from family and familiar carers and clear communication about all aspects of care and treatment is vital.

The following multicomponent interventions can reduce the symptoms and duration of delirium[1]:
- Daily medical review
- Daily orientation to time and space
- Early mobilization and maintaining function and normal routines
- Feeding assistance, good nutritional and regular drinks
- Therapeutic activities that engage the patient's brain
- Maintaining appropriate sleep patterns
- Ensuring that hearing and vision adaptations are in place.

Reference and Further reading

1. Cross J (2018). Nursing the patient with altered cognitive function. In: Hertz K, Santy-Tomlinson J (eds) *Fragility Fracture Nursing: Holistic Care and Management of the Orthogeriatric Patient*, pp. 109–23. Cham: Springer. https://www.springer.com/gb/book/9783319766805

Pressure ulcers

Pressure ulcers (PUs) are localized areas of soft tissue damage occurring in those who are immobile. They are avoidable breaches of patient safety in the orthopaedic patient. Tissue damage usually occurs because of a combination of pressure, shear and friction. Pressure is a perpendicular force that can occlude the blood supply to tissue by compressing the capillaries. Other external factors such as friction, shear, and moisture reduce the tolerance of the skin to pressure. Intrinsic factors such as the patient's general health status reduce the resilience of the skin to withstand these forces.[1]

Classification

Any skin redness over a bony prominence is a significant warning sign that further damage may be imminent and that intervention is needed. PUs are classified according to the NPUAP/EPUAP/PPPIA classification system[2] as follows:

- *Stage 1*—non-blanching erythema of intact skin, sometimes with blisters
- *Stage 2*—partial-thickness skin loss, involving the epidermis and/or dermis
- *Stage 3*—full-thickness skin loss involving a cavity
- *Stage 4*—full-thickness skin loss involving underlying structures and organs such as bone or muscle
- *Unstageable injuries*—those in which there is full-thickness tissue damage, but the base of the ulcer cannot be seen because it is filled with necrotic tissue such as eschar and slough
- *Deep tissue injury*—localized deep blue or black skin that indicates devitalized tissue but the full extent cannot be ascertained.

These stages enable clear assessment and documentation along with recording of the dimensions and appearance of the ulcer.

Risk assessment

Risk assessment considers the factors that contribute to PUs (Table 5.5). Risk assessment, on its own, does not prevent PUs, but recognition of the factors that can lead to PUs in individual patients is central to prevention through the management of specific risk factors.

Table 5.5 Common PU risk factors for orthopaedic patients

Intrinsic	Extrinsic
• Advanced age and frailty	• Pressure
• Medical conditions such as diabetes, Parkinson's disease, epilepsy, stroke	• Shear
• Malnutrition and dehydration	• Friction
• Medication and polypharmacy	• Reduced mobility
• Loss of sensation	• Moisture and faecal or urinary incontinence
• Dry or macerated skin	• Major surgery
• Pain	• General or regional anaesthesia

Prevention

Strategies for PU prevention should include[2]:

- At least daily risk assessment and documentation of the results informing a dynamic plan of care that is frequently evaluated
- Early mobilization and encouragement of the patient to move
- Frequent changes of position which include the *30° tilt*—turning a patient only partially onto their side so that their weight is resting on the side of the buttock rather than the sacrum or greater trochanter
- Avoiding sitting in a chair for long periods
- Frequent inspection of the skin for signs of PU development, such as redness and taking appropriate action
- Ensuring that patients' skin is kept clean, dry, and protected with emollients
- A balanced diet which includes plenty of protein and calories
- Maintenance of good hydration
- The use of high-quality foam mattresses and cushions which help to redistribute the pressure
- The use of dynamic support surfaces which have sequentially inflating and deflating cells while maintaining the above-listed interventions
- The patient needs to understand the causes and consequences of pressure ulcers so that they can actively participate in preventing them.

References

1. Donnelly J, Collins A, Santy-Tomlinson J (2014). Wound management, tissue viability and infection. In: Clarke S, Santy-Tomlinson J (eds) *Orthopaedic and Trauma Nursing: An Evidence-Based Approach to Musculoskeletal Care*, pp. 158–67. Oxford: Wiley-Blackwell.
2. National Pressure Ulcer Advisory Panel, European Pressure Ulcer Advisory Panel and Pan Pacific Pressure Injury Alliance (NPUAP/EPUAP/PPPIA) (2014). Prevention and treatment of pressure ulcers: quick reference guide. ℜ http://www.epuap.org/wp-content/uploads/2016/10/quick-reference-guide-digital-npuap-epuap-pppia-jan2016.pdf

Further reading

Hommel A, Santy-Tomlinson J (2018). Pressure injury prevention and wound management. In: Hertz K, Santy-Tomlinson J (eds) *Fragility Fracture Nursing*, pp. 85–94. Cham: Springer. ℜ https://www.springer.com/gb/book/9783319766805
NHS. Stop the Pressure. ℜ http://nhs.stopthepressure.co.uk/

Musculoskeletal conditions

Musculoskeletal disorders and conditions

This chapter provides an overview of common disorders and conditions of the musculoskeletal system, including aetiology, pathology, signs and symptoms, and principles of treatment. The treatment of non-traumatic musculoskeletal problems is often referred to as elective or planned orthopaedics. In Chapter 1 (see ➲ The orthopaedic patient, p. 120) an introduction to disease classifications was presented; musculoskeletal disorders can be further classified as follows:

- Bone and joint infections, e.g. osteomyelitis, septic arthritis, tuberculosis (TB)
- Arthritis and other joint disorders, e.g. rheumatoid arthritis (RA), ankylosing spondylitis (AS), osteoarthritis (OA), gout
- Tumours of the musculoskeletal system, e.g. osteosarcoma, chondroma
- Metabolic and endocrine disorders, e.g. osteoporosis, Paget's disease, rickets
- Degenerative conditions, e.g. osteonecrosis and osteochondritis
- Genetic disorders and malformations, e.g. osteogenesis imperfecta (OI), spina bifida.

Examples of common disorders

Bone and joint infections
See Fig. 6.1.

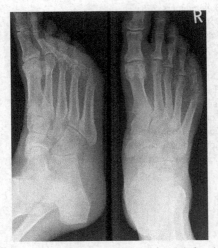

Fig. 6.1 Dorsoplantar (DP) and oblique radiographs of the right foot showing bony destruction in the right fifth metatarsal head of a patient with diabetes. On clinical examination, there was skin ulceration with surrounding redness over the area of radiographic abnormality, which was subsequently confirmed as acute osteomyelitis. Image courtesy of the Nottingham University Hospitals Radiology Department.

Arthritis and other joint disorders
See Fig. 6.2.

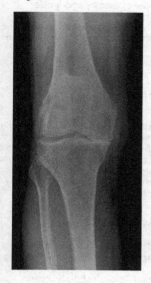

Fig. 6.2 AP radiograph of the right knee showing medial tibiofemoral compartment OA with secondary tibia varus deformity. Image courtesy of the Nottingham University Hospitals Radiology Department.

Metabolic and endocrine disorders
See Fig. 6.3.

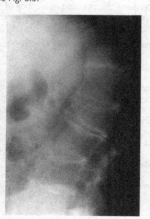

Fig. 6.3 X-ray of lumbar spine showing osteoporosis of the vertebral bodies. Reproduced from the *Oxford Textbook of Orthopaedics and Trauma*, with permission from Oxford University Press.

Osteoarthritis

Symptomatic OA is the commonest cause of disability among older people in the UK and the Western world. The impact of this disease on society is considerable in terms of lost working days, inability to work, and use of healthcare resources. The impact on the individual is also significant and includes[1]:

- Coping and living with pain
- Altered body image
- Inability to carry out everyday activities
- Inability to socialize with friends and family.

Causes

The exact cause/s of OA are not fully understood, but it is known that it is a complex metabolic process and not simply a wear and tear process associated with ageing. The most likely causes are mechanical, due to abnormal load distribution on weight-bearing joints due to an unstable or incongruent joint, or abnormal load bearing through the joint due to obesity and/or cumulative excessive exposure to overuse, e.g. work involving ascending/descending ladders leads to OA of the knee joints.

Pathology

The changes within the joint due to OA comprise five stages:

- Breakdown of the articular cartilage
- Irritation of synovial membrane and production of degradative enzymes
- Ineffective remodelling of the cartilage and increased density of the subchondral bone
- Eburnation of bone and cyst formation—erosion of the articular surface exposing subchondral bone, microfractures in the trabeculae of underlying cancellous bone, and loss of joint space
- Disorganization of the joint, enlargement of osteophytes, wearing of the bone surface, and joint stiffness and deformity, e.g. varus deformity of the knee and laxity of the joint capsule and ligaments.

Each affected joint may demonstrate two or more stages simultaneously within different areas.

Signs and symptoms

It is important to remember that there can be disparity between the symptoms reported by the patient and the signs evident on X-ray, i.e. there may be only minor changes visible on X-ray, but the patient reports significant pain and reduced movement. Signs include:

- Crepitus
- Restriction of range of movement
- Shortening due to lost joint space
- Gait alteration, e.g. positive Trendelenburg for patients with OA of the hip
- Deformity of the joint, e.g. flexion deformity of the hip and varus deformity of the knee

- Muscle wasting
- Signs visible on X-ray include loss of joint space, osteophytes, subchondral cysts, and sclerosis, spurs at the joint margins, laxity of the joint.

  Symptoms experienced include:
- Pain at rest, during activity, and night pain
- Joint stiffness
- Reduced mobility
- Joint instability.

The signs will depend on the stage of the disease and symptom reporting will be dependent upon the patient's coping mechanisms and previous experience of pain (see ➲ Pain management, p. 142 for further details).

Diagnosis and treatment options

Diagnosis of OA is made based on patient history, clinical examination, and radiographic findings. Treatment options will depend on the severity of the disease process and patient preference and include:
- Conservative measures—see ➲ Symptom management of OA, pp. 230–231
- Joint replacement—see ➲ Joint replacement surgery, pp. 286–287
- Intra articular joint injections—see ➲ Intra-articular injections, pp. 284–285
- Osteotomy—see ➲ Arthrodesis and osteotomy, pp. 308–309
- Arthrodesis—see ➲ Arthrodesis and osteotomy, pp. 308–309
- Arthroscopic procedures—see ➲ Arthroscopy, pp. 300–301
- Cartilage surgery and transplantation—see ➲ Autologous chondrocyte transplantation, pp. 302–303.

Reference

1. Parsons G, Godfrey H, Jester R (2009). Living with severe osteoarthritis, while awaiting hip and knee joint replacement surgery. *Musculoskeletal Care* 7:121–35.

Symptom management for osteoarthritis

There are several non-surgical interventions that can provide symptom relief and improve function for patients with OA. Conservative options are useful in the earlier stages of the disease process while patients are waiting for a surgical intervention such as joint replacement surgery or for patients who are not able to undergo surgery due to severe comorbidity rendering them high risk for anaesthesia and surgery.

Self-management programmes (SMPs)

SMPs have been found to be highly effective in empowering patients to take control of their symptom management and to become the expert in how the disease affects them as an individual. SMPs should adopt a problem-based learning approach and include the following key elements[1]:
- Skill development in problem-solving
- Development of clinical judgement
- Self-efficacy building
- Belief modification and symptom reinterpretation.

SMPs focus on increasing the patient's knowledge of their condition, how to develop coping and adaptation strategies, and how to effectively access healthcare resources.

Other methods of symptom relief

There are several non-surgical measures that can help with symptom relief including:
- Use of an appropriate walking aid to relieve some of the load bearing through the affected joint, e.g. a walking stick in the opposite hand
- Provision of aids to daily living such as raised toilet seat, stair rails, long-handled shoe horn, etc. to promote independence
- Health education and support regarding obesity—reduction of the patient's weight will reduce the load through the joint/s
- Pain assessment and management—regular review of the effectiveness of analgesia and review of concordance
- Intra-articular corticosteroid injections should be considered as an adjunct to core treatments for the relief of moderate to severe pain in people with OA.[2] Muscle weakness should be corrected as it leads to increased pain and joint instability.

Symptom management is, in the main, carried out by the primary care team with support from the orthopaedic team. Patients require an individual assessment to identify the particular impact of OA and the related symptoms and then a bespoke package of conservative measures can be planned and regularly evaluated for its effectiveness.[3] Psychological support is an important aspect of symptom management, specifically to develop coping and adaptation strategies.

References
1. Jester R (2007). Supporting people with long-term conditions. In: Jester R (ed) *Advancing Practice in Rehabilitating Nursing*, pp. 158–70. Oxford: Blackwell Publishing.
2. NICE (2014). Osteoarthritis: care and management. Clinical guideline [CG177]. ℜ https://www.nice.org.uk/guidance/cg177
3. Finney AG, Porcheret M, Grime J, et al. (2013). Defining the content of an opportunistic osteoarthritis consultation with primary health care professionals: a Delphi consensus study. *Arthritis Care Res* 65:962–8.

Osteochondritis

Osteochondritis is a term describing a group of musculoskeletal conditions where a piece of bone has become detached from its normal articulation. The causes include loss of, or reduced, blood supply to the area of bone resulting in necrosis, e.g. Perthes' disease of the hip or Kienbock's disease of the lunate bone of the hand. This type of condition is most common at times of rapid skeletal growth in adolescents. The presenting signs and symptoms will vary depending on the location of the condition, but usually involve locking followed by effusion within the joint, swelling, and pain. However, the presence of loose bodies can often be asymptomatic. Osteochondritis dissecans (OCD) is a common form of osteochondritis and an overview of the condition is presented here.

Osteochondritis dissecans

OCD most commonly occurs in the knee or elbow joints with the medial aspect of the knee being the commonest presentation. It involves interruption of the blood supply to a segment of subchondral bone with its adjacent articulating cartilage, e.g. the medial femoral condyle necroses, detaches itself and becomes a loose body within the knee joint. It is most prevalent in adolescent males who are athletic and is thought to be associated with trauma although its exact aetiology is unclear. The resulting cavity formed by the detachment of the fragment fills with fibrous tissue and thus the articulation of the joint surfaces can become subtly misaligned, leading to a predisposition to OA of the knee joint in later years. Diagnosis is made by review of X-ray revealing the cavity in the original articulating surface of the bone and a floating fragment. MRI scanning will give a more accurate view of the size of the fragment.

Signs and symptoms

Signs and symptoms include:
- Vague, aching pain in the joint worsened by activity
- Locking, catching, and giving way of the knee joint
- Effusion of the joint
- Range of movement is usually normal
- The avulsed medial femoral fragment may be palpable when the knee is flexed to 90°.

Principles of treatment

Before the fragment breaks away and has become compromised due to reduced blood supply, treatment will comprise rest, usually in a cast, reduced weight bearing, and cessation of sporting/athletic activity for several months.

Surgical options once the fragment has avulsed include arthroscopic surgery to remove the loose body or reattachment using a pin. For details of care of patients in casts (see ➜ Care of casts, pp. 372–373) and pre- and postoperative care (see ➜ Preoperative assessment and preparation, pp. 128–131 and Postoperative care, pp. 132–133).

Rheumatoid arthritis

What is RA?

RA is a relatively common autoimmune inflammatory condition that affects the synovium that lines the joints and tendon sheaths of the body. RA is classically characterized by symmetrical small joint polyarthritis involving the hands and the feet although larger joints can also be affected. The chronic systemic inflammation attacks the synovial tissues of moveable joints causing pannus formation and cartilage and bone degradation. RA is a chronic progressive disease which often leads to increased mortality.

What causes RA?

Although the cause is unknown, various factors might act as initiating factors in people with a genetic disposition including
- Infection
- Stress
- Trauma.

Who does RA affect?
- One million people in the UK
- Prevalence is 1:200 for women and 1:600 for men with the distribution more evenly distributed among the sexes over the age of 60
- RA can present at any age, although the peak age of onset is between 35 and 50 years

How does RA manifest?

RA can present in various ways:
- The most common form of presentation occurs typically in the fourth or fifth decade of life and manifests as an insidious onset of symmetrical small joint polyarthritis, affecting the MCP and PIP joints in the hands and the MTP joints in the feet. As the condition progresses, other joints can be affected
- Diffuse swelling is more commonly seen in older people
- A monoarticular form affects larger joints such as the knees or shoulders. The symptoms may be confined to these areas or become more generalized, affecting other joints
- RA has a rapid or insidious onset
- The presence of inflammation in the joints (especially the small joints of the hands and feet) should prompt early referral for diagnosis

Common symptoms patients with active RA can experience

These include:
- Joint pain
- Joint swelling
- Stiffness (often more marked on waking)
- Fatigue
- Low mood.

RA has extra-articular and systemic manifestations including:
- Anaemia
- Weight loss
- Vasculitis
- Rheumatoid lung and interstitial lung disease
- Ocular involvement—episcleritis, scleritis
- Haematological—Felty's syndrome, lymphomas
- Cardiovascular disease—pericarditis, myocarditis
- Lymphadenopathy
- Sjögren's syndrome
- Subcutaneous nodules
- Exocrine, salivary, and lachrymal gland involvement
- Entrapment neuropathies
- Increased risks of malignancies.

Diagnosing RA

RA can be difficult to diagnosis. The American Rheumatism Association's (ARA) revised criteria for the classification of RA includes:
- Morning stiffness in and around the joints lasting at least 1 hour
- Arthritis in three or more joint areas with swelling and fluid
- Arthritis of hand joints
- Symmetrical arthritis

(All those criteria listed above must be present for at least 6 weeks).
- Subcutaneous nodules
- Radiological changes
- Positive rheumatoid factor (RF) (although there is now a move to use the anticyclic citrullinated peptide (CCP) serology tests instead of the RF as it has a higher specificity and sensitivity in terms of diagnosis and a raised anti-CCP indicates more aggressive disease).

The ARA criteria may not be sensitive enough to identify early disease and the use of ultrasound is being advocated to identify early erosions, synovitis, ganglion cysts, or osteopenia to promote early treatment.

Management of rheumatoid arthritis

The aims of treatment include:
- Managing symptoms including pain and stiffness
- Suppressing the inflammatory process to prevent joint damage and deformity
- Educating patients on how to manage their symptoms and understand their treatment
- Optimizing physical, psychological, and social function.

As the aims of treatment are multifaceted, a multidisciplinary approach to care management is required which involves having access to a range of health professionals including:
- Specialist nurses to educate patients about their condition and monitor their drug therapy
- Physiotherapists to help maintain joint function, muscle tone and strength, gait assessment, and mobility
- Occupational therapists to assess daily activities that are hindered by having RA, help maintain hand function, teach self-management strategies, goal setting, joint protection, and relaxation techniques
- Podiatrists for foot health.

Managing pain and stiffness

A combination of pharmacological and non-pharmacological interventions can be employed:
- Simple or compound analgesia
- NSAIDs; Due to the risks associated with the use of NSAIDs, patients need to be assessed on a regular basis to establish whether they still require this medication or if the dosage can be reduced
- Neither analgesics nor NSAIDs influence the progression of the RA, they treat the symptoms only
- Corticosteroids can be administered via various routes including oral, IM, IV, or intra-articular (IA)
- Use of cold/ heat packs
- Exercises to reduce stiffness and maintain muscle strength
- Relaxation
- Pacing activities.

Suppressing the disease process

DMARDs are used to suppress the disease process and prevent the development of deformities and erosions. Clinical evidence supports early and aggressive treatment with DMARDs and recommends combination therapy—the use of two or more DMARDs at the same time—as an effective treatment strategy. Commonly used DMARDs include:
- Methotrexate
- Sulfasalazine
- Leflunomide
- Azathioprine
- Hydroxychloroquine.

If a patient fails to respond to DMARDs biologic treatment should be considered. Biologic therapies are often prescribed with a DMARD, usually methotrexate, and include:
- Antitumour necrosis factor alpha, e.g. adalimumab, etanercept, infliximab, certolizumab, golimumab
- IL-6 receptors, e.g. tocilizumab
- CD80 and CD86 receptors, e.g. abatacept
- B-cell depletion therapies (rituximab).

Patient education

This can be provided through a variety of sources:
- Booklets
- Videos
- Internet programmes
- One-to-one sessions with a specialist practitioner
- Group programmes to learn skills such as exercises and relaxation
- Support groups such as the National Rheumatoid Arthritis Society (NRAS): ◌ http://www.rheumatoid.org.uk.

Other types of rheumatology conditions

There are >200 different kinds of rheumatological conditions. The following are covered:
- Seronegative spondyloarthropathies
- Septic arthritis (see ➲ Septic arthritis, pp. 276–777)
- Crystal arthropathies
- Polymyalgia rheumatica (PMR).

Seronegative spondyloarthropathies

What are these?

A group of chronic inflammatory conditions that have a number of shared characteristics. Spondyloarthropathies include:
- Ankylosing spondylitis (AS)
- Psoriatic arthritis
- Reactive arthritis
- Enteropathic arthritis (EA)
- Undifferentiated spondyloarthropathies
- Enthesitis-related juvenile inflammatory arthritis (JIA).

What are the shared characteristics?

- Peripheral inflammatory arthritis, usually asymmetrical
- Radiological evidence of sacroiliitis
- Enthesopathic pain
- Strong association with HLA-B27.

How are these conditions managed?

- Relieving symptoms—analgesia, NSAIDs, hot/cold packs, pacing activities. Caution with NSAIDs in EA as this may precipitate a flare of the bowel disease
- Suppressing the disease process—DMARDs, biologics
- Maintaining function—exercise, physiotherapy, and hydrotherapy. Regular exercise is of particular importance to patients with AS
- Education about the condition and self-management strategies.

Crystal arthropathies

These are inflammatory joint disorders that result from the formation of crystals in the joints or periarticular tissues. The three major crystal arthropathies include:
- Gout (monosodium urate crystals)—often seen in peripheral joints
- Pseudogout (calcium pyrophosphate deposition)—seen in knees, wrists, hips, shoulders, and the symphysis pubis
- Acute calcific periarthritis (calcium hydroxyapatite crystals)—predominantly in the shoulders.

What investigations need to be performed?

- Joint aspiration and microscopy to locate crystals
- Blood tests, FBC, uric acid, ESR, U&Es, creatinine
- Additional blood tests to consider triggering factors, e.g. alcohol, glucose, and lipids
- X-rays—soft tissue swelling may be present with gout.

What is the management?
- Drug therapy: analgesia, NSAIDs, colchicine, allopurinol (but not in the acute phase) and febuxostat
- Joint aspiration and steroid injection if required
- Education regarding lifestyle, e.g. weight, alcohol intake.

Polymyalgia rheumatica

What is polymyalgia rheumatica (PMR)?

PMR is a common inflammatory joint condition seen in older people. It is characterized by pain and stiffness especially in the hips, pelvis, and shoulders and is often accompanied by fatigue and low-grade fever.

What investigations need to be done?
- ESR, CRP, LFTs, FBC
- Immunology (RF and antinuclear antibodies)
- Protein electrophoresis and Bence Jones urine to exclude myeloma
- Creatine kinase to exclude myositis
- Thyroid function test to exclude hypothyroidism
- Chest X-ray to exclude malignancy.

What is the management?
- Oral prednisolone (typically 15–30 mg with dose reduction dependent on the patient's symptoms)
- Bone protection medication, e.g. a bisphosphonate and calcium and vitamin D
- Analgesia
- Exercises to help the joint stiffness.

Connective tissue disorders

This is a complex autoimmune group of conditions which include:
- Systemic lupus erythematosus (lupus). The commonest of the connective tissue disorders, manifestations vary from skin rashes to life-threatening multisystem organ failure
- Sjögren's syndrome causes dryness of the eyes, mouth, vagina, pharynx, oesophagus, and skin
- Primary systemic vasculitides, e.g. granulomatosis with polyangiitis, eosinophilic granulomatosis with polyangiitis (formerly known as Churg–Strauss syndrome), microscopic polyangiitis, and polyarteritis nodosa. These are a group of rare, potentially life-threatening conditions characterized by inflammation and necrosis of blood vessel walls
- Behçet's syndrome characterized by oral and genital ulcers, eye inflammation, and arthritis
- Scleroderma caused by excessive collagen leading to fibrosis of the skin; in the systemic form internal organs are affected.

Further reading

Adebajo A, Dunkley L (2018). *ABC of Rheumatology*, 5th edn. Oxford: Wiley-Blackwell.

Ankylosing spondylitis

Definition: both words are Greek in origin, ankylosing means fusing and spondylitis means inflammation of the spine.

What is AS?

AS is a form of chronic rheumatic disease; it affects mainly the bones, muscles, and ligaments of the spine. However, it can also affect other joints, tendons, and ligaments as well as other structures such as the lungs, eyes, heart, bowel, and skin.

- Inflammation occurs at the site where certain ligaments or tendons attach to bone (enthesis) which is evident on X-ray as a 'squaring' of the vertebrae.
- This is followed by some damage to the bone at the site of the attachment and, as the inflammation reduces, healing takes place and new bone develops.
- Repetition of this process leads to further bone formation and the individual bones of the vertebrae then fuse together. This fusing makes the spine less flexible and can result in a hunched forward position which is often seen in patients.
- Commonly, the pelvis (sacroiliac joint) is affected first, but the lower back, chest wall, and neck may be involved at different times.
- AS can lead to arthritis developing in the large joints such as the hips and knees.

Causes of AS

It is an autoimmune disorder. There is some evidence that 96% of people with AS in Britain have a genetic cell marker—HLA-B27. It is thought that a harmless organism which the immune system cannot fight comes into contact with the HLA-B27 and an adverse reaction occurs. Not all patients with the B27 antigen develop AS.

Symptoms of reactive arthritis may also lead to AS. They include:

- Iritis/uveitis—inflammation of part of the iris causing rapid onset eye pain, sensitivity to light and blurred vision
- Conjunctivitis—red, painful, gritty eyes
- Urethritis—inflammation of the urethra.

AS can also run in families and the HLA-B27 antigen can be inherited. If there is a close family member with AS there is 3× more chance of developing it. However, AS is relatively rare so the overall likelihood of developing it is very small.

Who is at risk?

Anyone can suffer from AS and the onset is typically in the late teens and 20s with an average age of 24 years. It is 3× more common in men than women. In men, the pelvis and spine are more affected and in women and children, the pelvis, hips, and knees are the most commonly involved.

Signs and symptoms of AS

The signs and symptoms of AS vary from person to person and progresses gradually. Typical symptoms include:
- Back pain and stiffness—slow gradual onset
- Joint inflammation
- Early-morning stiffness and pain
- Pain improves on exercise and is worse on rest
- Weight loss
- Fatigue
- Compression fractures
- Fevers and night sweats.

Diagnosis

Because of the gradual progression of AS diagnosis can be difficult, but should include the following:
- History
- Blood tests:
  - FBC, ESR, CRP, HLA-B27
- Imaging:
  - X-rays—will only show AS late on in the disease
  - MRI scan—highlights changes in the joints
  - Ultrasound scan—to look for inflammation of the tissues.

Treatment and care

There is no cure for AS and it is a long-term condition. The aim should be to relieve the patient's symptoms, slow down its progress, and minimize the impact on the quality of life for the individual affected. AS treatment is most effective before bone damage has occurred.

Principles of treatment include:
- Referral to a rheumatologist
- Education—about AS and how the patient can help themselves with lifestyle changes
- NSAIDs—to help with the pain and inflammation unless they suffer from inflammatory bowel disease then other analgesics will be preferable
- Physiotherapy—to improve posture and to increase the range of movement in certain joints
- Alternative therapies—some patients find that this helps them
- Surgery—will only be used as a last resort to help manage the condition, e.g. hip replacement to relieve pain.

Complications of AS

- Uveitis—needs treating quickly as it could affect the patient's vision
- Osteoporosis—common in the spine of AS sufferers
- Cardiovascular disease—the risk is slightly higher in AS sufferers. Lifestyle changes will help
- Stiffening of the rib cage causing restricted lung capacity and function
- Spinal fractures—increased risk of fractures due to stiffness and poor movement

- Cauda equina syndrome—a very rare complication of AS where the nerves at the bottom of the spine become compressed, causing numbness and weakness in the lower limbs
- Fixed posture—this is rare but pain and stiffness can develop in the upper back decreasing mobility of the spine making it difficult to move and may give a bent posture.

Prognosis

The natural course of AS is very variable and there can be times of remission. However, patients can lead a productive life despite an AS diagnoses.

Further reading

Bond D (2013). Ankylosing spondylitis: diagnosis and management. *Nursing Standard* 28:52–9.

Haroon N (2015). Ankylosis in ankylosing spondylitis: current concepts. *Clin Rheumatol* 34:1003–7.

National Ankylosing Spondylitis Society (2020). About axial SpA (AS). ℘ http://www.nass.co.uk/about-as/

Patient UK (2018). Ankylosing spondylitis. ℘ https://patient.info/bones-joints-muscles/back-and-spine-pain/ankylosing-spondylitis

Prolapsed intervertebral disc

The spinal column is formed of 33 individual vertebrae which form a protective casing around the spinal cord. The spinal cord and brain form the central nervous system (CNS), which is responsible for receiving and transmitting messages to the rest of the body.

Between each vertebra there is an intervertebral disc—these are circular pads of connective tissue composed of two main components: the annulus fibrosus—the tough outer ring of fibrocartilage, and the nucleus pulposus—a soft gelatinous inner filling. Tears in the annulus can allow the nucleus pulposus to prolapse or herniate. If the prolapse is central, towards the spinal canal, bladder or bowel function can be affected. If the prolapse is lateral, pressure on a spinal nerve can affect movement and sensation (see Fig. 6.4). The lumbar and cervical areas are the most commonly affected.

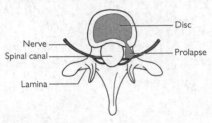

Disc
Nerve
Spinal canal
Prolapse
Lamina

Fig. 6.4 Prolapsed intervertebral disc.

Signs and symptoms

Signs and symptoms will depend on the site of the disc prolapse and the nerves involved. This may include:
- Pain in the lower back or neck—intermittent in both severity and frequency but made worse by activity
- Pain down one or both legs (sciatica) or in the shoulder or arm
- Increased pain on coughing, sneezing, or straining to go to the toilet
- Pain on straight leg raising
- Bladder or bowel dysfunction
- Paraesthesia/loss of sensation—depending on the nerve root affected
- Motor weakness and/or drop foot
- Lack of normal movement
- If the cauda equina is involved, this is a medical emergency—it needs immediate treatment to avoid permanent damage.

Assessment and investigations

The history taken from the patient is crucial and should include:
- Exact signs, symptoms, and location
- Duration of the symptoms
- A history of any injury sustained and any previous surgical treatments
- Social and financial impact and coping
- Any personal injury litigation pending.

Investigations will depend on the severity of the patient's symptoms and may include:
- Full physical and neurological examination
- Observation of gait, reflex testing, motor strength, toe touching, and pulses
- Radiography—although this will not show a disc prolapse but will show any degeneration and other skeletal abnormalities
- CT or MRI scanning (see ➔ Other types of diagnostic imaging, pp. 110–111)—will provide a clear picture of the prolapse
- Differential nerve blocks—can identify difficult nerve root problems in some patients.

Management

Management may either be conservative or surgical.

Conservative management

This is the first course of action once serious pathology has been eliminated. Conservative management may include:
- Bed rest—but for a short period of a few days maximum. Once acute pain subsides, the patient should be mobilized and return to normal activities
- Analgesia—muscle relaxants and NSAIDs
- Exercise programme—supervised by a physiotherapist
- Corsets and orthoses—may be used to assist pain relief for a short period of time
- Epidural steroid injections—in a limited number of cases injections of either local anaesthetic or steroids can help relieve pain
- Rehabilitation—once pain relief is achieved then rehabilitation programmes such as 'back schools' are vital. This provides the patient with education to decrease the probability of reoccurrence. Exercises are used to strengthen the spine and regain mobility, and muscle tone this can prevent further disability and can help to restore as much function as possible. This enables the patient to return to normal activities. If this is not possible, the patient is given education on adapting to new lifestyles so they can reach their maximum potential.

Surgical management

If symptoms persist surgery may be recommended if there is:
- Bladder or bowel dysfunction
- Loss of perianal sensation
- Neurological weakness that continues even following bedrest
- Pain that does not go away with abnormal neurological signs
- Obvious muscle weakness.

Surgical options (see ➔ Spinal surgery, pp. 310–311) can include any of the following:
- Percutaneous nucleotomy
- Removal of the disc—either by laminectomy or partial laminectomy
- Removal of the disc and fusion of the affected segment.

Small endoscopic discectomy (called nano endoscopic discectomy) is not invasive and does not cause post-laminectomy syndrome.

Complications

- Failed back syndrome (post-laminectomy syndrome)—a significant, potentially disabling result that can arise following invasive spine surgery
- Cauda equina syndrome—a medical emergency requiring immediate attention and possible surgical intervention.

Practitioners can help patients to understand that in the majority of cases pain improves and resolves after a few months following conservative treatment. Only a small percentage of patients may continue to have chronic back pain even after treatment or surgery and may need to develop coping strategies for their pain and may need psychological intervention to help them (see ➜ Psychological aspects of care, pp. 168–169).

Further reading

Gugliotta M, da Costa BR, Dabis E, et al. (2016). Surgical versus conservative treatment for lumbar disc herniation: a prospective cohort study. *BMJ Open* 216:e012938.

NICE (2016). Low back pain and sciatica in over 16s: assessment and management. NICE guideline [NG59]. ⅊ https://www.nice.org.uk/guidance/ng59

Spondylolisthesis

Spondylolisthesis

Spondylolisthesis ('vertebral slippage') is a common condition of the spine that involves forward subluxation (slipping) of one vertebra over another. It can occur at any level of the spine but is most common in the lumbar region.

The condition is usually classified as congenital (*dysplastic*), spondylolytic (*isthmic*—fatigue fracture), *degenerative* (due to OA), *traumatic* (following bony or ligamentous injury to the spine), or *pathological* (due to tumour or bone disease). Dysplastic and isthmic spondylolisthesis are more common in children and adolescents while other aetiologies are most common in adulthood. See Fig. 6.5.

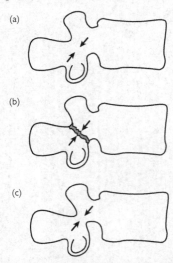

Fig. 6.5 (a) Isthmus (pars interarticularis) of the vertebral arch (arrows). (b) Isthmus defect (spondylolysis). (c) Isthmus elongation. Reproduced from the *Oxford Textbook of Orthopaedics and Trauma*, with permission from Oxford University Press.

Symptoms, assessment, and diagnosis

A large proportion of the population are thought to have some spondylolisthesis which may be asymptomatic and does not need any treatment—for those who have symptoms the following are the most common:

- The symptoms of spondylolisthesis usually include low back pain which can radiate into the buttocks. The pain is often brought on by strenuous activity and long periods of standing. Pain is worsened by activity and relieved on resting

- There may also be sciatic pain (affecting the leg) if the condition is severe and is causing nerve root pressure. This and other neurological symptoms such as weakness of the legs and bladder or bowel symptoms indicate an urgent need for medical assessment and possible surgery
- On examination and palpation, a step can sometimes be felt at the affected level of the spine
- Excessive curvature of the spine (kyphosis)
- The deformity can usually be clearly seen on radiographs—these should be taken with the patient standing as some slippages are less apparent when the patient is lying down.

The forward slippage of the vertebra can be described as a grade of severity of I–IV according to the percentage of slippage.

Management and care

Management and care can involve a combination of the following:
- Short periods of rest and restriction of any activity that causes pain, particularly strenuous activity, is advised. However, this restriction should not be complete and for long periods of time as this will lead to stiffness and muscle wasting and the complications of immobility. Gentle mobilization is recommended.
- A combination of different types of analgesics, including NSAIDs, are used to reduce inflammation and muscle spasm as well as general pain.
- Physiotherapy is recommended to reduce stress on the spine. Gentle exercise is used to help strengthen the extensor muscles of the back and the abdominal muscles that support the back.
- Lumbosacral support can be used when there is pain to provide some stability and protection to the back muscles. It is usually recommended that support devices such as braces and corsets are used when the patient is active and mobilizing and can be removed when they are at rest as long-term use may lead to weakness of the spinal muscles.
- Weight loss may be helpful in those patients who are overweight or obese as obesity can affect posture.
- Patients whose condition is not progressive are more likely to be managed conservatively. When symptoms are severe and conservative measures have not been helpful or the condition is worsening, a spinal fusion including bone grafting can resolve the problem (see ➲ Spinal surgery, pp. 310–311).

Spinal conditions, particularly those that result in back pain, are distressing and worrying for patients. Information, reassurance, and support are essential for patients with this condition. Advice needs to be based on a sound understanding of the condition following thorough assessment by medical practitioners. This includes education to help the individual and their family to understand their condition and those activities which are likely to relieve the symptoms and prevent the condition from worsening.

Spinal deformities

The normal curvatures of the spine enable strong support of the body and facilitate movement. These normal curvatures include cervical and thoracic curves and lumbar lordosis and sacral curves. Disruption to these curves can lead to pain and disability. This can cause significant chronic pain and disability as well as body image issues.

Cervical spine

Deformities of the cervical spine are uncommon. A head which is thrown forward will diminish the normal cervical curve. This can be indicative of mechanical problems in the cervical spine such as spondylosis. Cervical deformity is most commonly seen in AS.

Thoracic spine

Deformities of the thoracic spine are more common.

Scoliosis

This is a rotational deformity of the spine which can be seen when viewed from the rear and on bending. Asymmetry of the shoulders, trunk, and/or pelvis with a 'rib hump' as well as lateral spinal curvature can be seen. The deformity usually develops in adolescence and the cause is unknown, usually commencing during an adolescent growth spurt and the deformity continues to increase until growth stops—resulting in mild to severe deformity. The deformity also often involves some twisting of the spine. A mild deformity may cause no obvious problems, but severe deformity can result in altered body image, compromise of cardiac and/or respiratory functions, and progressive pain and degeneration of the spinal joints. See Fig. 6.6.

The child/adolescent should be followed up on a regular basis to assess the progression of the deformity with physical and radiographic examination. The patient and their family will need considerable support from practitioners with knowledge of the condition during this period so that they can understand the likely progression of the problem, outcomes, and management options.

Most mild deformities do not require treatment. Conservative treatment for scoliosis typically includes exercise, corrective casts, and/or braces which may halt or reduce the progression of the deformity. The evidence supporting the use of casts and braces, however, is controversial. Where the deformity is severe, surgery to correct the curvature should be considered. Surgery involves corrective release of the deformity and instrumented fusion (see ➲ Spinal surgery, pp. 310–311). Such surgery is major and carries a risk of serious complications such a paraplegia.[1,2]

Kyphosis

This is the anterior curvature of the thoracic spine, often caused by multiple compression fractures and collapse of the vertebral bodies of the thoracic spine due to osteoporosis. This deformity not only results in loss of height, but can lead to severe and chronic pain, with significant disability and reduced quality of life along with respiratory and gastric problems in severe cases.

In addition to the treatment for osteoporosis (see ➋ Osteoporosis, p. 252) the management of vertebral compression fractures and kyphosis involves the following:

• Pain management is the most important aspect of care. Once the acute pain of a fracture has subsided, this is often followed by chronic back pain which is both severe and long lasting and may be referred into other areas of the spine and thoracic region. When pain is severe it may be necessary to judiciously use opioid analgesics in long-acting/slow-release forms as well as muscle relaxants and NSAIDs. Referral to a chronic pain service may be beneficial, including potential treatment with nerve blocks.

• Conservative treatment involves rest balanced with activity and specific but gentle exercise to strengthen the supporting muscles of the spine carried out under supervision by a physiotherapist. Sometimes bracing of the spine may be prescribed.

• Kyphosis deformity results in a change in the centre of gravity for the patient and can lead to falls. Prevention of falls (see ➋ Falls, pp. 326–327) is a significant factor in preventing further deterioration of the vertebral stability.

• Surgical procedures known as *vertebroplasty* (the injection of plastic polymer into a partially collapsed vertebral body) and *kyphoplasty* (similar to vertebroplasty but a catheter balloon is inserted into the vertebral body before it is filled with polymer) can be performed. The aims of these procedures are to support and stabilize the fractures and decrease pain.

• Pain, disability, loss of independence, and altered body image can lead to depression and anxiety. The nurse has an important role in assessing patients' psychological well-being and providing emotional and psychological support.

Lumbar spine

The normal anterior curve of the lumbar spine (lordosis) can be exaggerated by scoliosis (see earlier) and other mechanical problems such as disc prolapse and vertebral body collapse caused by osteoporosis. Scoliosis can also be seen in the lumbar spine.

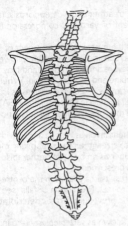

Fig. 6.6 Scoliosis: the spine curves and rotates.

References

1. Dandy DJ, Edwards DJ (2009). *Essential Orthopaedics and Trauma*. Edinburgh: Churchill Livingstone/Elsevier.
2. Simon M, Halm M, Quante M (2018). Perioperative complications after surgical treatment in degenerative adult de novo scoliosis. *BMC Musculoskelet Disord* 19:10.

Metabolic bone disease

Metabolic bone disease is a term that refers to conditions resulting in diminished bone density and reduced bone strength which is the result of deficiency in bone mineral content. These are an important category of skeletal diseases as they lead to an increased likelihood of pathological fractures of bones, resulting in significant complications and disability.

Causes and pathology

There is a complex relationship between bone and metabolism. Because bone is an extremely dynamic tissue and plays such an important part in growth, it is constantly being renewed and regenerated. Significant metabolic activity is required to do this. The constituents of bone and other minerals which are responsible for its strength, growth, and regeneration, such as calcium, phosphorous, magnesium, and vitamin D, play an important role in bone strength and its ability to resist injury and deformity. Vitamin D and sunlight are responsible for uptake of calcium in bone. Bone is constantly being formed and reabsorbed and there is a continuous turnover of calcium within the skeletal system. The cells which mediate this activity are osteoblasts (which build bone) and osteoclasts (which break down bone). This activity is metabolically controlled by hormones including parathyroid hormone (PTH), growth hormone, steroids, cytokines, and calcitonin. When the mechanisms producing these hormones malfunction, the ability of the body to maintain adequate calcium levels needed for bone strength can be lost or depleted, resulting in metabolic bone disease.

Bone density

Bone density (the amount of material per area of bone) is most often assessed as *bone mineral density* (BMD). This is usually measured using a radiological procedure called *densitometry*. There are a variety of forms of densitometry. The most commonly used is the DXA (or DEXA) scan; dual-energy X-ray absorptiometry, which uses X-rays with different energy levels to work out the density of bone (see ➔ Other types of diagnostic imaging, pp. 110–111).

Osteopenia

This is a term used to describe the appearance of bone on radiographs that is depleted in density and is often seen when radiographs are undertaken for other reasons such as a fracture or for a chest X-ray. This is usually a sign that there is already significantly reduced BMD due to metabolic bone disease or malignant pathology.

Conditions

The most common metabolic bone diseases are:

Osteoporosis

This is a disorder of bone density in which there is decreased bone mass and structural depletion of trabecular bone leading to subsequent bone weakening. This commonly leads to fractures. It is most common in postmenopausal women when oestrogen depletion inhibits both the formation and resorption of bone and resorption outpaces bone formation. Osteoporosis is discussed in more detail on ➔ Osteoporosis, pp. 252–253.

Paget's disease

This is also a relatively common disorder of bone density where there are focal increases in bone turnover, leading to deformity. This is discussed in more detail on → Paget's disease, pp. 258–259.

Osteomalacia and rickets

These are disorders of bone mineralization, mainly caused by hypocalcaemia, often as a result of a dietary deficiency of vitamin D which is essential for the uptake of calcium from the diet. Rickets is the juvenile form of osteomalacia. Rickets commonly occurs in children in communities where diet is poor. Common manifestations include bone pain and deformity, retarded bone growth, bowing of bones, pathological fractures, and translucent areas of bone on radiographs. Fractures and deformity are common in both adulthood and childhood.

Assessment and management

Assessment of metabolic bone disease involves identification of the cause of the metabolic bone disease and patients are usually referred to specialist services. The following options for management can then be considered:

- Metabolic bone disease is usually treated by focusing on the underlying deficit/deficiency—using medication to halt or slow down the loss of bone density
- Dietary supplements of calcium and vitamin D are best achieved by adapting the diet. Patients may be asked to complete a calcium diary so that the sources of the deficiency can be assessed. If the patient can't or won't eat dietary calcium, this can be supplemented in tablet or liquid form
- Microfractures and deformity can be very painful so pain management is a central aspect of care
- An essential aspect of care is fracture avoidance and protection from injury. This can be achieved by focusing on health promotion and health improvement, physical fitness, and falls prevention (see → Falls, pp. 326–327).

It is essential that the practitioner has an understanding of how the disease affects the individual so that they can provide support in helping patients and their families understand the condition and be concordant with, and be motivated to apply, health education and health promoting advice. The nature of metabolic disease is often not well known within communities. Such conditions may have familial links and ensuring that families understand this link and what can be done to avoid disease in other members of families can be very important.

Osteoporosis

Osteoporosis means bones that are too porous, i.e. a reduction in bone density, and because of this they are susceptible to fracture. PBD is achieved at skeletal maturity in the healthy individual and then a number of factors can reduce the density of the skeleton. These include:

- Reduced levels of oestrogen following the menopause
- Prolonged or excessive use of corticosteroids
- Alcohol abuse leading to reduced osteoblastic function and reduced absorption of calcium due to liver failure
- Smoking leading to reduced osteoblastic activity
- Disuse—e.g. lack of weight-bearing exercise and activity
- Hyperparathyroidism.

Women are affected by osteoporosis much more than men and Afro-Caribbean people are less likely to develop the disease than Caucasians because they achieve a stronger bone density at skeletal maturity.

Clinical manifestations

The whole skeleton can be involved, but the spine and distal and prox-imal ends of long bones are usually more affected because cancellous bone loses density more rapidly than compact bone. Osteoporosis is sometimes known as a silent disease because people are usually asymptomatic and the first sign is a pathological fracture, e.g. Colles' fracture or hip fracture. Patients with osteoporosis of the spine will often experience a dull back pain, deformity can develop in the form of a kyphosis, and compression fractures can occur.

Diagnosis

Osteoporosis is visible on X-ray most obviously in the vertebral bodies. Bones, particularly the cortices, will appear rarefied. The most effective in-vestigation is bone densitometry (see ➔ Other types of diagnostic imaging, pp. 110–111).

Prevention and treatment

There is no cure for osteoporosis at this time and prevention is the main strategy. Nurses have an important role in preventative education from the young child to the older adult. Preventative strategies include:

- Achieving a good PBD at skeletal maturity by a healthy diet including vitamin D and calcium and regular weight-bearing exercise
- Slowing down the loss of bone density after skeletal maturity by regular weight-bearing exercise, not smoking, avoiding excessive alcohol consumption, and hormone replacement therapy during and following the menopause if not contraindicated.

For older people with osteoporosis the main strategy is to prevent patho-logical fractures through prompt detection of the disease, falls prevention, assessment, and planning. Drug treatments include:

- Bisphosphonates—inhibit osteoclastic activity
- Selective oestrogen receptor modulators (SERMs), e.g. raloxifene, which mimic the positive functions of oestrogen on bone tissue while avoiding the harmful effects on breast and uterine tissue
- Calcium and vitamin D supplements.

Further reading

Royal Osteoporosis Society: ♒ http://www.theros.org.uk.

Van Oostwaard M (2018). Osteoporosis and the nature of fragility fracture: an overview. In: Hertz K, Santy-Tomlinson J (eds) *Fragility Fracture Nursing: Holistic Care and Management of the Orthogeriatric Patient*, pp. 1–13. Cham: Springer. ♒ https://www.springer.com/gb/book/9783319766805

Paget's disease

Paget's disease is also known as *osteitis deformans* and is the second most common bone disorder (after osteoporosis). The causes of the disease are unknown. Geographically, it is most common in the UK, North America, and Australasia, indicating a possible racial, genetic, or familial link. It is speculated that viral activity and environmental stimuli may also be implicated. The incidence of the disease increases with age and is most common in both men and women >55 years. There has been a considerable reduction in the incidence of the disease since the latter part of the twentieth century.

The disease occurs at a cellular level where the normal process of skeletal remodelling is disturbed—osteoclasts break down bone more quickly and osteoblasts create new bone more rapidly. Bone cells increase in number but are larger and activity within them is increased, resulting in abnormal, weaker, disorganized new bone formation. There is also an increase in blood supply to affected parts of bones. The bones most commonly affected are the skull, spine, pelvis, femur, and tibia. Rarely, Paget's lesions can become malignant tumours.

Symptoms and diagnosis

Often Paget's disease is asymptomatic. Where symptoms do occur, some of these include:
- Pain—specifically felt within the bone itself
- Areas of increased heat around affected bones
- Deformity of bone resulting in asymmetry—including bowing of long bones
- Weakness in deformed bone can lead to fractures
- Painful arthritic changes in joints near to diseased bone
- Hearing problems and nerve compression syndrome can also occur.

A diagnosis of Paget's disease will most likely be confirmed by radiographs or isotope bone scan. Where the bone is affected, radiographs will show enlarged and sclerotic bone and cortical thickening. A bone scan will show the extent of disease throughout the body. Increased blood alkaline phosphatase levels are also found.

Management

Asymptomatic Paget's disease requires no treatment. Management of Paget's disease with symptoms aims to relieve pain, slow down the disease, and prevent complications. Strategies include:
- Pain can be persistent, severe, and difficult to manage. It also frequently occurs at rest, often at night. Pain management involves trial and error to find an analgesic regimen that works for the individual patient. Complementary therapies are reported to be helpful by some patients.
- The mainstay of treatment is the use of bisphosphonate (oral or IV) drugs such as zoledronic acid, pamidronate, alendronate, and risedronate[1] to control the abnormal bone cell activity, resulting in bone structure that is less abnormal and causes less pain and deformity. This treatment helps to control the disease and may be necessary over long periods of time. Even with this treatment other pain-relieving medication may be required.

- An essential role of the orthopaedic practitioner is in helping patients to understand their medication and increase concordance with treatment. Oral bisphosphonates are not easily absorbed and must be taken correctly, and gastrointestinal side effects can be experienced.
- Where the disease is associated with significant OA, for example of the hip or knee, joint replacement surgery can be helpful (see ➔ Joint replacement surgery, pp. 286–287). Surgery may also be required to correct severe deformities.
- Paget's disease can contribute to non-union of fractures, so fracture management must be considered carefully.

Paget's disease can have a significant impact on the patient's health-related quality of life. The orthopaedic practitioner is central in ensuring that patients and their families are well informed about the disease and its effects as well as ensuring they receive accurate advice regarding management of the disease. There is a need for support in ensuring that patients' worries are allayed—particularly about the progression of the disease as they get older.

Reference

1. Kravets I (2018). Paget's disease of bone: diagnosis and treatment. *Am J Med* 131:1298–303.

Further reading

Paget's Association website: ℛ https://www.paget.org.uk
Sutcliffe A (2010). Paget's: the neglected bone disease. *Int J Orthop Trauma Nurs* 14:142–9.

Osteogenesis imperfecta

Osteogenesis imperfecta (OI)—also known as 'brittle bone disease'—is a genetic bone disorder in which there is low bone mass that results in bones which are fragile and fracture easily. This bone fragility is the result of a disorder of collagen synthesis which is caused by genetic mutation of either autosomal recessive or autosomal dominant genes. The disorder is present at birth and is diagnosed by general examination and history along with radiographs, bone densitometry, and collagen testing.

OI is often classified according to severity, the four most common types being:

- *Type 1*—the mildest form. Fractures occur in childhood but less frequently with age. There can be light blue discoloration of the sclera of the eyes and hearing loss can occur in adults
- *Type 2*—the most severe form. Fractures may occur *in utero* and stillbirth may occur. There are multiple fractures at birth
- *Type 3*—a severe form in which there are frequent fractures in childhood and adults. Short stature, hearing loss, and blue sclera. Often with developmental problems of teeth (dentinogenesis imperfecta)
- *Type 4*—a moderate form which occurs in childhood and adulthood. Sclera often not affected, but hearing frequently is, short stature, and possible teeth problems.

The severity of the effects of the disorder can be manifested in three ways:

- There are multiple fractures during childhood and deformities and bowing of bone occurs
- The individual suffers few fractures during childhood and the bone reaches normal strength when growth is complete
- The individual is so severely affected that they have multiple fractures *in utero* and do not survive birth.

Other problems include muscle weakness, bone malformation, and joint laxity. Depending on the severity of the disorder life expectancy may be hardly affected or significantly shortened.

Management

There is no cure for OI, so management strategies focus on preventing fractures and on independence and include:

- *Health promotion*—this includes weight-bearing exercise programmes from early childhood onwards which helps bone mass to be built. This can also help to maintain and improve cardiovascular and respiratory health
- *Management of fractures*—because bone weakens further with immobility this is best done using conservative management options which enable mobilization as early as possible
- *Orthotics*—various splints and braces can be used to support joints and weak bones
- *Surgery*—this can include the use of implants to correct deformities and prevent fractures in bones which are particularly prone to fracture
- *Medication*—this can involve oral calcium in high doses along with vitamin D, fluoride, and calcitonin. Bisphosphonates are increasingly being used and do reduce long bone fracture rates and support vertebral re-shaping following vertebral fracture.[1] Research is still underway in this field, particularly for new antiresorptive and anabolic agents.

Patient- and family-centred care

The care of the individual with OI is complex and involves specialist support. Individuals and their families spend a great deal of time interacting with healthcare services and this includes:

- Physiotherapy and exercise interventions
- Health promotion assessment, advice, and activities
- Care, management, and prevention of fractures
- Fitting and application of splints and braces
- Medication and treatment reviews.

A number of important aspects of care need to be considered:

- Initially, parents and families need support in understanding the need for the child to remain as active as possible and balancing precautions combating the risk of fracture against the need to maintain normal functioning.
- Health professionals also need to be aware that children who have OI are prone to bony injury significantly more than other children and it is important to make sure that this is not inappropriately labelled non-accidental injury.
- As it is a lifelong condition, patients with OI and their families often know a great deal about the condition and its impact on their lives. They often know best how they should care for themselves and their knowledge and wishes should be respected by practitioners.
- Parents of children and adults with OI are increasingly well informed because of the wide availability of information on the Internet and from other sources. Practitioners need to be aware of the latest information so that they can support patient and families in selecting the best information to inform their decisions about daily life and important aspects of their care and treatment. Various organizations around the globe provide information and facilitate networks of individuals and families with OI.

Reference

1. Palomo T, Vilaca T, Lazaretti-Castro M (2017). Osteogenesis imperfecta: diagnosis and treatment. *Curr Opin Endocrinol Diabetes Obes* 24:381–8.

Bone tumours

Introduction

Primary tumours of the musculoskeletal system can originate in bone, cartilage, fibrous tissue, or their origin may be unknown. Tumours of soft tissue origin are discussed on ➜ Soft tissue tumours, pp. 266–267. Within this topic, tumours originating from bone tissue and uncertain tissue origin will be discussed. Primary bone tumours and those of uncertain origin are uncommon and this can lead to either delays in diagnosis or misdiagnosis as pattern recognition for GPs is difficult due to the infrequency with which they will encounter the conditions. When a malignant bone or tumour of unknown tissue origin is suspected, prompt referral to a specialist bone tumour unit is essential. Tumours can be benign or malignant and a summary of classifications is as follows:

- Bone origin/benign—osteoma, osteoid osteoma, osteoblastoma, osteoclastoma (giant cell tumour)
- Bone origin/malignant—osteosarcoma
- Uncertain origin/benign—simple bone cyst, aneurysmal bone cyst
- Uncertain origin/malignant—Ewing's sarcoma, adamantinoma.

The signs and symptoms of bone tumours and those of unknown tissue origin will vary considerably depending on their location. Therefore, the commonest tumours from the listed categorization will be presented individually.

Osteoma

This is a benign growth originating from an osteoblast. It usually occurs in long or flat bones or the skull and is seen most commonly in the second decade of life. They are usually asymptomatic and quite often will not be visible or palpable unless on the skull. No treatment is needed, unless excision is required by the patient for cosmetic reasons.

Osteoclastoma (giant cell tumour)

This benign tumour is found in the epiphysis of long bones, most commonly at the proximal end of the tibia/fibula. It occurs in the age group of 20–40-year-olds and the patient presents with a tender, palpable bony swelling which is often painful. The pathology of the tumour, although benign, is aggressive with rapid growth and expansion up to the articular cartilage and can often result in a pathological fracture. The tumour is filled with maroon-coloured vascular tissue surrounded by a thin outer shell of bone. X-ray followed by biopsy will be used to diagnose the tumour and treatment is usually curettage and bone grafting, removal of the bone if possible, e.g. the fibula, or resection of the affected bone and replacement with a metal prosthesis.

Osteosarcoma

This malignant tumour usually originates in the metaphysis of long bones and affects men more than women—2:1. It most commonly develops around the knee and proximal end of the humerus. The aetiology is unknown, but those exposed to therapeutic radiotherapy are more at risk and in the older age group the tumour may develop secondary to Paget's disease. The signs and symptoms include pain which will gradually worsen as the tumour grows and lifts the periosteum and tiny stress fractures occur. Swelling is often, but not always apparent because the mass in the metaphysis is hidden by soft tissue. As the tumour grows and metastasizes, if left undetected the patient will develop weight loss, fever, loss of appetite, and pallor. Diagnosis is made on X-ray findings which will show irregular destruction of the metaphysis and new bone growth. There may be destruction or breaching of the cortex of the bone in very aggressive/advanced tumours. Treatment involves surgery to either remove the affected bone and replacement with a prosthesis or amputation of the limb preceded and followed by a course of multiagent chemotherapy.

Ewing's sarcoma

A Ewing's sarcoma is a highly malignant tumour that usually occurs in the diaphysis of bones, usually the femur and pelvis, although potentially any bone can be susceptible. It usually affects children and young people between 5 and 20 years of age. Its exact tissue origin is unknown but is thought to originate in the endothelial elements of bone marrow. The signs and symptoms are similar to those noted earlier for osteosarcoma. Surgical treatment is the same, but the chemotherapy regimen differs from that used in the treatment of osteosarcomas.

The role of the nurse

Malignant tumours such as osteosarcomas and Ewing's sarcoma are difficult to detect and diagnose and often this results in patients presenting late in the disease trajectory to a specialist centre. This is a devastating experience for the patient and their family and they require specialist support throughout diagnosis and treatment. The orthopaedic and oncology teams need to work collaboratively to ensure optimal care and treatment of the patient. Although prognosis for this patient group has improved significantly over the last decade with the use of more effective chemotherapy regimens and surgical techniques, a significant percentage will not survive and the support of the palliative care team should be instigated. See ➲ End of life issues, pp. 24–25.

Further reading

Hamblen D, Simpson H (2010). Bone tumours and other local conditions. In: *Adams's Outline of Orthopaedics*, 14th edn, pp. 104–33. Edinburgh: Churchill Livingstone/Elsevier.

Bone metastases

Bone metastases are much more common than primary bone tumours, with ~30% of patients with a malignant disease developing secondaries in the bony skeleton. There are a number of primary tumours that commonly metastasize to bone including:

- Lung
- Breast
- Prostate
- Thyroid.

Cancer spreads by direct invasion or via the lymphatic or blood systems therefore the bones most commonly affected by secondary cancer are those with vascular marrow, i.e. areas with significant presence of cancellous bone such as:

- Vertebral bodies
- Ribs
- Flat bones of the pelvis
- Proximal/distal ends of long bones such as the femur and humerus.

Signs and symptoms

The patient may present in a variety of ways to trauma and orthopaedic services, i.e. the patient may present with pain in the pelvis/spine/limbs which has resulted from a pathological fracture due to metastatic disease. Alternatively, the patient may present with pain in these areas without the presence of a fracture, but with radiological evidence of metastatic disease. Involvement of the intervertebral bodies and/or spinal compression can lead to patients experiencing neurological problems. Also, patients may present with local swellings without the presence of pain. Most patients who present with bone metastases have a diagnosis of a primary tumour and are receiving treatment, but occasionally their presentation with metastases may be the first indication of cancer. Hypercalcaemia may develop which can inhibit muscle function.

Investigations

Those presenting with the described signs and symptoms with or without a history of a primary cancer should have the following investigations to identify bone metastases:

- X-ray of the spine/pelvis/sternum etc. depending on presenting symptoms and history—X-rays can appear normal and abnormality can present as either osteolytic or sclerotic lesions
- X-ray of the chest to exclude lung secondaries
- Bone scanning is a very accurate method of detecting bone secondaries
- MRI scan of the spine if spinal metastases are suspected
- Blood test to detect hypercalcaemia.

Principles of treatment

The orthopaedic and oncology teams need to work in close collaboration to optimize patient outcomes. The principles of treatment are to relieve pain and preserve mobility/movement and may include:

• Internal fixation of pathological fractures
• Palliative radiotherapy
• Prophylactic fixation or prosthetic replacement of diseased bone which is susceptible to fracture
• Bisphosphonates to inhibit bone reabsorption and subsequently to reduce pain
• Spinal decompression when cord compression has occurred.

A significant number of patients presenting with bone metastases will need to be supported by the palliative care team. See ⊃ End of life issues, pp. 24–25 for principles of end of life care.

Soft tissue tumours

Soft tissue tumours in relation to the musculoskeletal system include tumours that originate in cartilage, muscle, fibrous tissue, and fat. This topic provides an overview of the types of tumour, signs and symptoms, and principles of management. Tumours can be benign or malignant and a summary of classifications is presented here:

- Cartilage origin/benign—chondroma and osteochondroma
- Cartilage origin/malignant—chondrosarcoma
- Muscle origin/benign—myoma
- Muscle origin/malignant—leiomyosarcoma and rhabdomyosarcoma
- Fibrous tissue/benign—fibroma
- Fibrous tissue/malignant—fibrosarcoma
- Fat tissue/benign—lipoma
- Fat tissue/malignant—liposarcoma.

The signs and symptoms of soft tissue tumours will vary depending on their location within the musculoskeletal system. The commonest tumours from the above-listed categorization are presented as follows.

Osteochondroma

This is the commonest type of benign tumour of the musculoskeletal system and is sometimes known as an osteocartilaginous exostosis. The tumour occurs in children and young adults and originates in the growing epiphyseal cartilage plate.[1] The tumour comprises a cartilage cap and a bony stalk protruding from the cortex of the bone and therefore is said to resemble a mushroom in its structure. The tumour will continue to grow until skeletal maturity is reached and in severe cases may interfere with growth. The signs are usually a hard swelling near the joint, which is not usually painful unless it interferes with adjacent nerve structures. In the case of multiple growths, the term diaphyseal aclasia is used. Treatment comprises excision of the lump if symptomatic and if the tumour continues to grow after skeletal maturity, a biopsy is needed to exclude malignancy. It is estimated that 10% of osteochondromas become malignant.

Chondrosarcoma

This is a malignant tumour that originates from cartilage cells and usually presents in adults 40–60 years old. Chondrosarcomas originate in the central bone (medullary) typically in long bones such as the femur or humerus or peripherally in the flat bones of the pelvis. The tumour will present differently on X-ray depending if it is central or peripheral in its location. Patients will present with pain and local swelling and may have a history of a benign tumour in the same region. This type of tumour does not respond well to radiotherapy or chemotherapy and treatment is focused on the surgical excision of the affected bone/soft tissue and replacement with a prosthesis or amputation of the limb.

The role of the nurse

Soft tissue tumours are rare and it is important that if they are suspected there is prompt referral to specialist centres for investigation and treatment. Within these centres, nurse consultants/advanced nurse practitioners work as expert members of the MDT to support the patient/child and their family through the journey of diagnosis/treatment and follow-up. The prognosis for chondrosarcomas is better than that for malignant bone tumours, but still a significant number of patients will not be cured and will require timely referral to palliative care teams. Rehabilitation will be required following either endoscopic prosthetic replacement or amputation and the nurse has an important role to play in pain management, wound care, psychological support, and integrating all aspects of skills learnt in therapy into the patient's activities of daily living.

References

1. Hamblen D, Simpson H (2010). Bone tumours and other local conditions. In: *Adams's Outline of Orthopaedics*, 14th edn, pp. 104–33. Edinburgh: Churchill Livingstone/Elsevier.

Tuberculosis of bones and joints

Background

TB of the bones and joints is a localized destructive disease caused by *Mycobacterium tuberculosis* (tubercle bacillus). The primary focus of TB is mainly located in the lungs or lymphatic system with haematogenous spread to the bones or joints as a secondary condition. TB is spread from person to person by air-borne cross-infection. Before 1985, primary TB (often known as consumption) had declined due to improved living conditions and the use of early and aggressive drug therapies and the development of antibiotics. However, in the last 30 years it has made a resurgence due to the increase in international travel, the arrival of immigrants from lower income countries, an increase in HIV infection, an increase in homelessness, and patients not completing their course of treatment. Since this resurgence there have been outbreaks of TB that would have originally been successfully treated with complex drug combinations but now there are some strains that can no longer be treated and are drug resistant. TB that is drug resistant is often fatal. TB is not, however, highly contagious compared to some other infectious diseases. Only about one in three close contacts of a TB patient are likely to become infected and fewer than 15% of more remote contacts. As a rule, close, frequent, or prolonged contact is needed to spread the disease.

Bone and joint tuberculosis

TB of the bones and joints usually occurs in the spine (Potts disease), the bones and joints around the hips and knees (weight-bearing surfaces), and the thoracic and cervical vertebrae. It is often referred to as extrapulmonary tuberculosis (EPTB). Skeletal TB onset is insidious and may not be diagnosed for years with destruction of the bones and joints continuing undiagnosed and because it is often unrecognized, it can cause long-term disability. It can occur at any age but the young and the old are at particular risk.

Pathology

TB of the bones and joints is a secondary disease spread from a primary infection. TB of the spine will cause a cavity in the vertebral body which will then collapse, causing a wedge fracture; the infection can then cross the disc spaces to adjacent vertebrae. If the pressure continues to build without diagnosis it will lead to compression of the spinal cord and subsequent neurological impairment. When the tubercle bacilli reach the long bone metaphysis, the infection causes bone destruction centrally and produces a cavity that can be seen on X-ray. Once this has occurred, the bone does not regenerate and very little new bone is formed. As the disease continues, necrotic material and exudate is produced causing a build-up of pressure in the bone or joint leading to a 'cold' abscess. Without treatment the abscess can burst through the skin (a sinus) and the infection is termed as 'open' making other patients at risk, as infectious bacteria can leak through the sinus.

Presentation and diagnosis

Clinical features will reflect the areas of the body involved. If the lungs are involved there will be a persistent non-productive cough. In bone and joints there may be some redness and warmth over the area involved. Pain will be localized and some patients experience muscle spasm. Typically, the pain is worse at night with low-grade pyrexia. Diagnosis is confirmed by thorough assessment, as well as laboratory and radiological findings.

Assessment

Clear questions need to be asked about:
- The patient's history and family history of TB
- Housing and living conditions
- Substance misuse
- History of migration/travel from a country where TB is prevalent
- Joint examination—patients with joint involvement will find it difficult to tolerate active or passive movements of the joints. If the lower limb is involved, they will be unable to weight bear. It may also be red, swollen, and painful to touch. If the spine is involved, there may be signs of spinal deformity and/or neurological involvement
- Examination of any wounds—this may indicate seepage from a sinus
- History of night pain, malaise, and pyrexia.

Investigations

- FBC—this may show hypochromic anaemia and a small increase in WBC count
- ESR and CRP will be elevated
- Blood cultures
- Mantoux test—a strong positive will indicate either early BCG vaccination or active TB
- Early-morning specimens of urine and sputum—this may show evidence of the bacilli
- Biopsies of the synovium, sinus, bony lesion, or lymph nodes to identify the bacilli
- Chest X-rays—for evidence of the TB in the lungs
- Skeletal X-rays but they may not show any early changes to bones or joints
- CT or MRI—will show abscess formation and the degree of bone destruction.
- CT-guided biopsies.

Treatment of tuberculosis

Treatment of patients with bone and joint TB needs to be holistic and involve all of the MDT in order to assist the patient while in hospital and to continue their care at home. Treatment priorities are to eliminate the underlying disease, improve the patient's general health, minimize deformity, and drug therapies to eliminate the causative organism. Surgical intervention is not advocated unless to drain a joint or bone using needle aspiration or arthroscopy, or for cases of advanced joint involvement.

Management

Drug therapies are multimodal and usually include four drugs: isoniazid, rifampin, pyrazinamide, and either ethambutol or streptomycin. The drugs must be continued for at least 12 months. Recovery following skeletal TB takes at least 18 months to 2 years as the disease has often been present for many years before treatment. Surgery may be indicated in the long term to correct or replace damaged joints and bones, but not when the disease is active. Effective pain relief is essential and also liaison with public health experts in managing the infectious aspects of the disease in relation to protection of the affected patient's immediate family and the wider community (it is a communicable disease).

Physiotherapy

Physiotherapy will be required for patients with impaired physical mobility. This will ensure they maintain their joint function at the optimum. Patients may need to be immobilized initially to rest the joint, followed by physiotherapy to mobilize the joint to its full potential.

Recovery

TB of the bones and joints can be completely cured if treatment is started as soon as possible. As most of the patient's recovery takes place at home, their home environment needs to be assessed to ensure optimum recovery. Patient education is also crucial to ensure they maintain their drug regimens. This could also have financial implications for the patient, and they need to be supported in this as this could contribute to non-adherence with treatment. The patient needs a healthy diet and rest is essential. The patient must not be discharged without thorough assessment of all areas of their life so that all the resources possible are offered to help them achieve and maintain their optimum health status.

Further reading

Clarke S, Santy Tomlinosn J (2014). *Orthopaedic and Trauma Nursing: An Evidence-Based Approach to Musculoskeletal Care*. West Sussex: John Willey and Sons Ltd.
Zimmerli W (2015). *Bone and Joint: From Microbiology to Diagnostics and Treatment*. West Sussex: John Willey and Sons Ltd.

Osteomyelitis

Osteomyelitis is an infection of bone. It is commonly caused by bacterial or (rarely) fungal infection, the most common bacterium being *Staphylococcus aureus*. The infection occurs most commonly in long bones in children and in the pelvic and vertebral bones in adults. However, it can occur in any bone. Osteomyelitis begins as an acute condition but if not treated promptly can develop into a chronic condition.

Causes
- Via the bloodstream—bacteria can enter the blood from an infection in another part of the body and then travel to bone, e.g. from a skin or wound infection
- Following injury—bacteria can spread to bone if there is a surgical or traumatic wound or following an open fracture.

Risk factors
Anyone of any age can develop osteomyelitis. However, the risk factors include:
- Recent fracture of bone
- Prosthetic orthopaedic implants (hip, knee, or screws and plates)
- Recent orthopaedic surgery
- Diabetes
- IV drug use
- Renal dialysis
- Immune system compromise (e.g. HIV, sickle cell disease)
- Previous episode/s of osteomyelitis.

Signs and symptoms
- Pain and tenderness over the area of bone affected
- Swelling and redness of the joint next to the affected bone
- Fever
- Oedema
- Warmth of the overlying skin
- Reduction in the use of an extremity
- Fatigue
- Generally feeling unwell
- Purulent discharge following an open fracture.
- A child may not want to use an arm or leg.

Diagnosis
- A full history and physical examination should look for any of the earlier listed signs and symptoms
- Blood samples should be taken for FBC, ESR, and CRP, which if raised will indicate signs of infection and raised inflammatory markers
- Blood cultures should also be taken to detect the bacteria involved
- If the blood tests show no bacteria then a needle aspiration of the area will also be taken as this will identify the bacterium. A bone biopsy may also be performed
- A bone scan would be needed to confirm the diagnosis. Radiographs are not generally helpful as they will only show well-advanced infection.
- Occasionally, a biopsy will be required.

Treatment

The objective of treating osteomyelitis is to eliminate infection and to prevent the development of chronic osteomyelitis. If the infection is treated quickly then osteomyelitis can be resolved.

- Antibiotics intravenously should be commenced as soon as blood cultures have been acquired (they can be changed later if necessary). These will need to be continued intravenously for at least 4–6 weeks depending on the patient's symptoms and then orally for up to 12 weeks
- Pain relief
- Drainage—if there is an open wound or abscess this may need to be drained
- Splinting or cast immobilization—this may be necessary to immobilize the affected bone and nearby joints to assist healing and to avoid further trauma to weakened bone
- Surgery—if the infection affects other structures, e.g. spinal cord, or a prosthesis becomes loose and infected, then surgery may be needed.

Complications of osteomyelitis

- Septicaemia
- A sinus may form between the bone and the skin—there may be purulent discharge
- Resistant strains such as MRSA are difficult to treat with antibiotics
- Non-union of a fracture
- Amputation—rarely needed and only if infection persists
- Chronic osteomyelitis occurs when acute osteomyelitis is not treated quickly enough. Resultant poor blood supply to the bone may lead to necrosis. Necrotic bone must be removed, with associated bone grafting
- There is some evidence that the use of hyperbaric oxygen may help recovery but further research is needed.

Prognosis

If the infection is treated quickly there is a chance of a complete cure. Once you have had osteomyelitis, the risk of further occurrences is higher than average.

Further reading

Conterno LO, Turchi MD (2013). Antibiotics for treating chronic osteomyelitis in adults. *Cochrane Database Syst Rev* 6:CD004439.

Haemarthrosis

Definition

Haemarthrosis is the term for bleeding into a joint or joint cavity. It can occur in any joint or joint cavity but most commonly in the knee.

Classification

- Traumatic:
  - Anterior or posterior cruciate ligament injury
  - Chondral fractures
  - Dislocation of the patella
  - Meniscal tears
- Non-traumatic:
  - Bleeding disorders, e.g. sickle cell disease, haemophilia, or anticoagulants
  - Neurological disorders
  - Tumours
  - Vascular damage
  - OA.

Causes of traumatic haemarthrosis

- In the young—sporting injuries are the most common, e.g. skiing, netball
- In older people—falls.

Signs and symptoms

- Joint pain and tenderness
- Joint swelling (within 4–6 hours of injury if traumatic)
- Limited movement
- Warmth.

Investigations

- Physical examination of the joint for tenderness, range of movement, deformity, swelling
- X-ray may show a fracture or an increased fluid level
- MRI—shows damage to soft tissue within the joint and the presence of blood
- Blood tests to exclude infection and clotting abnormalities
- Synovial fluid analysis—reddish colour to the fluid indicates blood in the sample

Management of non-traumatic haemarthrosis

- Adequate medical prophylaxis for patients with a bleeding disorder— this will prevent ongoing damage within the joint
- Rest
- Splints may help to prevent further damage
- Pain relief.

Management of traumatic haemarthrosis

- Initial—the aim of the initial treatment is to alleviate the symptoms, make a diagnosis, and plan the treatment:
  - Pain relief
  - Aspiration—allows for better clinical examination and lets the surgeon know what is in the aspirate, e.g. fat globules may indicate a fracture
  - If examination is inadequate, e.g. due to pain, then further investigations may be required such as MRI, examination under anaesthesia (EUA), or arthroscopy
  - Treatment options will be decided when the cause of the haemarthrosis has been identified, e.g. surgical repair of a torn ligament (see ➲ Soft tissue injury 2, pp. 358–359).

Arthroscopy

Arthroscopy (see ➲ Arthroscopy, pp. 300–301) during the acute phase is notoriously difficult but does let the surgeon make a more accurate diagnosis. There are times, however, when an acute arthroscopy needs to be performed these include:

- Locked knees
- Osteochondral fractures
- Severe grinding on the Lachman test
- Fat in the aspirate.

Further reading

Iorio A, Marchesini E, Marcucci M, et al. (2011). Clotting factor concentrates given to prevent bleeding and bleeding-related complications in people with hemophilia A or B. *Cochrane Database Syst Rev* 9:CD003429.

Septic arthritis

Septic or infective arthritis is an uncommon condition, but potentially fatal and associated with significant mortality and morbidity if treatment is delayed or inadequate.[1] It is characterized by infection occurring within a joint. Usually it is due to the blood-borne seeding of infection into the joint from another site, often unknown. Most often it is isolated to a single joint, but can occasionally occur in multiple joints. The most common infecting organisms are bacterial, classically *Staphylococcus* and *Streptococcus*, and there is also an increasing incidence of MRSA. *Salmonella* is often seen in patients with sickle cell disease.

The characteristic signs are pyrexia, and a hot, tender, swollen red joint which is painful to move and thus has a decreased range of motion. In children signs of systemic infection such as fever and generally feeling unwell may also be evident.

Types

Paediatric type

This is a critical emergency. There is a bacterial infection usually of the hip, where the child is clinically very unwell with a high temperature and will not walk on the affected limb. Pain in the hip can sometimes be referred to the knee. WBC count and CRP (indicating the presence of inflammation) are commonly significantly raised. Usually the hip is held in a flexed position and the child will not permit it to be moved. A child with a fever, groin or leg pain, and an inability to weight bear on the limb has septic arthritis until proven otherwise. Immediate assessment and investigation is essential. It is paramount that the joint is drained and washed out as soon as the diagnosis is made; delay in this can cause irreversible joint damage due to chondrolysis, the rapid destruction of articular cartilage. Immediate assessment should be carried out by an experienced surgeon.

Gonococcal

Most commonly seen in young adults due to infection with *Neisseria gonococcus*, and can be associated with a history of recent travel or sexual activity. This is often associated with a pustular rash and generalized joint pain. This often does not require drainage and IV antibiotic therapy is usually sufficient.

Adult type

This only usually occurs in either a previously damaged joint, e.g. a severely arthritic knee, or in an immunocompromised patient, such as a transplant recipient, or those taking immunosuppressive medication, patients with multiple medical problems, and those with diabetes. The joint may be swollen but have no warmth or tenderness because of the lack of immune response and resultant inflammation. As a consequence, there may be a delay in diagnosis, and often a poor outcome.

Arthroplasty type

Either an acute or more indolent infection can occur in patients who have a joint arthroplasty; the definitive management of these patients is often more difficult due to chronic infection of the implant and the possible need to revise this in a staged surgical procedure. It is vital that an experienced orthopaedic surgeon be consulted about the possibility of this at the earliest stage, as early washout and debridement can prevent the need for revision.

Management and care

Definitive diagnosis is made by the presence of the bacteria in the synovial fluid or following culture of the pathogen.[1] Dependent on the type, immediate surgical intervention is often required. Needle aspiration of the joint is carried out, and if pus is present then septic arthritis is confirmed. The joint is surgically opened and copiously irrigated with saline. A drain may be left in place for 1–2 days afterwards.

Broad-spectrum antibiotic therapy (usually high-dose penicillin) is commenced as soon as joint aspiration has been performed for microbiological culture. After the culture results have been obtained, more specific antibiotics can be administered. Treatment continues for a minimum of 6 weeks.

In the acute phase the joint is extremely painful on movement and splintage is used for pain relief and joint protection Due to the inflammation and damage which has occurred in the joint, there is a significant risk of severe stiffness because of inflammation and scarring within the joint. Early mobilization is encouraged as soon as pain allows. This will be supported by an active physiotherapy programme. Weight bearing should not be allowed in the first 1–2 months.

Pain management is an essential aspect of care. This involves the gradual but progressing reintroduction of range of motion in the joint. There must be careful observation of the temperature and the limb to ensure that the infection continues to settle.

General information and reassurance are vital due to the significant pain on motion and the rapid of onset of the condition. The limb is often painful and swollen for many weeks, and there is a significant psychological impact.

Severe complications can occur following a delay in diagnosis, with secondary arthritis and joint dislocation/destruction being the most frequent. Many patients will require further surgery to the affected joint later in life.

Reference

1. Garcia-Arias M, Balsa A, Mola E (2011). Septic arthritis. *Best Pract Res Clin Rheumatol* 25:407–21.

Common foot conditions 1

The foot is a very complex structure of bones, ligaments, muscles, and soft tissues. As a complex structure the foot is prone to developmental problems and problems related to overuse or misuse often associated with poor footwear. This can affect people's lives in the short and long term through pain and disability.

Hallux valgus (bunions)

This is a deformity of the foot involving the big toe (hallux) and the first metatarsal. The big toe deviates laterally and the first metatarsal often deviates medially and an exostosis (bunion) forms on the metatarsal head. It can occur through degenerative conditions within the joints, during rapid growth periods in adolescence, or remodelling of the metatarsal head through pressure usually associated with poor footwear. More women than men suffer with the condition.

Diagnosis
- On examination there will be a distortion of the patient's shoe over the big toe
- History of difficulty finding shoes to fit
- Pain and a tender prominence on the first metatarsal head
- Callus formation found under the second and third toe due to the shift in weight bearing
- Weight-bearing X-rays will show a bony misalignment which would be missed on non-weight-bearing views.

Conservative treatment
- Education and advice on correct shoe wear and its fitting
- Education and advice on correct socks and stockings
- Orthosis may help—referral to podiatry/orthotics
- Surgery may be necessary.

Hallux rigidus

This condition results in pain and restriction of the big toe and is associated often with OA. It also is associated with lateral foot pain as weight bearing is shifted off the big toe. The condition is more common in men.

Diagnosis
- On examination there will be pain on plantar and dorsiflexion of the big toe
- There may be evidence of osteophytes on examination
- The patient may recall trauma to the big toe before developing symptoms

X-ray may show flattening of the head of the big toe, narrowing of the joint space, and osteophytes.

Conservative treatment
- Education and advice on correct shoe wear and its fitting, e.g. shoes with rigid soles
- Orthosis such as rocker bottom soles may help—referral to orthotics/podiatry
- Surgical fusion may be necessary.

Pes planus (flat foot)

In this foot disorder the head of the talus is displaced medially and up-wards from the navicular. Mobile flat foot is very common and familial. It is usually symptom free although it may impact the patient's gait. Problems arise when there is flattening of the medial longitudinal arch that was once normal.

Diagnosis
- Examination of the foot will reveal flattening of the medial longitudinal arch on weight bearing
- Callus formation under the first metatarsal head
- Pain along the medial border of the foot
- Loss of mobility of the foot
- Weight-bearing X-rays will show sagging of the talonavicular joint and deviation of the head of the talus.

Conservative treatment
- Exercises may help—referral to physiotherapy
- Orthosis may also help—referral to podiatry.

Hammer toe

This is a deformity of the second toe (usually) which can occur due either to a bunion overcrowding the second toe, or an abnormally long toe being compressed by footwear. This results in a flexion deformity at the PIP joint, which develops a painful callus overlying it. The DIP joint may then flex, causing a claw toe, or hyperextend, creating a hammer toe.

Diagnosis
- Examination of the foot to detect the deformity
- Pain when wearing shoes
- Callus formation on the toes.

Conservative treatment
- Education and advice on correct shoe wear and its fitting
- Padding to the affected toes and trimming of the callus—referral to podiatry
- Surgical fusion of the affected joint may be necessary.

Common foot conditions 2

Onychocryptosis (ingrowing toe nails)

A toenail is considered ingrowing when the side of the nail cuts into the skin next to it and soft tissue overgrows it. It can happen to any toe, but most commonly occurs in the big toe. Ingrowing toenails can be acute and caused by injury to the toe or damage to the nail, causing the nail to imbed deeply into the skin. Less severe are chronic ingrowing toenails, which usually occur over a long period of time, due to nail neglect, improper footwear or incorrect cutting of the toenails.

Diagnosis
- Examination of the foot will show redness and sometimes infection; pus may also be present
- Swelling
- Pain (paronychia) on side-to-side pressure of the nail
- Surgery may be required.

Conservative treatment
- Education and advice on correct shoe wear and its fitting
- Education and advice on correct socks and stockings
- If infection is present, drainage of the area and antibiotic therapy
- Referral to a podiatrist for advice on foot care and ongoing care.

Gout

In 90% of patients who suffer with gout the big toe IP joint is affected. Repeated attacks can lead to progressive destruction of the articular surface of the joint. See ➲ Crystal arthropathies, p. 234 for investigations and treatment of gout.

Diagnosis
- Examination of foot will show red and shiny skin over the joint of the big toe, swelling, and pain
- Pain on plantar and dorsiflexion of the big toe
- Blood tests will show uric acid levels raised (cannot be done until 6 weeks after an acute attack).

Conservative treatment
- Education and advice on diet and exercise
- In the acute phase (3–10 days)—rest and elevation
- Anti-inflammatory drugs in the acute phase.

Plantar neuroma (Morton's metatarsalgia)

This condition is found mainly in middle-aged women and athletes. A swelling forms on the planter digital nerve where it splits to go to the toes. It is most common between the third and fourth toe but can occur between the second and third as well. The exact cause is unknown, but there is some evidence to suggest it occurs because the nerve becomes intermittently trapped between the metatarsal heads.

Diagnosis
- Pain on palpation of the swelling and in the ball of the foot
- There may be some loss of sensation on the nerve pathway
- A history of wanting to remove the shoes and rub the metatarsals.

Conservative treatment
- Education and advice on shoes, socks, and stockings
- A pad behind the metatarsal heads
- Local anaesthetic injections may help
- Surgical excision is the definitive treatment.

Common hand conditions 1

Hand function is essential for most activities of living and therefore any deformity or reduced movement can have a major impact on the patient's quality of life and ability to be independent. The following topics provide an overview of common hand conditions.

Tenosynovitis

This is inflammation of the tendon sheaths of the hand and is a common occurrence. The cause is unknown, but has been attributed to repetitive trauma or overuse. It can occur as a secondary problem from an underlying disease such as RA.

Trigger finger (flexor stenosing tenosynovitis)

This is the most common tendon entrapment of the hand. It is caused when a nodule forms on the tendon as it passes through the proximal end of the tendon sheath. The enlargement of the tendon causes it to catch and give way as it passes through the sheath and as the patient actively flexes or extends the IP joint there is a characteristic snapping sound. This can occur in any finger.

Diagnosis
- The patient will have pain in the affected finger
- The patient will complain of popping or catching on flexing the finger
- On examination there may be inflammation of the finger and a nodule will be felt on the affected tendon sheath
- The patient will also have difficulty extending the finger once flexed and this may only be achieved on passive extension only to lock again on flexion.

Conservative treatment
- Rest of the finger involved which could include referral to occupational therapy for splinting
- NSAIDs may help
- Surgical release is recommended.

De Quervain's tenosynovitis

This condition is caused by irritation at the base of the thumb. This traps the abductor pollicis longus and the extensor pollicis brevis tendons (see ➲ The wrist and hand, pp. 68–69) as they pass through the first dorsal compartment of the wrist. It is caused by repetitive motion of the wrist.

Diagnosis
- The patient will have pain at the base of the thumb and there may be swelling
- On examination, if the thumb is flexed across the palm of the hand and the wrist forced into ulnar deviation the patient complains of severe pain (Finkelstein's test) see ➲ Chapter 3 for further information on testing of tendon stability and tears.

Conservative treatment
- Limiting of activities that cause the pain
- Resting of the thumb which could include referral to occupational therapy for splinting
- NSAIDs may help
- Steroid injections and physiotherapy usually settle the symptoms.

Common hand conditions 2

Dupuytren's contracture

A progressive condition where there is thickening of the soft tissue and formation of nodules just below the skin in the palm of the hand (palmar fascia). Joint contractures eventually occur and pull the fingers in towards the palm of the hand. Males are affected 10 × more than females and the condition seldom presents below the age of 40. The ring and middle fingers are the most commonly affected. Onset and progression is typically gradual, but occasionally can occur rapidly.

Diagnosis
- The patient will have pain-free nodules in the palm of the hand and the skin will be puckered
- There may be contractures of the fingers with impairment of hand function.

Conservative treatment
When the nodules are small and there are no contractures, reassurance about the diagnosis is needed with advice to the patient only to seek treatment when the contracture begins to impede hand function. See ⮕ Hand surgery, pp. 306–307 for surgical intervention.

Carpel tunnel syndrome

This condition is caused by increased pressure on the median nerve of the wrist and is often attributed to work-related activities. It is 4× more common in women than men and more prevalent in diabetic patients and during pregnancy.

Diagnosis
- The patient will have pain in the hand and numbness and tingling over the thumb
- The patient will complain of paraesthesia in the distribution of the median nerve
- The patient will complain of sleeping for 3–4 hours then waking with the paraesthesia which is relieved on shaking the hand
- On examination, the nerve is tapped over the carpel tunnel continually (Tinel's test): a positive sign causes the patient pain
- If the wrist is flexed for 60 seconds and causes tingling in the fingers (Phalen's test) this is also a positive test
- X-rays will rule out any bony pathology
- If the diagnosis is in doubt, nerve conduction studies will be used to assess the velocity and amplitude of signals transmitting through the nerve.

Conservative treatment
- Resting of the wrist in a splint at night in a neutral position will reduce symptoms
- Advice re: adjustments to the work place if work related
- For surgical intervention, see ⮕ Hand surgery pp. 306–307.

Ganglion

This is the most common soft tissue mass in the hand. It usually presents as a hard swelling in the dorsum of the hand. However, it can occur in other places. The swelling typically enlarges during activity and recedes after rest.

Diagnosis

The patient will have a tense swelling on the hand, which is usually painless.

Conservative treatment

- Many ganglions will resolve spontaneously and the patient will only require reassurance
- Sometimes aspiration of the ganglion is appropriate and, if causing distress to the patient, surgical removal is appropriate.

Chapter 7

283

Elective interventions

Intra-articular injections 284
Joint replacement surgery 286
Hip replacement and resurfacing 288
Revision joint replacement 290
Knee replacement 292
Shoulder replacement 296
Small joint replacement 298
Arthroscopy 300
Autologous chondrocyte transplantation 302
Foot surgery 1 303
Foot surgery 2 304
Hand surgery 306
Arthrodesis and osteotomy 308
Spinal surgery 310
Elective limb amputation 312

Intra-articular injections

IA injections are used to relieve pain, reduce inflammation, and restore function in synovial joints affected by OA or RA. The effect varies between individual patients, but ranges from several weeks to many months. More than three injections into the same joint within a 12-month period is not recommended due to concerns over risks of degeneration of the surrounding tissue.

The procedure

Common sites for successful injections include the knee, ankle, spine, shoulder, elbow, hands, feet, and, rarely, the hip joints. The administration of IA injections is often carried out by a specialist/advanced nurse or physiotherapy practitioner who has completed a specialist training programme and is working within an approved protocol. The procedure can be undertaken in several settings including primary care, outpatient department, pain clinic, or within the day-case surgical unit. The decision on where the procedure takes place depends largely on if image intensification/X-ray is needed during the procedure. The patient does not require a general anaesthetic for the procedure, but either a local anaesthetic by SC injection prior to the procedure and/or sedation to provide relaxation is usual.

The procedure involves an injection of a long-term steroid preparation, sometimes with the addition of a local anaesthetic into the joint space. The patient gives written consent to the procedure before proceeding. It is essential that the skin is cleaned prior to commencing the procedure and that strict aseptic technique is applied. The practitioner may inject the drugs into several areas of the joint space, depending on the nature of the patient's symptoms and the impact of the disease process. There are several contraindications for IA injections including:

- Bleeding/clotting disorders
- Anticoagulant therapy such as warfarin
- Local infection in or around the joint
- IA fracture.

Aftercare and potential complications

Initially following the procedure the patient may experience increased pain within the joint due to the pressure of the injected drugs. The patient should be advised to rest the joint for at least 24 hours and be given information about pain relief, including the appropriate use of ice packs (see ➔ Pain management, p. 142). Patients should be observed for any potential reaction to the steroid for 30 minutes following the procedure. Complications include:

- Reaction to the steroid preparation, e.g. facial flushing
- Skin atrophy
- Infection in the joint
- Bleeding within the joint
- Tendon rupture
- Damage to articular cartilage.

Patients should be advised to seek prompt attention if they develop any signs or symptoms related to these complications.

Joint replacement surgery

Joint replacements (arthroplasties) have revolutionized the treatment of joint disease. They are one of the most common elective procedures in the UK NHS, with 91,698 primary hip replacements and 102,177 primary knee replacements being performed in 2017 in England and Wales.[1] Hips and knees are the most common joints to be replaced, but nearly all other joints can also be replaced. The aim of joint replacement is to alleviate pain and restore function. The number of hip and knee replacements being performed continues to increase globally due to increasing demographics of older people and rising rates of obesity. General principles of preoperative preparation, postoperative care, and rehabilitation will be discussed here. See ➔ Elective interventions, pp. 283–313 for detail of specific joint replacements, i.e. the hip, knee, shoulder, and small joints.

Preoperative preparation

Patients who are undergoing a total joint replacement (TJR) must give informed written consent. This is a legal requirement and necessitates the patient receiving both verbal and written information about the procedure, alternative treatment options, potential risks and benefits, aftercare, and rehabilitation. There is also evidence to support the fact that well-informed patients are more likely to be concordant with advice and treatment regimens. Providing information does not necessarily equate to understanding and the nurse has an important role in ensuring information is provided in a way which suits the individual patient's needs (see ➔ Communication, pp. 166–167). Information can be provided either on a 1:1 basis or within a group session followed by an individual consultation to allow the patient to raise any specific issues related to them as an individual. The patient will also be required to have a preoperative assessment to ascertain their fitness to undergo anaesthesia and surgery; see ➔ Preoperative assessment and preparation, pp. 128–131.

The National Joint Registry (NJR)

Many countries have developed national joint registries in the last decade. In England and Wales, patients undergoing TJR have been asked to give consent to their details being given to the NJR. The NJR provides a central data base of all procedures carried out and provides useful statistics on outcomes and complications.

The procedure

TJR involves removing the diseased articulating surfaces of the joint and replacing them with an artificial prosthesis. The orthopaedic surgeon decides on the most appropriate type of prosthesis depending on the condition of the joint, e.g. the knee joint being affected uniformly or worse on the medial aspect leading to consideration of total or unicompartmental knee replacement. The weight and activity levels of the patient are also taken into consideration. Prostheses are made from a variety of materials including:

- Stainless steel
- Chrome/cobalt
- Titanium alloy
- High-density polyethylene (HDP).

Typically, prostheses will comprise an alloy stem and a corresponding articulating surface made from HDP. Since 2012 there has been a dramatic reduction in the number of MoM replacements and resurfacing procedures due to increasing concerns regarding metallosis and adverse reactions to migrating chromium and cobalt ions (see ➲ Soft tissue reactions to the wear debris associated with MoM hip articulations, pp. 210–211). Prostheses can be cemented or un-cemented into position, the function of bone cement is to fill the spaces between the bone tissue and the prosthesis—it does not fix the prosthesis in place. During the procedure the patient's joint is dislocated and significant physical force is needed to ream (scrape) off the diseased bone and insert the prosthesis; this inevitably means that the patient will experience swelling and bruising following the procedure and elevation and appropriate pain relief is essential to manage this.

Postoperative care and rehabilitation

➲ See pp. 132–133 for general principles of postoperative care. Specific postoperative care following TJR includes:

- Effective pain assessment and management
- Application of evidence-based practice to minimize the risk of complications such as VTE (see ➲ Venous thromboembolism, pp. 194–195), infection (see ➲ Wound infection, pp. 206–207), dislocation of prosthesis (see ➲ Hip replacement and resurfacing, pp. 288–289), haemorrhage (see ➲ Haemorrhage, pp. 192–193), and skin blistering (see ➲ Wound blistering, pp. 208–209)
- Check X-ray to ascertain positioning/stability of the prosthesis prior to mobilization/movement
- Early mobilization PWB (typically initially with a frame or elbow crutches) following hip and knee replacement
- Regimen of mobility and exercise to optimize function (including stair safety).

Typically, patients will be admitted on the day of surgery and then remain in hospital for 2–4 nights. Many countries now have well-established fast-track programmes which facilitate even shorter hospital stays (see ➲ Models of service delivery: enhanced recovery/fast-track, pp. 30–31 for information on fast-track/enhanced recovery pathways). It is important that discharge planning is started prior to admission at the preoperative assessment stage and special adaptive aids and any social or nursing support organized well in advance of discharge. Decisions about discharge should be made in liaison with the patient and their family. Patients are usually followed up in outpatients at 6 weeks, 6 months, and then annually.

Reference

1. National Joint Registry for England, Wales, Northern Ireland and The Isle of Man (2018). 15th Annual Report: 2018. ℘ https://www.hqip.org.uk/wp-content/uploads/2018/11/NJR-15th-Annual-Report-2018.pdf

Hip replacement and resurfacing

A total hip replacement (THR) is one of the most commonly performed elective orthopaedic procedures. Its primary function is to treat hip pain caused by diseases such as OA and RA with a secondary function to improve function and mobility. THR is also recommended as the best surgical option for intracapsular hip fractures when the patient was independently mobile out of doors prior to the fracture, does not have cognitive impairment, and is medically fit for the procedure.[1] THR involves the replacement of the femoral head and acetabular articulations with a two-part prosthesis. There are many types of hip prosthesis, but one of the most commonly used is the Charnley prosthesis which comprises a metal femoral stem component and an acetabular cup made from HDP (see Fig. 7.1). However, there is an increasing trend in the use of hybrid prostheses, particularly ceramic-on-polyethylene. The hip prosthesis may or may not be cemented (see ➲ Total joint replacement, pp. 286–287).

A THR may eventually need revision (see ➲ Revision joint replacement, pp. 290–291 for revision surgery), but depending on the weight and activity levels of the patient, the prosthesis should not become loose for at least 10–15 years.

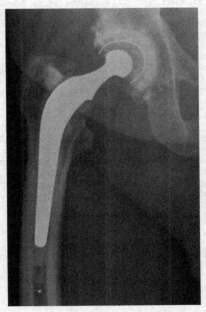

Fig. 7.1 AP radiograph of the right hip showing a cemented total hip replacement—Charnley type. Image courtesy of the Nottingham University Hospitals Radiology Department.

Preoperative preparation

General principles of preoperative preparation can be found on
→ Preoperative assessment, pp. 128–129. Specific advice for patients
undergoing THR will need to be given about limitations to their movement
and activities following the procedure to minimize the risk of dislocation of
the prosthesis. These include:

* Not flexing the hip beyond 90° until reviewed at 6 weeks
  postoperatively, i.e. not sitting on low chairs or toilets, not bending over
  to reach below their knees to put on their sock/shoes, etc.
* Advice about resuming sexual activity and positioning
* Not to adduct the hip, i.e. not to cross their legs or lie on the affected
  side until 6-week review.

To assist the patient in avoiding these risks, the occupational therapist will
arrange for the following equipment to be loaned/provided to the patient
prior to their discharge:

* Raised toilet seat
* Armchair of suitable height with sturdy arms or adjustment to existing
  furniture using chair blocks
* Assessing the height of the patient's bed and providing bed-raising
  blocks if needed
* Long-handled shoe horn and stocking aids.

Postoperative care and potential complications

General postoperative care and complications following TJR are provided
on → Joint replacement surgery, pp. 286–287. Specific to THR is potential
dislocation of the hip prosthesis which, although relatively rare (13% of all
primary THRs), is a serious complication resulting in a great deal of discomfort necessitating readmission to hospital and reduction of the dislocation
under anaesthetic. NICE guidelines[2] recommend that, to minimize the risk
of VTE following THR, patients should receive SC LMWH daily for 28 days
following surgery (requiring patients or a carer to be taught SC injection
techniques). In addition mechanical methods may be employed such as foot
pumps and/or full length antiembolic stockings to be *in situ* for 6 weeks
postoperatively unless there are contraindications.

Hip resurfacing

Resurfacing of the femoral head with a titanium shell protects the articulating surfaces of the joint and slows down the destruction caused by OA.
This procedure is essentially a time-buying option for younger patients with
OA of the hip joint aiming to reduce pain, restore function, and stave off
the need for THR for several years. The number of hip resurfacing procedures performed has dramatically decreased since concerns regarding
metallosis were raised for some types of re-surfacing components in 2012.

Reference

1. NICE (2011, updated 2017). Hip fracture: management. Clinical guideline [CG124]. https://
   www.nice.org.uk/guidance/cg124
2. NICE (2007). Venous thromboembolism: Reducing the risk of thromboembolism (deep vein
   thrombosis and pulmonary embolism) in in-patients undergoing surgery. Clinical guideline
   [CG46]. https://www.nice.org.uk/guidance/CG46

Further reading

Pivec R, Johnson A, Meers S, et al. (2013). Hip arthroplasty. *Int J Trauma Orthop Nurs* 17:65–78.

Revision joint replacement

As the number of joint replacements performed increases as well as longer life expectancy then the number of revision procedures will continue to increase. It is important that patients are informed about the possibility of failure and its potential causes at the time they make the decision to undergo primary TJR. The revision rate at 14 years postoperatively for knee replacements is 4.47% and for hip replacements, 7.4%; this figure is influenced by much higher rates of revision for MoM hip prostheses (19–22%).[1] The commonest reasons for revision surgery are[1]:

- Infection
- Dislocation (hip)
- Aseptic loosening
- Adverse reaction to particulate debris (metallosis) (hip)
- Pain
- Periprosthetic failure
- Instability (knee)

Infection

Infection is a serious complication following TJR and is categorized into early infection (at the time of surgery or through the surgical wound in the early postoperative phase) or late sepsis (occurring 6–24 months after surgery). Postoperative wound infection following TKR occurs in ~0.2% of cases.[2] Late sepsis around a TJR is estimated to occur in 1.67% of cases 2 years following hip replacement.[3] Infection around the TJR typically presents as:

- Pain
- Swelling
- Localized redness and warmth
- Loss of function
- Occasionally a discharging sinus tracking from the prosthesis to the skin.

Patients may present with all or some of these signs and symptoms. The MDT have an important role in minimizing the risk of infection through sterile/aseptic adherence intra- and postoperatively, judicious use of antibiotic prophylaxis, and advising patients to seek prompt treatment if they suspect they have developed a blood-borne infection. Patients should also be advised to request prophylactic antibiotics if they are to undergo invasive dental treatment following their TJR. Depending on the virulence of the infection and quality of the bone stock, there are several approaches to revision:

- Low virulence and good bone stock—one-stage procedure to remove the prosthesis and replace with new components
- High virulence—requires a two-stage procedure; first stage to remove the infected prosthesis followed by a period of ~6 weeks of antibiotic therapy and either NWB or PWB through the joint and then replacement of the components
- Poor bone stock—may necessitate removal of the infected joint and an arthrodesis of the joint (see ⊃ Arthrodesis and osteotomy, pp. 308–309).

Stiffness

Postoperative stiffness following TJR is more common in the knee and shoulder than the hip. It occurs either because of excessive scar formation within the joint or due to poor alignment and sizing of the prosthesis, causing abnormal strain on the ligaments and joint capsule. Excessive scar formation may be caused by patients not being concordant with postoperative exercise regimens; the physiotherapist and the nurse have an important role in supporting and educating patients about this. The primary symptoms, apart from stiffness of the joint, are loss of function and pain. Revision surgery may involve removal of the excessive scar tissue or a revision prosthesis if the cause is poor alignment and sizing.

Loosening

Loosening may occur either with time, breakdown of the bone–cement interface due to debris from wear, abnormal forces due to poor surgical technique, or implant design or infection. Mechanical loosening is rare before 10 years, but increases steadily after this, particularly with cemented components. When a prosthesis loosens, the patient presents with increasing pain and instability of the joint. X-ray findings will include one or more of the following:

- Increasing radiolucency around the prosthesis
- Fracturing of the bone cement
- Movement of the prosthesis
- Bone reabsorption around the prosthesis.

The procedure

The procedure of revision is much more complex than primary TJR and should be carried out by very experienced orthopaedic surgeons within specialist centres. The procedure involves opening the joint and removing the prosthetic components and any residual bone cement, followed by a reconstruction of the joint using new prosthetic components augmented by bone grafting if needed. The procedure takes much longer than a primary TJR, there is more blood loss, and the hospital length of stay and rehabilitation process will be longer than for a primary procedure. Potential complications following a revision procedure are the same as after a primary procedure (see ➲ Revision joint replacement, pp. 290–291).

References

1. National Joint Registry for England, Wales, Northern Ireland and The Isle of Man (2018). 15th Annual Report: 2018. ♫ https://www.hqip.org.uk/wp-content/uploads/2018/11/NJR-15th-Annual-Report-2018.pdf
2. Woon C, Piponov H, Schwartz B, et al. (2016). Total knee arthroplasty in obesity: in-hospital outcomes and national trends. *J Arthroplasty* 31:2408–14.
3. Dale H, Skråmm I, Løwer HL, et al. (2011). Infection after primary hip arthroplasty: a comparison of 3 Norwegian health registers. *Acta Orthop* 82:646–54.

Knee replacement

A total knee replacement (TKR) is one of the most commonly performed elective orthopaedic procedures. Its primary function is to treat knee pain caused by diseases such as OA and RA, with a secondary purpose to improve function and mobility. The procedure involves the removal of the damaged articulating surfaces of the tibia and femur and replacement of the tibial plateau and the femoral condyles with metal components (see Fig. 7.2 and Fig. 7.3). A TKR uses a polyethylene insert to act as a low-friction bearing surface and avoid MoM articulation. The patella is not usually replaced, but if there is damage to the posterior surface the surgeon will smooth the surface or, in severe cases, replace with a patella button. A TKR will eventually need revision (see ➋ Revision joint replacement, pp. 290–291 for revision surgery), but depending on the weight and activity levels of the patient, the prosthesis should remain stable for between 10 and 15 years.

Partial knee replacements

In some patients only part of their knee joint may be affected by arthritis, usually this is the medial compartment. In such cases a partial knee replacement, also known as unicompartmental replacement, may be offered to the patient, particularly if they are younger and want to delay undergoing a TKR. The procedure is less invasive than a TKR and recovery tends to be quicker, but there is always the risk of the patient developing arthritic changes in the remaining aspects of the knee and requiring a conversion to a full replacement.

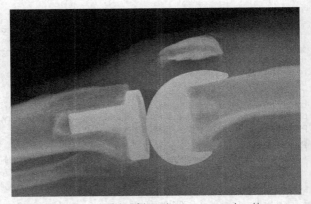

Fig. 7.2 Lateral radiograph of the left knee showing a cemented total knee arthroplasty with patellar resurfacing. The spacer device can again be seen correctly sited between the prosthetic articular surfaces. There is also fluid in the joint (an effusion), notable as abnormal soft tissue density in the suprapatellar recess of the joint. Image courtesy of the Nottingham University Hospitals Radiology Department.

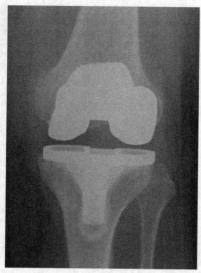

Fig. 7.3 AP radiograph of the left knee showing a cemented total knee arthroplasty. The slightly more lucent (blacker) spacer devices can be seen between the prosthetic articular surfaces. Image courtesy of the Nottingham University Hospitals Radiology Department.

Specific considerations and care following TKR

The general principles of preoperative preparation found on ⊃ Pre-operative preparation, pp. 130–131 are applicable to patients undergoing TKR; a procedure that is technically much more difficult than a THR with even a slight misalignment of the prosthesis can result in poor outcomes. It is expected that patients should be able to achieve 90° of active flexion following TKR. Patients are required to actively adhere to postoperative exercise regimens to optimize knee extension and flexion and this often involves attending outpatient physiotherapy for several sessions following discharge from hospital. Many patients, due to OA of the knee, develop severe deformities including fixed flexion and valgus deformities; although TKR can often help to correct these deformities it should be made clear to them prior to the procedure that this is not always possible and the patient, for example, may not reach 0° of extension. Swelling following TKR can be significant and prolonged, taking several months to resolve. Advice regarding taking regular prescribed analgesia, elevation, and appropriate use of ice packs (see ⊃ Pain management, p. 142) should be given to the patient prior to discharge. It takes several months following surgery for the patient to be able to assess the true impact/benefit of having a TKR, whereas patients undergoing THR often report almost instantaneous improvement.

This is an important issue to talk through with patients and their families as they often report regretting having the procedure in the first few months due to unrealistic expectations at that stage. To minimize the risk of VTE, NICE guidelines[1] recommend that LMWH be given daily by SC injection for 10 days following TKR plus mechanical methods of prophylaxis such as foot pumps and/or antiembolic stockings for 6 weeks following the procedure.

Reference

1. NICE (2018). Venous thromboembolism in over 16s: reducing the risk of hospital-acquired deep vein thrombosis or pulmonary embolism. NICE guideline [NG89]. ॐ https://www.nice.org.uk/guidance/ng89

Shoulder replacement

There are three main types of shoulder replacement:
• 'Reverse' polarity total shoulder arthroplasty
• Humeral hemiarthroplasty
• Total shoulder arthroplasty (glenohumeral)

Shoulder arthroplasty is performed for degenerative joint disease (OA), rotator cuff tear arthropathy, and trauma. It is the third most common joint replacement performed. It is much less common than hip and knee arthroplasty because OA in the shoulder is relatively uncommon and usually secondary to previous injury.

The glenohumeral joint can be described as like a golf ball upon a golf tee; it is inherently unstable and requires the correct functioning and tensioning of several ligaments and tendons in order to function correctly. As a result of joint degeneration and bone loss, the function of the shoulder dramatically decreases alongside an increase in pain.

The procedure can be successful in reducing the pain from arthritis. However, due to the complexity of the stabilizing structures in the shoulder, and the fact that scar tissue can hinder movement, the result in terms of function is often less favorable than that of hip and knee arthroplasty, with elevation of the arm rarely reaching >120°.

The surgery is carried out via an anterior incision, the shoulder joint is opened, and the humeral head resected and replaced with a hemispherical head attached to a stem which may be either cemented or press-fitted into place (see Fig. 7.4). If possible, the glenoid is prepared and a small polyethylene bearing often with a metal keel is cemented into place. The surgeon pays attention to the tension of the muscles and ligaments of the shoulder in order to optimize the correct tracking of the prostheses.

Surface replacement arthroplasty, in the form of a small metal cap placed over the humeral head, is gaining popularity as a less invasive treatment for earlier stages of joint degeneration.

Preoperative preparation

Due to the degenerative conditions of the shoulder, patients may have lost considerable range of motion in the joint prior to surgery. Preoperative physiotherapy and exercise can be helpful in improving the range of motion and strengthening the supporting muscles of the joint and can facilitate and speed up postoperative rehabilitation.

Postoperative care

Like any joint replacement, the main concern postoperatively is the prevention of infection. Wound care and antibiotic prophylaxis are central in this aim. Postoperative pain can be significant, and either an IA or perineural catheter in place for regional analgesia administration (see ➲ Pain management, pp. 142–143) is used.

The shoulder is very prone to significant scarring and joint contracture, so range of motion exercises are commenced immediately and progressed aggressively. As the rotator cuff muscles are usually partly detached to allow the arthroplasty to be performed, these must be protected during the healing period, so passive and active-assisted exercises are advised during the first 6 weeks. It is important to keep the hand and elbow mobile,

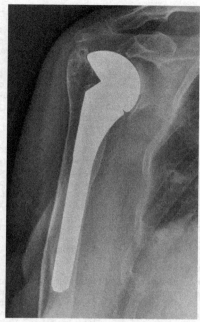

Fig. 7.4 AP radiograph of the right shoulder showing an uncemented hemiarthroplasty. Image courtesy of the Nottingham University Hospitals Radiology Department.

as significant oedema can occur in the upper limb following shoulder arthroplasty. Dislocation of the arthroplasty is possible, particularly in the first 6 weeks, but once the surgical approach has healed the risk decreases significantly.

'Reverse' polarity shoulder arthroplasty

If a rotator cuff tear has not been treated successfully, a condition called cuff arthropathy can occur. This is due to the abnormal movement of the humeral head over other parts of the scapula and is a devastating problem for the patient which is characterized by chronic, often constant, pain and significant loss of function. Because the rotator cuff is necessary for correct functioning of the glenohumeral joint, a standard shoulder replacement is usually unsuccessful in terms of improving function.

In this situation, a replacement which comprises a large ball screwed into the glenoid, and an articulating socket on a stem inserted into the humerus is used. This allows the deltoid to act as the primary shoulder stabilizer and can allow much better pain relief and greater postoperative function. The postoperative management remains the same as with conventional shoulder replacement.

Small joint replacement

The small joints of the hands and feet are prone to both OA and RA (see
➋ Osteoarthritis, pp. 228–229 and Rheumatoid arthritis, pp. 234–235).
Surgery aims to improve the function of the hand or foot (which can be
severely restricted by joint degeneration) and to relieve pain. The tendons
which move across small joints can also be damaged by the degenerative
processes. Pain, swelling, stiffness, and deformity in the joints of the fingers
result in difficulty in gripping and other fine movements required for daily
life such as doing up buttons on clothing and preparing food. Painful joints
in the feet can severely restrict mobility and lead to a loss of independence.
Joint surgery is considered when pain and disability are severe. Surgical options include:

- *Excision* of the joint to remove spurs and smooth roughened surfaces—
  more often performed when joint disease is in the earlier stages
- *Joint fusion*—the joint is surgically removed so that it becomes
  permanently fixed and immobile; this serves to reduce the pain in the
  joint for patients for whom arthroplasty is not advised—e.g. if they are
  young and therefore likely to put the joint under considerable strain,
  resulting in failure of the prosthesis
- *Joint arthroplasty*—more suitable for older patients who are less active
  and therefore less likely to place undue pressure on the new joint; this
  option can significantly improve hand function.

General issues

The development of arthroplasty of the small joints of the hands and feet
has been fraught with problems difficulties of the pressure these joints are
under during daily life and the concentration of problems in a very small
area. Many prostheses developed in the past have been prone to fracture
and loosening. The surgery is also technically difficult and postoperative
problems common. For these reasons arthroplasty of these small joints
tends only to be used where joint disease is severe and for older patients
who are less active.

Hand and finger joints

Specific consideration for surgery to the hand and fingers include:

- The smaller joints of the hands and feet such as the DIP joints are
  technically more difficult to replace and joint fusion tends to be more
  beneficial
- The PIP joints are more likely to benefit from arthroplasty
- The MCP joints of the hand are sometimes affected by RA and benefit
  from silicone implants
- The joint at the base of the thumb is a saddle joint and is therefore
  very mobile and under great pressure—joint reconstruction can be
  performed using tendon grafts to interpose and stabilize the joint.

Modern implants for the joints of the hand are mostly made from silicone or
autograft material made from the patient's own tendon tissue.

Joints of the feet and toes

Joint replacement of the toes is relatively uncommon. Arthritic conditions often affect the MTP joint at the base of the big toe, so arthroplasty is most common in this joint.

Postoperative care

Postoperative care aims to regain use of the fingers or toes as soon as possible while avoiding complications. The most significant issues in the care of the patient following small joint arthroplasty are pain, swelling, preventing infection, and regaining mobility of the joints.

- Elevation of the foot or hand is essential in the first 24–48 hours to enable swelling to subside—in small joints this can be a significant problem and can lead to wound healing problems and additional pain. In the hand, elevation will involve the use of slings and splints. A Braun frame is helpful to achieve elevation in foot surgery.
- Following foot surgery, remobilization should begin within 24 hours of surgery and may involve heel weight-bearing to protect the implant for the first 6 weeks.
- In the immediate postoperative period, adequate analgesia is essential as surgery to the sensitive small joints can be particularly painful.
- Because the joints of the hand may be unstable until soft tissue healing has taken place, the use of flexible splints to control movement postoperatively is likely to be recommended for the first 10 days to 3 weeks. Gradual return to use of the fingers is executed through physiotherapy and exercises.
- Minimizing the risk of infection is essential. It can be particularly devastating for small joints and leads to failure of the implant. Protection of the foot following surgery is particularly important as this area is more likely to be exposed to pathogens. Wound drains should be removed after 24 hours. It is essential that wounds, particularly in the foot, are protected from exposure with sterile dressings and bandages until wound healing has been achieved.

Further reading

NICE (2005). Artificial metacarpophalangeal and interphalangeal joint replacement for end stage arthritis. Interventional procedures guidance [IPG110]. ℘ https://www.nice.org.uk/guidance/IPG110

Arthroscopy

Arthroscopy is used for diagnostic and treatment purposes. The procedure involves the filling by injection of a joint with saline followed by insertion of a scope through a small incision. The scope is fitted with a fibreoptic light for illumination and is usually attached to a viewing screen. The procedure is performed under a general anaesthetic or a regional block. Arthroscopy can be performed in most joints within the body, but most commonly it is used for the following joints:

- Shoulder
- Knee
- Ankle
- Hip
- Wrist.

Arthroscopy as a diagnostic procedure

The arthroscope can be inserted via various approaches, e.g. medial or lateral anterior, and then manipulated to view various structures which are suspected as being damaged. However, the procedure is not without risk and is not a replacement for physical examination and clinical investigations such as X-ray and MRI scanning. Therefore, arthroscopy is seldom used as a purely diagnostic aid, but as a means of conducting minimally invasive surgery.

Minimally invasive surgery

This type of procedure involves the insertion of the arthroscope through a small incision as detailed earlier while various surgical instrumentation is inserted through another small incision/s. The types of procedure that can be carried out include[1]:

- Removal of loose bodies
- Meniscus repair or meniscectomy (the knee)
- Rotator cuff repair/rotator cuff decompression (the shoulder)
- Trimming of cartilage or scar tissue
- Synovectomy (wrist or knee)
- Arthroscopic washout and debridement as part of treatment for OA of the knee, but only in cases where the patient has a clear history of mechanical locking, as opposed to morning stiffness, giving way, or X-ray evidence of loose bodies.[1]

The benefits of minimally invasive surgery over traditional surgical methods include:

- Reduced length of stay (most cases are performed as day surgery)
- Less postoperative swelling
- Reduced risk of haemorrhage
- Very small incisions (i.e. thumbnail size) not sutured, but steri-strips applied.

Specific considerations and care following minimally invasive surgery

- The procedure is usually carried out as a day case, but patients need to be assessed for their suitability in terms of comorbidity and having a capable adult at home on the night of surgery
- Specific postoperative instructions in terms of mobility/movement restrictions will depend on the nature of the procedure carried out, e.g. a period of PWB following meniscectomy
- Potential complications include haemarthrosis, infection, VTE, and joint stiffness
- Patients need to be given effective pain relief both in the immediate postoperative period and to take home
- Written and verbal instructions regarding care of the incisions, mobility, and who to contact in case of complications.

Reference

1. NICE (2014). Non-pharmacological management. In: Osteoarthritis: care and management. Clinical guideline [CG177]. ℘ https://www.nice.org.uk/guidance/cg177/chapter/1-Recommendations#non-pharmacological-management-2

Autologous chondrocyte transplantation

There are several procedures beside joint replacement surgery that are used to treat damaged or missing articular cartilage within the joints, most commonly the knee. These include:
• Autologous chondrocyte transplantation (ACT)
• Microfracture technique.

Autologous chondrocyte transplantation

ACT is a relatively new treatment and currently there are only a few specialist centres carrying out the procedure to treat loss of articulating cartilage in the knee joint which is seen as an alternative for knee replacement surgery in younger/more active patients. There have also been some early examples of ACT being used for damaged cartilage in the ankle joint. ACT involves a two-stage procedure: harvesting and transplantation. The first stage involves the harvesting of cartilage cells (chondrocytes) from a non-weight bearing aspect of the joint; these cells are then sent to a laboratory and are grown within a culture medium and multiplied. The second stage is carried out approximately 6 weeks later and involves opening the joint and preparing the area where cartilage is missing or damaged and then applying a collagen film and inserting the new cells underneath. The new cells anchor themselves to the bone and will generate new articular cartilage within several weeks/months.

Microfracture technique

This procedure is performed arthroscopically (see ➲ Arthroscopy, pp. 300–301) and involves the removal of any loose, unstable, or damaged cartilage and thoroughly preparing and cleaning the surface of the bone. Multiple holes or microfractures are then made in the bone about 3–4mm apart. A large clot then forms as a result of this damage and will, after several months, develop into firm tissue providing an articulating surface between the bone ends. It can take between 2–6 months for the patient to feel the benefit of the procedure.

Postoperative care

Both ACT and microfracture procedures usually require a hospital stay of 1 night. The patient will be mobilized PWB for 6–8 weeks following surgery, and will need a course of outpatient physiotherapy focusing on early optimization of knee extension and flexion. In the immediate postoperative period continuous passive motion may be used until the patient embarks upon active exercise.

Foot surgery 1

If conservative measures for foot conditions are unsuccessful (see
➔ Common foot conditions, pp. 278–279) then surgery is advocated.

Hallux valgus (bunions)

Surgery will depend on the deformity that is present, the amount of
valgus, and how much the patient's function is disrupted. There are several surgical procedures that may be considered, but the most commonly
performed are:

- *Exostosectomy*—this procedure will be undertaken when there is minor
  deformity; it involves removal of the bony prominence on the medial
  side of the big toe, streamlining the side of the foot. It does not correct
  any valgus deformity
- *Keller's arthroplasty*—this involves removal of the prominence as for
  exostosectomy and excision of the base of the big toe. This means that
  the toe can then be splinted in the correct position with a wire down
  the length of the toe until there is formation of a fibrous joint between
  the phalanx and the metatarsal. The big toe, however, is permanently
  shortened and its function is impaired
- *Mitchell's osteotomy*—again the prominence on the big toe is removed
  and then it is incised with an osteotomy at the first metatarsal head and
  realigned using internal fixation. The toe is then splinted in alignment
  until the osteotomy is healed usually in a plaster cast.

Hallux rigidus

There are four forms of surgery used for hallux rigidus:
- Keller's arthroplasty (discussed in 'Hallux valgus')
- Cheilectomy—trimming of the upper part of the joint and then washing
  out of the joint space
- Fusion of the joint—the proximal and distal articulating bone ends are
  removed and then the bones are repositioned. They are then usually
  held together with a pin placed in the bone
- Replacement joints—some surgeons perform a joint replacement
  (see ➔ Joints of the feet and toes, p. 299).

Pes planus (flat foot)—often called fallen arches.

This is when the arches of the foot collapse, so the sole of the foot is in
complete or near complete contact with the floor. Most are asymptomatic
and do not cause pain and require no treatment.

If the patient does have pain and their activities are limited, then orthotics or surgery may be considered. Orthotics are used in conjunction with
exercises. This increases arch flexibility and strength. If surgery is required
it is usually a subtalar joint fusion (sometimes called triple arthrodesis). This
involves releasing the soft tissues to mobilize the talar joint, preparation of
the bones, repositioning, and fixation with screws. A cast is applied, and the
patient will be NWB for a period of 2–6 weeks following the procedure.

Foot surgery 2

Hammer toe

The surgery for this condition is IP joint fusion, involving resection of the bone from the middle phalanx and the head of the proximal phalanx. The bones are then fixed with Kirschner wires (K wires) so that the toes will fuse. The wires protrude from the end of the toe and will require removal 3–4 weeks following the procedure.

Onychocryptosis (ingrowing toe nails)

The surgery for ingrowing toenails is partial or total nail removal. This is usually done by phenolization—controlled application of phenol and alcohol, or by Zadek's procedure—removal of the toenail and nail bed.

Plantar neuroma (Morton's metatarsalgia)

The surgery for plantar neuroma is removal of the neuroma (growth).

Complications

There are many complications that can occur following foot surgery:
• *Infection*—any surgical procedure can leave the patient susceptible to infection. The incidence of infection can be reduced by providing advice on foot care, dressings, and foot hygiene. Prompt detection and treatment of infection is important to avoid the development of osteomyelitis
• *Recurrence of the deformity*—usually due to unsuccessful surgery or the patient not being compliant with postoperative mobility instructions/advice about footwear
• *Limitations of movement*—usually due to adhesions or scar tissue
• *Paraesthesia*—due to prolonged swelling or scar tissue which may compromise nerve function for up to a year postoperatively
• *Delayed wound healing*—can occur when patients have an underlying medical condition such as diabetes or a vascular condition
• *Chronic regional pain syndrome*—an extremely uncommon condition that can occur following tissue injury (including surgery). The exact process is not fully understood, but it appears that the nervous system overreacts to the surgery and becomes extremely sensitive and painful. Even the lightest touch or movement is unbearable and for the patient this can be disabling. Early diagnosis significantly improves successful treatment. Treatment by a specialist pain clinic is required. The condition can lead to amputation if it does not resolve as the patient is worn down by the constant pain.

Postoperative care

The postoperative care following foot surgery will depend on the surgery performed but some of the principles apply to all foot surgery:
• *Pain*—the patient needs good pain relief as foot surgery is often very painful. The foot will also need elevating above the level of the sacrum to help with pain and swelling
• *Swelling*—ice may help to reduce swelling and pain (see ➲ Pain management, p. 142)

- *Neurovascular assessment*—this needs to be done quarter-hourly for an hour, half-hourly for 1 hour, and then 2-hourly. Any changes need reporting (see ➲ Neurovascular compromise, pp. 196–197)
- *Dressings*—need to be monitored for excess discharge and reported if this occurs. In foot surgery there will always be a small amount of oozing due to the inflammatory response
- *Mobility*—once recovered the patient needs to be taught how to mobilize. Depending on the type of surgery performed, the patient may be required to either heel walk or PWB/NWB with crutches. It is important to ensure patients are able to use their walking aids safely and correctly before discharge
- *Dressings*—the patient will need advice on keeping the dressings clean and dry and what to do about having them changed
- *Pin care* (Keller's arthroplasty)—advice will need to be given on care of the pin, prevention of injury, and infection. Sterile corks are often used to protect the end of the pin
- *Cast care*—if the patient has a cast then verbal and written instructions need to be given to the patient (see ➲ Care of casts, pp. 372–373).

Hand surgery

If conservative measures for hand conditions are unsuccessful (see
→ Common hand conditions, pp. 282–283) then surgery is advocated.

Tenosynovitis

Surgery is rarely needed for this condition but if it is, it involves the release of the tendon. However, a new treatment is being used to help this
condition:

- *Shockwave therapy*—this uses high-energy sound waves; a special device
  allows the shockwaves to be passed through the skin to the affected
  area. Local anaesthetic may be given, as sometimes the shockwaves can
  be painful. This procedure does appear to be safe but it is not clear yet
  exactly how well it works, and more research is needed.

Trigger finger (flexor stenosing tenosynovitis)

If surgery is required, surgeons can use one of two methods:

- Percutaneous trigger finger release with a needle—in this method the
  tight mouth of the tendon tunnel is released using a needle inserted
  under a local anaesthetic injection
- Surgical decompression of the tendon tunnel. The anaesthetic may be
  local or a general. Through a small incision, the pulley overlying the
  thickened flexor tendon is divided longitudinally.

De Quervain's tenosynovitis

The surgery that may be required for this condition is decompression of
the tendon tunnel under local or general anaesthetic. Through a transverse
or longitudinal incision, the surgeon widens the tendon tunnel by slitting its
roof. The tendon sheath will heal following the procedure, but more space
will have been created for the tendons to move without causing pain.

Dupuytren's contracture

In this condition, if the fingers can be fully straightened surgery is not required. When the patient finds it impossible to put their hand flat on a table,
surgery is the only option. There are several different types of operation
and they may be carried out under local, regional, or general anaesthetic.

- *Fasciotomy*—this is a simple cut in the palm, in the finger, or both, to
  release the Dupuytren's contracted cord. It is done using a small knife or
  a needle
- *Partial fasciotomy*—as much of the diseased tissue as possible is removed
  although not all of it may be removed as it is hard to identify the
  diseased tissue in the early stages
- *Open fasciotomy*—this means cutting through the skin and then cutting
  the thickened tissue. The skin is then stitched back together or if a lot of
  skin has had to be removed, a skin graft may be used.

Carpel tunnel syndrome

This involves cutting the ligament over the front of the wrist to ease the
pressure in the carpal tunnel under local anaesthetic or via an endoscope.

Ganglions

If conservative measures are not successful then the ganglion can be aspirated using a needle in the first instance and if this does not work, then it is surgically removed.

Potential complications

- *Infection*—all surgery has the potential for infection as there is opening up of the skin creating a potential portal for entry of organisms
- *Numbness of the hand or fingers*—if nerves are disturbed during the surgery or affected by postoperative swelling, then numbness can occur and last several weeks. However, this could be due to the bandages being too tight so they need to be checked regularly.
- *Finger stiffness*—this can be more disabling than the original condition and is usually due to pain, inflammation, swelling, and immobility
- *Scarring*—this will be worse in the first few weeks and the patient will need to be advised about this and reassured that it will fade with time
- *Incomplete correction of the deformity*—this is either due to poor surgery or not all the diseased tissue being removed
- *Reoccurrence of the condition*—if this happens further surgery will be required
- *Complex regional pain syndrome*—a rare condition where there is severe pain, loss of sensation, and loss of movement in the hand.

Postoperative care

The postoperative care will depend on the surgery performed but some of the principles apply to all hand surgery:

- *Pain*—the patient needs good pain relief as hand surgery is painful. The hand will also need elevating above the level of the heart to help with pain and swelling (see ➔ pp. 142–149)
- *Swelling*—elevation and ice help to reduce swelling
- *Neurovascular assessment*—this needs to be done quarter-hourly for an hour, half-hourly for 1 hour, and then 2-hourly. Any changes need reporting promptly
- *Dressings*—need to be monitored for excess discharge and reported if this occurs. In hand surgery there will always be a small amount of oozing
- *Exercises*—once recovered, the patient needs to be taught how to exercise both the operated hand and arm and the unoperated. They will need written instructions to take home with them
- *Dressings on discharge*—the patient will need advice on keeping the dressings clean and dry and what to do about having them changed
- *Splinting*—some surgical procedures will require the patient to wear a splint for a temporary period
- *Discharge*—check how the patient will manage at home with only one hand, particularly the elderly or those that live alone.

Arthrodesis and osteotomy

Arthrodesis

Arthrodesis means fusion of a joint. This can occur as the end stage of a grossly arthritic or damaged joint but is more usually undertaken electively to deal with a grossly deformed or damaged joint, when arthroplasty is not a viable option.

The commonest sites for arthodeses are the foot and ankle, small joints of the hand, and the wrist. Arthrodesis of a large joint other than the ankle is very poorly tolerated and is associated with poor quality of life, due to the restriction of movement at the joint. Situations such as chronic osteomyelitis and infected joint arthroplasty are the main reasons for large joint arthrodesis, while OA is the main indication for the majority of arthrodesis of other joints. The success of joint replacement in the hand and foot is often poor and has a limited lifespan, thus an arthrodesis is often an acceptable long-term solution [1].

The surgical technique requires the removal of all remaining cartilage and burnished bone, down to a bleeding surface, sometimes with the addition of bone graft, and the stabilization by compression of the joint, either by internal or external fixation. Fusion takes a minimum of 6 weeks, more commonly 12, and unless external fixation is used, weight bearing must be avoided. Failure in the form of non-union of the bone ends is a serious risk, and can occur in up to 20% of fusions, requiring additional surgery.

Function following arthrodesis is usually excellent, the joints adjacent to the fusion develop a greater range of motion (and thus are at risk of developing arthritis sooner, particularly in the hindfoot) and as the patient has lost the pain from the arthritic joint, greater functional capacity results despite the loss of the remaining few degrees of motion from the damaged joint.

Osteotomy

Osteotomy refers to the surgical division of a bone. This is performed for several different reasons: (1) malunion (a fracture which has healed incorrectly) may require surgical correction, due to pain, cosmetic deformity, or abnormal distribution of load in the lower limb; (2) both developmental and degenerative disorders can cause deformity which requires correction to increase quality of life; (3) an arthritic joint can be improved by redistribution of the weight to a less worn portion, in particular at the knee, where arthritis more commonly affects the medial side, although with developments in unicompartmental knee replacement prostheses this is seldom carried out in the developed world.

Osteotomy is carried out by surgically incising the bone, either with a saw, or more usually with osteotomes to avoid heat injury to bone from a saw. Wedges of bone can be taken out to correct an angular deformity. The correction can either be achieved immediately, and the bone secured and compressed with internal or external fixation, or can be performed progressively, most commonly using an Ilizarov external fixator (see ➲ Fig. 9.7, p. 391). The same technique is used to surgically lengthen bones in the case of short stature or limb length inequality. As with a fusion, healing of an osteotomy takes 2–3 months.

Surgical wounds associated with fusions and osteotomies often have poor healing properties, due to either their anatomical location and/or presence of medical comorbidities (age, diabetes, peripheral vascular disease), or related to the underlying reason for the deformity or arthritis, such as prior trauma. As such, careful attention to wound care is critical; the nursing care for the patient must pay particular attention to the appearance of the wound, swelling must be minimized by elevation, and correction of nutritional status and reduction of risk factors are important. Careful attention to the pin sites of an external fixator and patient education regarding pin site care and care of the limb is necessary (see → Pin site care, pp. 394–395).

Mobility of the patient undergoing fusion or osteotomy can be poor due to other comorbidities or OA, and thus both the nurse and physiotherapist have an important role in ensuring that the patient is safe and independent with walking aids, particularly when NWB status is essential and must be maintained.

References

Beldner S, Polatsch D (2016). Arthrodesis of the metacarpophalangeal and interphalangeal joints of the hand: current concepts. J Am Acad Orthop Surg 24:290–7.

Spinal surgery

There are several spinal conditions that may necessitate surgery when conservative measures fail to relieve symptoms including:

- Spondylolysis (➲ Ankylosing spondylitis, pp. 240–241)
- Spondylolisthesis (➲ Spondylolisthesis, pp. 248–249)
- Spinal stenosis
- Herniated/prolapsed intervertebral discs (➲ Prolapsed intervertebral disc, pp. 244–245)
- Spinal deformities (➲ Spinal deformities, pp. 250–251).

This section will explain the principles of care following spinal surgery and gives brief details on specific procedures including:

- Spinal decompression
- Spinal fusion
- Disc decompression.

Spinal decompression

The aim of this procedure is to remove the source/s of compression of the spinal nerves and their blood supply which may be a prolapsed disc and/or bony deformity, e.g. osteophytes. The surgery can be complex with the surgeon having to do several specific procedures to ensure there is enough space for the spinal nerves. Specific surgical procedures include:

- Discectomy—removal of a herniated disc that is causing compression
- Laminectomy—opening up space to relieve the compression.

Spinal fusion

This procedure is carried out to stabilize the spine and restore alignment, with the aim of improving back pain and associated disability. It is estimated that 60% of patients report pain relief, 48% report improvements in function and disability, and 89% are satisfied with the outcome of the procedure.[1] It involves the release of stretched nerves or compressed nerves which may include removal of any protruding disc material and bridging the vertebrae with bone grafts taken from donor sites such as the ilium or allografts may be used. There are three approaches to spinal fusion: anterior, spinal, or lateral. The approach taken depends on the specific pathology of the spine. It is important to check the patient's surgical notes to ascertain which approach has been taken and where any bone grafts have been harvested from to allow checking of the wounds for haemorrhage. Patients may be required to wear a spinal brace or support following surgery to limit certain movements of the spine until fusion is established.

Disc decompression

Many herniated discs can be treated with conservative approaches (see ➲ Prolapsed intervertebral disc, pp. 250–251). However, central disc prolapses that manifest with neurological dysfunction (known collectively as cauda equina syndrome) include:

- Bilateral motor weakness or loss of sensation to the lower limbs
- Bladder or bowel sphincter dysfunction
- Loss of perianal sensation.

These require urgent medical attention including a MRI scan and prompt decompression surgery to avoid permanent damage to the spinal nerves.

Also, when conservative approaches to chronic disc herniation fail to relieve symptoms such as unrelenting leg pain then surgery is indicated. Specific surgical approaches include:

- *Percutaneous nucleotomy*—the disc is decompressed by laser or instrumentation passed into the disc under X-ray control. It is less invasive so patients are mobile much earlier
- *Removal of the disc (discectomy)*—either by laminectomy or partial laminectomy. Again, the patient will be mobilized quickly
- *Removal of the disc and fusion of the affected segment*—this will be used if the structures following removal of the disc are unstable. Recovery will obviously be longer, and the patient may need to wear a corset or orthosis postoperatively.

Principles of care following spinal surgery

- Careful observation for possible neurological complications, e.g. altered or loss of sensation and/or movement to the lower limbs, paralysis of anal or bladder sphincters
- Observe for signs of chest infection as the patient may have been lying in the face-down position for several hours during surgery
- Observe the spinal wound site and any graft sites for sign of haemorrhage, haematoma, or infection
- Mobilize the patient as per surgeon's instructions—usually to lie with one pillow only, and not stand or sit for sustained periods of time. The patient may have a spinal support or brace *in situ* until stability is established
- Good pain relief and early mobilization to avoid complications such as DVT and pressure sores
- Teach the patient how to rise from a lying position by turning onto their side, lowering their legs over the edge and using their hands to push to a sitting position before attempting to stand.

There is a high rate of failure and patient dissatisfaction following spinal surgery due to the following issues:

- Incomplete decompression
- Failure of bony fusion
- Recurrent disc herniation
- Loosening of instrumentation.

These may necessitate revision surgery. Patients need to be given appropriate information about the potential benefits/disadvantages/complications of spinal surgery compared to non-surgical interventions prior to consenting to any procedure. Often patients with chronic back disability have suffered depression and anxiety because of their condition and may often have unrealistic expectations of the outcome of surgery and psychological support is essential.

References

1. NICE (2017). Lateral interbody fusion in the lumbar spine for low back pain. Interventional procedures guidance [IPG574]. ℘ https://www.nice.org.uk/guidance/ipg574

Further reading

Butler-Maher A (2016). Neurological assessment. *Int J Trauma Orthop Nurs* 22:44–53.
Damsgaard J, Jørgensen L, Norlyk A, et al. (2017). Spinal fusion: from relief to insecurity. *Int J Trauma Orthop Nurs* 24:31–9.

Elective limb amputation

There are three main reasons for the amputation of a limb in the ortho-paedic setting:

- Traumatic limb amputation at the scene of an accident (see ➲ Crush injuries and traumatic amputation, pp. 362–363)
- Surgical amputation of a severely damaged limb in which there is severe vascular damage (see ➲ Crush injuries and traumatic amputation, pp. 362–363)
- Elective amputation of a limb for other reasons following discussion between the patient, their family, and the medical team.

Elective amputation will be the focus in this section. There are several reasons why a patient may decide to have such life-changing surgery per-formed. The main reason is that they have a limb which causes them chronic severe unresolvable pain (often in the joints of the foot or leg). Other reasons might be severe deformity or neurological deficit. One example is the patient who has a flaccid, unusable arm following brachial plexus injury (see ➲ Brachial plexus injuries, pp. 408–409) and some improvement in pain and disability is anticipated after the amputation. Less commonly, elective amputation may be performed due to malignant bone tumour (see ➲ Bone tumours, pp. 262–263). The most common reasons for elective lower limb amputation include vascular disease, diabetic foot ulcer, and chronic non-healing or recurrent leg ulcers.

Preparation and preoperative care

Limb amputation is significant, life-changing surgery. Prior to the patient being admitted to hospital for surgery they are likely to have undergone a long process of decision-making regarding their limb which has resulted in their planned surgery. They may have suffered pain and discomfort over several years and coming to the decision to have their limb amputated will have been a culmination of a great deal of discussion. One positive aspect of elective amputation is that the patient and family can prepare for the surgery and aftermath both physically and psychologically. The patient must also be aware that they may suffer 'phantom' limb pain postoperatively.

Preparation of the patient for surgery is extremely important. Although they and their family will have discussed the surgery in detail with the sur-geon, the importance of consent to the procedure must still be considered in the days and hours before surgery. Issues about the level of the ampu-tation and the need for a stump that will work well with a prosthetic limb must be considered. It is often helpful for the patient to have visited the limb prosthetist and met other patients with amputations before their own surgery.

Patients who are overweight may benefit from losing some weight before surgery and working on their physical fitness will help in the rehabilitation phase. Following lower limb amputation good upper body and arm strength is needed for using crutches and wheelchair transfers. It is helpful for patient to practise these manoeuvres prior to their surgery.

Psychological support and body image

Psychological support begins prior to surgery. Patients need to know that they will not be fitted for or use a prosthetic limb for some weeks or months following the surgery as the tissues in the stump will need time to recover from the swelling and inflammation caused by the surgery before weight can be borne on it. For patients who may have been suffering with chronic severe pain in the affected limb for many years, elective amputation can be a positive choice, leading to improvements in function and relief of pain. Clinicians who have been working with patients for many years trying to heal chronic wounds may view amputation as a failure, but this must not be the message given to patients and their families. Patients need to be prepared for changes to body image and referral to a clinical psychologist can be useful pre- and postoperatively.

Postoperative care

In additional to the usual postoperative care of the orthopaedic patient, wound care is an important aspect of practice following amputation. Wound drainage systems may be used in the first 48 hours after surgery to help prevent haematoma at the amputation site. The stump and wound should be inspected several times daily for signs of infection as this should be treated as soon as possible. The best conditions for good wound healing should be facilitated including good pre- and postoperative nutrition.

The stump should have been shaped by the surgeon to facilitate good fitting of a prosthesis this can be enhanced postoperatively by careful bandaging of the stump and use of pressure bandages. Once the surgical wound has healed, the stump can be moisturized and gentle massage performed to help prevent hard scar tissue from forming and affecting the fit of the prosthesis.

Rehabilitation

Gradual remobilization and rehabilitation involving adaptation of the patient's living environment (especially if a lower limb is involved) are important aspects of rehabilitation.

Phantom limb pain can be felt as continued sensation from the amputated limb which can manifest as severe pain. The pain is thought to be neurological in nature and a variety of chronic pain management strategies can be helpful.

Both local and national support groups are available across the world, many of which are accessible online as well as telephone and face-to-face meetings. Meeting and communicating with other amputees who are well adjusted to their lives can be very helpful in the first months after the amputation.

Further reading

Liu F, Williams RM, Liu H-E, et al. (2010). The lived experience of persons with lower extremity amputation. *J Clin Nurs* 19:2152–61.

Musculoskeletal trauma care

The nature of trauma

The term trauma is synonymous with injury. Trauma is commonly defined as relating to a *wound or injury caused by some event or assault to the human body* and which can have psychological and social implications as well as physical consequences. Injuries occur suddenly and without warning and can result in long-term disability and death associated with shock and other complications. Injuries account for 5 million deaths worldwide each year, are a leading cause of death among young people and the elderly and are a major cause of disability.[1]

The aetiology of trauma

Aetiology is the science and study of the causes of diseases, disorders, or conditions. Understanding the background to trauma is important when caring for the injured patient as the underlying causes can have a significant impact on care needs and management decisions.

The causes of traumatic injury can be both simple and complex but are largely the result of an unpredicted incident which may have been prevented (see ➲ Accident prevention, pp. 324–325). A significant feature of the sudden and unpredictable nature of traumatic injury is that there is no opportunity for pre-admission or preoperative preparation of the patient and their family, making the care process more challenging.

Traumatic injuries are usually caused by one or more of three 'impacts':
- The body, or part of the body, is in motion and collides with another, harder object
- An object, in motion, collides with the body or part of the body (e.g. blast material from an explosion)
- Organs within the body (e.g. the brain or abdominal organs) collide with the bony cavity (e.g. the skull or chest) in which they are contained.

Resultant injuries will depend on the nature and severity of the incident, the speed of movement, and the impact involved. The higher the velocity and the more violent the impact, the more severe the injury is likely to be. There are numerous events that can lead to traumatic injury which broadly fall into the following categories:
- Individual personal accidents and accidents in the home
- Falls, trips, and slips inside and outside the home
- Drug- and alcohol-induced injury
- Motor vehicle and pedestrian collisions/accidents
- Self-harm and parasuicide
- Deliberate harm/violence by others (e.g. gun shot, stabbing, punching)
- Industrial accidents
- Terrorist attacks
- War and conflict
- Natural disasters such as earthquakes and floods.

The incidence of trauma

Trauma is a leading cause of death and disability in all communities. For each death, several thousands more individuals are non-fatally injured often leading to permanent disability. The incidence of injury varies according to the risks within a community and the activities and risks taken by individuals and groups. Patterns of trauma vary across age groups with traumatic injury being the most common cause of death and disability in children and young adults. Children, pedestrians, cyclists, and older people are the most likely to be injured in motor vehicle incidents because of their physical vulnerability and lack of protection from being within a vehicle. Motor vehicle accidents continue to be a significant cause of injury in all societies. The pattern of injury, however, in drivers and passengers in motor vehicles has changed because of safety belt and child restraint laws, improvements in vehicle manufacture and in response to road safely measures.

The impact of trauma

The impact of trauma on both the individual and their families can be far-reaching and its effects can be felt well beyond those that might be considered physical. Trauma can impact every aspect of the patient's life. This impact can be affected by several factors:

- Age and general health status along with the severity of the injury
- Coping strategies: those which the patient can access within themselves
- Support available to the patient from a variety of sources including those with whom they live, their families, and local health and social services
- Social circumstances—the patient's home, financial, and employment circumstances can have a significant impact on recovery.

It is also important to consider the impact of traumatic events not only on those who have suffered injury but those who witnessed the traumatic event and those who provide care for injured individuals. High-quality trauma services must also include support for all individuals affected by trauma.

Reference

1. World Health Organization (WHO) (2014). *Injuries and Violence: The Facts*. Geneva: WHO.
ℛ https://www.who.int/violence_injury_prevention/key_facts/en/

Further reading

Bowden G, McNally M, Thomas S, et al. (2010). *Oxford Handbook of Orthopaedics and Trauma*. Oxford: Oxford University Press.

The physiological response to trauma

Tissue response

Because of damage to tissues and vital organs, traumatic injury can be life-threatening. It is essential that the practitioner understands the complex pattern of physiological response to injury so that such knowledge can inform the care provided to the injured individual to prevent deterioration and death and facilitate recovery. Close observation of vital signs is a central to recognizing life-threatening responses to injury and the need for emergency and intensive action.

Following traumatic injury the tissues damaged may include bone, soft tissue (muscle, tendon, ligament, and skin), and possibly vulnerable tissue of vital organs such as the lungs, brain, and intestinal system as well as nervous tissue making up the brain, spinal cord, and nerves. Each type of tissue reacts to trauma in a different way, but there is a general response to injury which has an impact on all homeostatic mechanisms and involves the sympathetic nervous and cardiovascular systems as well as endocrine functions. This response can include the following:

- *Vascular injury* to capillaries and other larger vessels resulting in blood loss. This includes bruising and contusion affecting superficial and internal tissues which may have collided with the bony skeleton during a severe traumatic event. The site and size of the blood vessel/s damaged will affect the amount of blood lost as well as the action of clotting mechanisms.
- Loss of blood from vascular and tissue injury may lead to *shock*. Depletion of the circulating volume of blood leads to reduced cardiac output and reduced supply to vital tissues and organs. Tissues become hypoxic and metabolites build up because low circulating pressure means that they cannot reach excretory organs to be excreted. Signs of shock include pallor, tachycardia, low BP, increased respiratory rate, shallow breathing, nausea, and disorientation. Because of shock and haemorrhage, the peripheral blood supply will start to shut down, diverting supply to vital organs such as the heart, lungs, and brain. The main aim of emergency treatment of shock and haemorrhage is the restoration of circulating blood volume, usually by administering IV fluid or blood replacement.
- Following injury and because of associated bleeding, *clotting* mechanisms are stimulated which are designed to reduce blood loss and form haematoma. In severe trauma and multiple injury, excessive demand on clotting mechanisms can lead to hypercoagulation (excessive blood clotting) and an increase in the risk of thrombi as well as excessive bleeding.
- The tissues at or around the injury will exhibit an *inflammatory* response to injury (mediated by both a vascular and a cellular response). This response is designed to facilitate the early stages of tissue repair and assist in the prevention of infection, but also contributes to additional stress on physiological functions.

- The body suffers a high level of *stress* when injury is severe because of the extra demand on tissues, organs, and their functions. This response is the result of hormonal and metabolic activity and can be extreme, resulting in organ failure and placing the individual at risk of death.
- All the responses to injury increase the need for *energy* and energy stored within the body (e.g. as fat) will be used up very quickly, resulting in energy being derived from lean muscle mass, leading to muscle wasting.

Numerous factors affect this response to injury, including:
- The age of the patient
- The patient's general health status and concurrent diseases
- The previous nutritional status of the patient
- The severity of the injury/ies.

Combating the effects of the physiological response to injury takes precedence over the management of musculoskeletal injuries in the early hours and days following trauma. The central role of the practitioner is in constantly monitoring and recording vital signs (see Box 8.1) and acting upon and reporting any abnormalities.

Box 8.1 Essential observations following traumatic injury

Blood pressure—both low and raised BP are significant

Pulse—observation for tachycardia

Respiratory rate and depth—increased rate or shallowness

Skin colour and condition—signs of pallor, blueness, sweating, rashes

Urine output/fluid balance—depletion of output indicates dehydration and/or renal complications

Nausea and vomiting—indicates reduced motility within the gut

Headache—indicates irritation of the central nervous system

Mental status—particularly confusion, disorientation, and restlessness may indicate hypoxia

Further reading

Heaney F, Santy-Tomlinson J (2014). The principles of trauma care. In: Clarke S, Santy-Tomlinson J (eds) *Orthopaedic and Trauma Nursing: An Evidence-Based Approach to Musculoskeletal Care*, pp. 200–20. Oxford: Wiley-Blackwell.

Psychological responses to trauma

Following any trauma, it is a normal human response to feel anxious and stressed by what has happened. The way individuals respond will vary depending on their coping strategies and support mechanisms (internal and external from family, friends, and healthcare professionals) and their personality traits. The stress response to trauma usually manifests in stages; initially, people may feel numb and dazed and then proceed to feelings of denial where they fail to acknowledge and accept the trauma they have experienced. However, with time, people's feelings can develop into one or more of the following:

- *Frightened* ... that the same thing will happen again, or that they might lose control of their feelings and break down
- *Helpless* ... that something really bad happened and they could do nothing about it; they feel helpless, vulnerable, and overwhelmed
- *Angry* ... about what has happened and with whoever is perceived to have been responsible
- *Guilty* ... that they have survived when others have suffered or died; they may feel that they could have done something to prevent it
- *Sad* ... particularly if people were injured or killed, especially if it was someone they knew
- *Ashamed or embarrassed* .... that they have these strong feelings they can't control, especially if they need others to support them
- *Relieved* ... that the danger is over and that the danger has gone
- *Hopeful* ... that their life will return to normal. People can start to feel more positive about things quite soon after a trauma.[1]

Supporting patients following trauma

Most patients will be able to resolve their feelings of stress following trauma with the help and support of healthcare professionals. The principles of psychological support include:

- Treating patients with dignity, kindness, and respect
- Offering information about support services available
- Open and honest communication with patients and their families
- Listening to patients' anxieties and concerns
- Empowering patients to actively participate in their own care and involving their families and friends
- Providing information at the right time and in an appropriate format.

(See ⮩ Communication, pp. 166–167 for further details.)

Post-traumatic stress disorder

Post-traumatic stress disorder (PTSD) can manifest anytime between several days and 6 months or longer after the traumatic event. It is particularly prevalent in those who have suffered trauma during assault, combat, or road traffic collisions/accidents. PTSD is officially classified as a mental health disorder and the signs and symptoms include:

- Nightmares and flashbacks
- Sleep disturbance
- Inability to concentrate
- Withdrawal from social life.

The condition can be successfully treated even many years after the traumatic event has occurred through counselling and psychological therapies such as cognitive behavioural therapy (CBT). Nurses need to talk to patients and their families about the possibility of PTSD and provide details of where they can seek support.

Reference

1. Royal College of Psychiatrists (2016). Coping after a traumatic event. ℜ https://www.rcpsych.ac.uk/healthadvice/problemsanddisorders/copingafteratraumaticevent.aspx

The principles of trauma care

Trauma care

To provide effective care for the individual following traumatic injury there must be well-organized and coordinated services including those at prehospital, hospital, and community levels. Trauma care is provided across a variety of settings including:

- At the scene
- During transport to a hospital or emergency care facility
- In an acute hospital setting
- In a formal or informal rehabilitation setting
- In the community/patient's home.

In the continuum of trauma care, a team approach to care is essential in ensuring that the patient receives appropriate and expert care at all stages during their recovery and rehabilitation[1]. Trauma practitioners work in settings where the arrival of work cannot be controlled or predicted and the ability to react quickly to sudden events is essential.

Care can be provided by a range of individuals including:

- The patient who self-cares
- Family and other informal carers
- Prehospital care professionals
- Nursing and medical practitioners from a variety of specialties including ED services, orthopaedics, intensive/critical care, operating departments, neurosurgical, plastic surgery, and vascular surgery
- Therapy services including physiotherapy, occupational therapy, dietetics, pharmacy, and clinical psychology.

The team involved in providing trauma management should be explicitly trained to carry out specific roles within well-organized systems of care which ensure that the most effective and up-to-date trauma care strategies are implemented in an evidence-based manner at a variety of levels including:

- Preventing incidents which lead to injury where possible
- Management of the incident and associated injuries at the scene
- Acute management of traumatic injury in the days or weeks initially following the traumatic event
- Long-term rehabilitation following traumatic injury and its social and psychological consequences
- Health promotion and secondary prevention of future injuries.

The quality and effectiveness of trauma management varies globally. In wealthier countries significant resources are available to provide systems of care which can lead to success in both the survival of the individual following trauma, and the prevention of long-term complications and disability. Such facilities are scarcest in rural areas of resource-poor countries. The proximity of trauma care centres to the site of the traumatic event and methods of transport from the scene to the hospital can also be significant factors in the success of interventions.

Trauma management has been described[1] as following five main phases:
- *Resuscitation*—measures taken to save life within the first hour following the traumatic incident. The importance of this first stage is discussed in more detail on ➔ Advanced Trauma Life Support (ATLS®), p. 328
- *Stabilization*—further assessment of the effects of the injury/ies and determination of a longer-term management plan
- *Support*—providing the required physical and emotional support and assistance to enable the individual to recover from their injuries
- *Rehabilitation*—assisting the injured individual to achieve a level of recovery that enables them to re-engage with their life
- *Integration*—enabling the individual to adapt to a changed life as a result of their injury/ies and achieve as much life satisfaction as possible.

Systems of trauma care have developed considerably over the last century, often in response to changes in society and following lessons learnt from major events such as wars, disasters, and other significant incidents. In many localities, specialist centres have been developed in which there is significant expertise in managing traumatic injury. Trauma care is about much more than physical trauma and potential physical disability. Injured individuals experience events beyond the realms of 'normal' experience. This can lead to psychological effects as well as have an impact on social issues. The rehabilitation phase of trauma care is often difficult and long but begins at the scene of the incident and requires skilled support from practitioners.

The orthopaedic (or musculoskeletal) injury on which this chapter focuses is often part of a much more complex pattern of injury and it is important that the practitioner is able to care for the patient holistically, taking into consideration the nature of, and the source of, the injury and its consequences as well as the physical and psychological effects so that expert orthopaedic trauma care can be provided.

Reference

1. Langstaff D, Christie J (2000). *Trauma Care: A Team Approach*. Oxford: Butterworth Heinemann.

Accident prevention

Practitioners must give clear advice to the general public about accident prevention. Following accidental injury, patients and their families are likely to be more receptive to accident prevention messages. Accidents can cost the lives of patients (many thousands of people a year die from accidental injury) and considerable suffering (there are millions of non-fatal accidents each year) as well as vast amounts of absence from work, interrupting production processes, and increasing costs. Accidents are often preventable.

The following factors affect accident rates:

- Human behaviour—people's attitude to risk and safety
- Social deprivation—e.g. people who are in poor health or homeless have more accidents
- Environmental hazards—e.g. property or equipment being poorly maintained
- Mental health—e.g. depression and stress can increase the risk of accidents
- Gender and age—men in the 19–24-year age range suffer more accidents than women as they are more likely to engage in risk-taking behaviour. Children and older people are also more prone to accidents due to vulnerability and impaired decision-making
- Drugs and alcohol—the influence of illicit substances and alcohol are implicated in up to 30% of accidents.

The most at-risk groups for accidents are children and the elderly.

Children

Most children are injured at home usually following falls. Children need thorough assessment to identify underlying social problems and careful questioning to ensure non-accidental injuries are identified.[1] Road traffic collisions cause the most deaths and more serious injuries outside the home. Some general advice that can be given to families includes:

- Scan the house on all fours to see it like children do
- Use covers on electric sockets
- Keep household cleaning fluids and other liquids etc. locked up
- Use stair gates, window guards, and fire guards
- Install smoke alarms
- Have car seats that meet safety regulations secured properly and correctly
- Bath water should never be left unattended.

Older people

Slips, falls, and trips are the most common type of accident involving older people. Associated injuries following falls can lead to long-term reductions in the patient's quality of life and increase their dependency on others. Careful assessment should identify any underlying causes and risk factors for further falls. A medication review may identify issues with polypharmacy. Simple advice may be helpful:

- Take your time to get out of the chair or off the bed
- Make sure carpets are secured to prevent tripping
- Don't rush to answer the doorbell or telephone
- Have regular eye checks

- Ensure there is plenty of light at night
- Wear well-fitting, sturdy footwear
- Keep walking areas, stairs, corridors, hallways, and landings clutter-free (see ➲ Falls, pp. 326–327).

When advising patients following an injury, offer links to carers or local and national services that can help. Help and support may include:
- Medical practitioners—GPs and elderly medicine specialists can identify and manage the reasons older people fall
- Social workers—can help the homeless and those living in inappropriate dwellings with accommodation, property maintenance, and finding temporary accommodation for those who need it in the short term. They may also be able to advise on useful support services
- Physiotherapists—can advise on individual and group activity to help maintain strength and mobility, as well as advising on correct footwear and aids to mobility
- Pharmacists—can help with medication reviews and suggestions for changes
- Occupational therapy—can ensure that the patient has the most appropriate environment and recommend equipment and adaptations that may help to maintain independence
- Dieticians—can provide advice on avoiding malnutrition that can increase the risks of falls.

Workplace accidents

Workplace accidents are a common cause of injury in adults. Employers must, by law, take all steps necessary to ensure the health and safety of workers through risk assessment, risk management, and monitoring. All hazards identified through risk assessment should be addressed. Depending on the circumstances, patients may be able to seek legal representation following an accident.

Reference

1. Clarke S, Liggett L (2014). Key issues in caring for the child and young person with an ortho-paedic or musculoskeletal trauma condition. In: Clarke S, Santy-Tomlinson J (eds) *Orthopaedic and Trauma Nursing*, pp. 279–89. Oxford: Wiley-Blackwell.

Falls

Falls are the leading cause of accidental death in older people and can result in serious injury such as hip fracture and head injury. All providers of health and social care should have a plan in place to work in an interdisciplinary way to reduce the number of falls and associated injuries. Trauma practitioners work daily with patients who have either sustained injury as a consequence of falling or are at risk of falling due to their injury and multiple underlying medical, social, and psychological factors. Although the risk of falling can never be completely eliminated, it can be reduced by assessment of risk factors and implementation of prevention strategies.

Risk factors

Risk factors can be classified as either *intrinsic* (internal to the patient) or *extrinsic* (environmental). See Table 8.1 for examples of risk factors.

Risk assessment tools

It is vital that every older person is holistically assessed for risk of falling, considering both intrinsic and extrinsic factors. There are several falls risk assessment tools available to assist practitioners in identifying the risk of falls, including, e.g.:

- Fall Risk Assessment Scale for the Elderly (FRASE)
- St Thomas's Risk Assessment Tool in Falling Elderly Inpatients (STRATIFY)
- Individual healthcare organizations may also have in place their own risk assessment tool.

Such tools focus on assessing the intrinsic risk factors and do not always include environmental issues. Many tools also lack predictive accuracy and have not been adequately tested to ensure they are valid and reliable. Post-fall analysis can provide valuable information about risk factors, such as what the patient doing when they fell, the locality, and relationship to timing of medication.

Preventative strategies and management

An individual prevention plan should be developed in collaboration with the patient, their family, and all members of the MDT. The plan must be based

Table 8.1 Intrinsic and extrinsic risk factors

Intrinsic factors	Extrinsic factors
Postural hypotension	Ill-fitting footwear
Altered balance and/or gait	Unfamiliar surroundings
Medication/polypharmacy	Poor lighting
Urgency/frequency of micturition	Loose floor covering/uneven flooring
Confusion/cognitive impairment	Inappropriate walking aids
Loss of muscle tone/mass	Staff-to-patient ratio
Sensory impairment	Experience of staff in identifying risk of falls
Previous history of falls	Lack or failure of equipment

on the information elicited during the assessment of intrinsic and extrinsic factors. Key preventative strategies include consideration of (1) environment, (2) exercise, (3) vision, (4) medication review, (5) footwear and foot care, and (6) fear of falling.

Interventions should include:

- Careful positioning of support rails, adequate lighting, and removal of obstacles that may lead to tripping
- Proximity to toilet from bed/seating area
- Orientation to unfamiliar surroundings by use of clear signage and colour coding for bathrooms etc.
- Accurate assessment of the type of walking aid needed and adjustment for the patient's height
- Medicines management, including regular review of effectiveness, concordance, and removal of all unnecessary medications.

Patients who have fallen should be referred to specialist falls services where a comprehensive assessment and investigations can be carried out and preventive measures planned. It is also important to provide psychological support to those who have fallen and/or who fear falling. Fear and anxiety can severely impact independence, mobility, and quality of life. Specialist practitioners can teach patients how to get up safely following a fall and provide information about getting help, personal alarms, and preventing hypothermia in the event of a fall at home. All fall-related incidents must be accurately recorded in the care records and the organization's incident reporting systems.

Further reading

NICE (2013). Falls in older people: assessing risk and prevention. Clinical guideline [CG161]. ⅋ https://www.nice.org.uk/guidance/CG161

Santy-Tomlinson J, Speerin R, Hertz K, et al. (2018). Falls and secondary fracture prevention. In: Hertz K, Santy-Tomlinson J (eds) *Fragility Fracture Nursing*, pp. 27–40. Cham: Springer. ⅋ https://www.springer.com/gp/book/9783319766805

Advanced Trauma Life Support (ATLS®)

ATLS® is a safe, reliable, and standardized method for the immediate assessment and management of the trauma patient both at the scene and in the ED. The system was developed in the USA in the 1970s and is now widely accepted as the standard of care for initial assessment and treatment of all trauma patients. The system is designed to treat the greatest threat to the patient's life first to ensure that treatment for life-threatening injuries is prioritized, enabling time-critical interventions to be implemented first. The process is designed to be conducted by one individual or by a full trauma team.

The primary survey

The first part of the process aims to quickly identifying life-threatening problems. This takes the form of the A, B, C, D, E approach to assess and treat the patient, ensuring that the most likely causes of death are treated first.

A: Airway maintenance
B: Breathing
C: Circulation
D: Disability (neurological evaluation)
E: Exposure

Airway

Rapid assessment for signs of airway obstruction. Patients who become unconscious often have airway obstruction which needs immediate attention. In most cases, opening, examining, and supporting the airway will identify any obstruction which can rapidly be resolved; 100% oxygen should be administered.

Breathing

Observation of the rate and depth of breathing for at least 10 seconds will identify respiratory distress. The cause can then be quickly sought and treated. Following multiple trauma this is often caused by chest injury (see ➜ Chest trauma, pp. 336–337). Pulse oximetry can be used to assess oxygenation levels. Oxygen saturation levels (SpO_2) of 95–100% are deemed normal.

Circulation

In most cases hypovolaemia due to bleeding will be the cause of post-injury death. Along with pulse rate and BP, skin colour should be assessed for signs of circulatory problems as well as observing for pallor, clamminess, cyanosis, and capillary refill. An IV cannula should be inserted to facilitate fluid replacement.

Disability

Focusing on neurological assessment, it is important to determine and record the level of consciousness, initially with a rapid assessment of alertness, voice response, response to pain, and for unconsciousness (A, V, P, U—alert, voice, pain, unconscious). This can then be compared to future assessments to identify deterioration and need for emergency action.

Exposure

To facilitate a full head-to-toe examination of the body, clothing will need to be removed. This must be done quickly, ensuring that the patient is covered again as quickly as possible and kept warm to prevent heat loss. Privacy and dignity should be maintained.

The secondary survey

When the primary survey is completed, resuscitation efforts are well established, and vital signs are stabilizing, the secondary survey can take place. In severely injured patients this may take several hours. The secondary survey involves a full head-to-toe physical examination and should include a history of the injury. All vital signs should be reassessed at this stage, including Glasgow coma scoring (see ➜ Head injuries pp. 332–333). At this point X-rays may be undertaken.

A urinary catheter and nasogastric tube should be inserted so that fluid input and output can be closely monitored. Decreasing urine output is an important sign of physiological deterioration.

Continuous monitoring, using an early warning tool, must be maintained as the patient's condition may deteriorate suddenly and at any point during the secondary survey. Should deterioration occur, another primary survey should be conducted.

Once the patient is stable, all medical and care records must be fully completed.

Traditional responses to critical illness have been 'reactive'. However, abnormal physiology is common following traumatic injury and regular frequent monitoring is essential to detect deterioration. EWS systems are now commonly used. If used frequently and consistently they can to identify early deterioration, and prevent critical illness and death (see ➜ Early warning scores, pp. 340–341).

Multiple injuries

The term multiple injury (often termed *polytrauma*) refers to major injuries occurring simultaneously in different parts of the body due to severe physical trauma to both skeletal and other tissues and organs. There may be more than one fracture and other anatomical structures may be involved. The presence of a complex pattern of injury indicates a severe traumatic event and, therefore, a major assault to physiological functioning brought about by significant tissue damage. An extreme inflammatory and immunosuppressive response, along with potential coagulopathy (abnormal clotting), can place the patient at risk of death. This situation, therefore, requires a 'total care' approach delivered by a highly skilled healthcare team from the time of injury until a stable recovery is achieved.

Multiple injuries include those to the:

• Head, face, and/or neck
• Chest, trunk, and/or abdomen
• Skeletal and or soft tissues of the limbs
• Major blood vessels and nerves
• Significant areas of skin with severe wounds.

Patients who have sustained polytrauma should receive immediate and subsequent care at a hospital with specialist trauma services including trauma intensive care facilities. The severe impact of major trauma on physiological functioning places patients at risk of life-threatening complications in the first few days after injury. Those who have sustained severe multiple injuries frequently need intensive care and monitoring with mechanical ventilation and circulatory support.

Care priorities and 'damage control'

Although the priorities of initial treatment of a severely injured person focus on the life-threatening aspects of cardiovascular (particularly uncontrolled bleeding as this is responsible for most trauma deaths in the first few hours after injury), respiratory, and neurological status of the patient, it has been recognized that the early stabilization of fractures plays a significant role in recovery. There is an urgent need to temporarily stabilize fractures and undertake surgery which prevents injuries to other tissues and organs from worsening the condition of the patient. However, conducting major surgery in patients who have sustained severe trauma puts additional stress on their physiological functioning, potentially leading to deterioration and death due to multiple organ failure (MOF) or adult respiratory distress syndrome (ARDS).

'Damage control' surgery involves the temporary stabilization of long-bone fractures, usually with an external fixation device or non-reaming internal fixation, along with debridement of any devitalized tissue. This may be conducted alongside surgery to repair any life-threatening damage to organs, vascular structures, and soft tissues.

Once the patient's physiological condition has been stabilized, definitive orthopaedic surgery can then be employed to permanently manage skeletal injuries. The early stabilization of major fractures of long bones and the pelvis results in less complications and increased survival, as this facilitates early mobilization and avoids the complications of immobility. Severely injured patients often deteriorate physiologically, suffering respiratory problems during the first few days following injury. The presence of unstable long-bone fractures contributes to this deterioration so it is recommended that temporary fracture stabilization takes place in the first 24 hours following injury.

Subsequent care

During the first few days following injury, the polytrauma patient should be cared for in an intensive care or high dependency setting where continuous cardiovascular and respiratory monitoring and support can be provided by staff with specialist skills. This may include mechanical ventilation and cardiovascular support, depending on the patient's physiological status. Once the patient's physiological condition is stable, transfer can take place to a general orthopaedic ward.

During this time, it is essential that close monitoring of the patient's vital signs are continued so that later complications, particularly fat embolism, compartment syndrome, and VTE, can be detected (see ➔ Venous thromboembolism, pp. 194–195). Patients with multiple injuries are also at significant risk of both superficial and deep infection due to the extent of their injuries and should be observed closely for any signs of infection. An EWS system (see ➔ Early warning scores, pp. 340–341) should be in place to help staff to identify patients who are deteriorating physiologically.

The patient and family will need considerable psychological support on transfer from an intensive care unit to a ward where the nursing presence is less obvious and they are likely to feel anxious when they have been used to the constant presence of a health professional in the critical care setting.

Further reading

White TO, Mackenzie SP, Gray AJ (2015). *McRae's Orthopaedic Trauma and Emergency Fracture Management*, 3rd edn. Edinburgh: Elsevier.

Head injury

Any trauma to the head may include injury to the brain. At least 1 million people attend EDs in the UK each year with a head injury which are associated with 50% of all traumatic deaths. Common causes are road traffic collisions, home and occupational accidents, falls, assaults, bicycle accidents, and non-accidental injury.

Types of head injury

Head injuries include injuries to the skull, brain and/or vascular structures of the brain. X-rays of the skull may show extensive injury but radiographic findings may not correlate with the injury to the brain.

Skull fractures

These can be closed or open. Closed fractures occur when the skull is intact and open fractures when the skull and dura mater is breached. Fractures can be linear or depressed, with depressed injuries more likely to cause brain injury. Leakage of CSF fluid from the nose or ears and 'Battle's sign' (periorbital bruising) usually indicate a basal skull fracture.

Brain injury

Brain injuries may be diffuse or focal and can be close to the site of the injury or on the opposite side of the skull due to what is known as a 'contrecoup' effect—the brain can move within the skull and collide with the skull on the opposite side to the impact. Types of brain injury include:

- Contusion—bruising of brain tissue
- Cerebral laceration—the brain tissue is cut or torn
- Focal injuries—the injury is localized to a specific part of the brain
- Intracerebral haemorrhage—when there is bleeding into the brain tissue
- Vascular injury—there is damage to the blood vessels in the skull and brain which can include:
  - Extradural haematoma—haemorrhage to the meningeal vessels between the skull and the dura mater
  - Subdural haematoma—blood gathers within the inner meningeal layer of the dura mater; usually from tears in veins which can cause compression of and damage to the brain
  - Subarachnoid haemorrhage—bleeding into the area between the arachnoid membrane and the pia mater.

Diagnosis

Signs and symptoms of traumatic head injuries depend on the type of injury and the part of the brain affected. There are some common symptoms including headache, visual disturbances, loss of consciousness, vomiting or nausea, dizziness, lack of motor coordination, tiredness, amnesia, and unconsciousness. Diagnosis of traumatic head injury will depend on obtaining the history of the injury so the mechanism of injury can be determined and clinical evidence gathered. The Glasgow Coma Score (GCS)[1] is used to determine the severity of the injury. X-rays are necessary if a fracture is suspected. A CT scan may be performed to confirm haemorrhage or haematoma. MRI may be used for patients with severe head injuries to determine the expected outcome in the long term or to help with clinical decision-making.

The Glasgow Coma Score

The GCS[1] is the most reliable of the various neurological assessment scales. It requires only a brief examination of the patient by any practitioner. As it is easy and quick to undertake, it can be repeated frequently to help identify deterioration very quickly as well as identify potential outcomes and the course of action needed. The GCS was designed to provide a standardized initial assessment. It includes three components (see Table 8.2): eye opening, best verbal response, and best motor response. The lower the score, the more severe the brain injury. The lowest score possible is 3. The highest score possible is 15. As a patient recovers from coma, the score rises.

Table 8.2 The Glasgow Coma Score

	Example	Score
Motor response		
Commands	Follows simple commands	6
Localizes pain	Pulls examiner's hand away when pinched	5
Withdraws from pain	Pulls a part of body away when pinched	4
Abnormal flexion	Flexes body inappropriately to pain	3
Abnormal extension	Body becomes rigid in an extended position when examiner pinches	2
No response	Has no motor response to pinch	1
Eye-opening		
Spontaneous	Opens eyes on own	4
To voice	Opens eyes when asked to in a loud voice	3
To pain	Opens eyes when pinched	2
No response	Does not open eyes	1
Verbal response (talking)		
Orientated	Carries on a conversation correctly and tells examiner where he is, who he is, and the month and year	5
Confused conversation	Seems confused or disoriented	4
Inappropriate words	Talks so examiner can understand him but makes no sense	3
Sounds	Makes sounds that examiner cannot understand	2
No response	Makes no noise	1

Reprinted from *The Lancet*, Vol 304, Teasdale and Jennett, Assessment of Coma and Impaired Consciousness: A practical scale, Copyright 1974 with permission from Elsevier.

Reference

1. Teasdale G, Jennett B (1974). Assessment of coma and impaired consciousness. *Lancet* 2:81–4.

Management of head injury

Treatment will depend on the severity of the head injury. Patients who have received primary head trauma are often admitted for observation because of the risk of 'secondary' injury. Such secondary injuries are potentially preventable or reversible and can be caused by hypoxia, hypercapnia, decreased cerebral perfusion due to hypotension, and haemorrhage.

• Minor injuries—a patient with a GCS of 13–15 who, following trauma to the head, has had a brief period of unconsciousness or none at all. Symptoms may include nausea, dizziness, impaired concentration, memory problems, tiredness, intolerance to light/noise, anxiety, and/or depression. If the patient can be observed by relatives, they may go home with written instructions for observation and action (see 🔊 Table 8.2, p. 333). The patient and relatives should be instructed to return if there are any changes that may indicate deterioration.

• Moderate head injuries—a patient with a GCS of 9–12 who has lost consciousness for between 15 minutes and 6 hours and had a period of post-traumatic amnesia for up to 24 hours. Admission is needed for close observation for signs of deterioration. The GCS must be undertaken frequently, and any changes reported to medical staff. Patients will need assistance with all activities of daily living initially and there may be changes in the patient's personality and behaviour.

• Severe head injury—the patient has a GCS of <9. There will be a coma for 6 hours or more or post-traumatic amnesia for >24 hours. There are often serious physical deficits. The practitioner needs to use the GCS to determine any improvement or deterioration in the patient's condition and admission to a critical care unit may be necessary for mechanical ventilation and monitoring if cardiovascular/respiratory function is affected. Assistance will be needed with all activities of daily living. MDT input will be needed for eating issues and passive exercises while unconscious. Support for families will be needed and they must be prepared for poor outcomes.

Prognosis

• Minor head injuries—most patients recover well, but less than half of all patients will be fully recovered after a minor head injury a year later. Patients with minor head injuries who have suffered other musculoskeletal injuries are often cared for in orthopaedic trauma units

• Moderate head injuries—residual problems can be physical/cognitive and/or behavioural. These may gradually improve over a period of 6–9 months

• Major head injuries—the outcome will depend on the extent of the injury and any secondary complications. There are usually residual problems which either never resolve or take many years to resolve.

Patients who suffer head injuries, particularly major head injuries, are at risk of other injuries such as spinal injury and these must be considered when planning care.

Patients with moderate and major head injuries may require neurosurgery and are usually cared for in a specialized regional neurosurgical unit. Staff and facilities in such units are set up to provide patients and their families with the best treatment, care, and support from the acute phase of injury through to rehabilitation.

Further reading

Woodward S, Mestecky A (eds) (2011). *Neuroscience Nursing: Evidence-Based Theory and Practice*. Oxford: Wiley-Blackwell.

Chest trauma

The skeletal structures comprising the chest wall—the ribs, sternum, and the thoracic section of the spinal column—form a protective cavity containing the lungs, trachea, bronchi, diaphragm, and heart, as well as several vascular structures and the oesophagus. The chest is vulnerable to both blunt and penetrating trauma. Significant trauma can result in injury to both the chest wall and the structures contained within it. As well as the impact itself, displaced skeletal injuries of the chest (see ➜ Chest trauma, pp. 336–337) can be responsible for damage to organs and other structures within the chest such as the lungs and heart. This can result in hypoxia, hypovolaemic shock, and respiratory failure, making it a significant cause of death following traumatic injury. Mechanical ventilation and/or tracheostomy may be needed.

There are several potential serious chest injuries which require emergency management:

- *Flail chest*—multiple rib fractures can produce a segment of the chest wall that is free floating and moves paradoxically with respiration
- *Closed pneumothorax*—partial or complete lung collapse occurs when air can enter the pleural space following lung injury, preventing the lung from expanding normally. This can also lead to *haemopneumothorax* if there is blood loss into the pleural space. If significant, the injury is treated with an underwater seal chest drain
- *Tension pneumothorax*—penetrating chest wounds allow air to enter the pleural space. The accumulation of pressure can cause partial or total lung collapse. Emergency decompression is conducted by inserting a needle into the intercostal space. This creates a simple pneumothorax which can then be treated as previously outlined
- *Pulmonary contusion*—damage to lung tissue may lead to haemorrhage and oedema and result in impaired respiratory function.

Assessment

Chest injuries may not be immediately apparent and careful early respiratory assessment of the injured individual is needed. Assessment for significant injury to the chest should include the following parameters:

- Airway obstruction must be resolved immediately before any other action
- Tachypnoea/any difficulty breathing/respiratory distress
- Hypoxia—including both oxygen saturation measurement and other signs such as confusion and/or agitation. Arterial blood gases should be assessed
- Full assessment of vital signs including temperature
- Signs of soft tissue injury to the chest such as bruising and lacerations
- Abnormal chest wall movements
- Chest pain—particularly on inspiration and expiration
- Auscultation and palpation of the chest identifying any abnormal sounds
- Chest X-ray and ECG with possible chest ultrasound scan.

Emergency care

Immediate care of the patient with suspected or actual chest injury should include:

- High-concentration oxygen administered via a face mask
- Close observation of vital signs and oxygen saturation levels
- Pain management should be considered early. Chest injuries are extremely painful and untreated pain can lead to increased respiratory distress. Opiate analgesia should be used while being vigilant for side effects, especially respiratory depression. Adjunctive pain management such as intercostal nerve blocks can be useful and help diminish the need for strong opiates with consequent respiratory depression. All patients with chest injuries should be cared for in an upright posture if possible, providing this does not compromise other conditions such as spinal injuries.

Subsequent care

Once the initial chest injury has been managed and the patient's physiological condition is stabilized, care should focus on the prevention of complications such as chest infection. This includes the facilitation of optimum breathing and gaseous exchange. The patient needs to be able to cough and expectorate to prevent the collection of secretions in the lower lobes of the lungs. The healthcare team should work closely with the physiotherapist in facilitating this. Adequate analgesia facilitates normal chest expansion, deep breathing, and physiotherapy. This can include continuous infusion of opiates and epidural blocks can be useful. Care and monitoring of chest drains and apparatus should continue until the drain is removed. Vigilant monitoring of the patient's vital signs along with humidified oxygen therapy should be continued until full recovery is achieved.

Further reading

Curtis K, Ramsden C (2016). *Emergency and Trauma Care for Nurses and Paramedics*, 2nd edn. Edinburgh: Elsevier.

Abdominal trauma

Abdominal trauma is a significant cause of death following major trauma, particularly from uncontrolled bleeding from injured abdominal organs and vascular structures. Unlike the organs of the chest and pelvis, the abdominal organs are not well protected with a bony cavity. Following injury to the trunk (commonly following high-speed road traffic collisions and pedestrian injuries), trauma to the abdomen can cause damage to internal structures such as the liver, spleen, kidneys, and intestines. 'Seat-belt' injury is often implicated, especially as the 'lap belt' lies across the abdomen. Blunt trauma can cause contusion or tears to the organs.

Abdominal organs have a rich blood supply and can bleed profusely so such injuries are often life-threatening due to haemorrhage. They can, however, be easily missed because they are not immediately visible and may be asymptomatic—especially if there are other more painful and obvious injuries. The patient may rapidly become critically ill due to severe bleeding, resulting in haemorrhagic shock. Splenic injury, for example, is a significant cause of death following trauma.

Later in the management of multiple injuries, abdominal trauma can result in sepsis. This demonstrates the importance of continued vigilant assessment of the polytrauma patient being cared for in the orthopaedic setting with abdominal trauma in mind, even when the risk of bleeding seems to have passed.

Assessment

Abdominal injury should be suspected in all cases of major trauma where the mechanism of injury indicates possible trauma to the abdomen. In the emergency setting, and in the first 24 hours following trauma, several signs should alert the practitioner to this possibility:

- Examination must include the back and sides of the abdomen as well as the front (from the lower ribs to the pelvis)
- Sometimes there is a distended or rigid abdomen
- If the patient is conscious, they may experience abdominal pain, but this can be masked by other injuries and analgesia
- There may be bruising, friction marks, or laceration to the abdomen which may indicate underlying injury
- Diagnostic peritoneal lavage conducted by experienced medical staff, may be used in the ED and, subsequently, by a surgeon to detect blood in the abdominal cavity
- Ultrasound scanning is also useful in detecting blood in the abdominal cavity
- If the patient's condition is stable, a CT scan of the abdomen may be performed to assess the degree of injury.

Management and care

Immediate surgical intervention under the care of a general or specialist surgeon will usually be required to undertake laparotomy to investigate and repair injuries causing abdominal bleeding and to achieve haemostasis. This may result in the resection of organs where damage is severe. Postoperative high dependency care may be needed, but if there is also significant skeletal injury, transfer to an orthopaedic setting may be preferred for definitive care and rehabilitation. The following care should be provided:

- Nil by mouth until gut motility returns. An IV fluid regimen will be required to maintain fluid balance. A nasogastric tube may be *in situ* as well as a urinary catheter and wound drain
- Regular observation of all vital signs until the patient is eating and drinking normally

Signs of later problems such as abdominal sepsis include careful observation for the following:

- Along with abdominal pain, the patient may feel generally unwell, unable to eat, and may be vomiting
- Unstable vital signs such as pyrexia and rapid pulse indicate possible sepsis.

These symptoms should be acted upon immediately and medical attention sought from a general surgeon.

Many patients are cared for in a high dependency/critical care setting for the initial period following abdominal injury and surgery. The orthopaedic trauma practitioner needs, however, to be aware of the later care of the patient following such surgery, including definitive care of wounds and drains. Recovery from musculoskeletal trauma may be complicated by abdominal surgery, not least because such surgery may result in nutritional depletion and low energy levels as well as an additional source of postoperative pain.

Early warning scores

An EWS system was first developed in Great Yarmouth from the Apache II scoring system and has been introduced widely in UK hospitals following recommendations by the Department of Health. The EWS is an approach to early detection of physiological deterioration to prevent seriously deterioration. The purpose is to avoid a 'reactive' approach by detecting clinical deterioration of patients at a much earlier stage so that a timely action can be taken to prevent further deterioration and hopefully prevent the patient from requiring admission to intensive care A physiological 'score' is derived from regular observations. The assessment is designed to be quick and simple to complete. This process is also sometimes called the 'patient at risk score' (PARS) or modified early warning score (MEWS)—adaptations of the EWS.

Indications for use

EWSs should be calculated for any patient who might be considered at risk of deterioration or who raises concern. It is common for hospitals to have guidelines in place which recommend that all patients have EWS conducted and that they are recorded a minimum of twice a day or more often if indicated. All patients admitted following trauma or surgery should be commenced on EWS monitoring on admission or transfer to make an initial assessment to be followed by continuous monitoring. The EWS is a reproducible indication of how at risk of deterioration a patient is that allows the patient's condition to be identified before physiological deterioration results in critical deterioration.

Once the patient is identified as deteriorating, either a medical/advanced practitioner or a member of a rapid patient assessment team, or critical care outreach team should undertake a detailed rapid assessment. The patient's subsequent management and further monitoring can then be modified to reflect the patient's condition.

As patients who are deteriorating are identified very early, relatively simple interventions, such as oxygen therapy, may prevent further deterioration or collapse. The EWS is designed to assist in effective clinical judgement and empowers practitioners to make confident decisions. It also aims to improve communication within the MDT—e.g. nurses can communicate observation findings to medical staff so that appropriate decisions can be made based on comparable and standardized data.

EWS calculation

EWSs are usually based on five physiological parameters: (1) mental response, (2) pulse rate, (3) BP, (4) respiratory rate, and (5) temperature. For postoperative patients or catheterized patients, urine output can be used as a sixth parameter. Of all the parameters, respiratory rate is deemed the most important as it is the most sensitive indicator of a patient's physiological well-being.

A score is given for each observation and the individual scores are then added to give the EWS. If most of the physiological parameters are normal the EWS will be <3. If the patient scores ≥3 they will 'trigger' action to be taken. Sometimes, a score >3 will be normal for that patient; this decision however, needs to be made by the whole team looking after the patient and should be documented in the patient's records.

Action

If the score indicates action is required, the next steps will depend on a standard response. In most cases, a score of ≥3 indicates the need for an immediate review by the ward doctor. The frequency of observations should be increased. If no improvement is seen when rechecked at 30 minutes and the doctor has not attended, they must attend in the next 30 minutes to review the patient. If the patient is still not improving, the practitioner should request attendance of a more senior doctor. If the patient does not improve or there is further deterioration, referral to the intensive/critical care team may be required.

The use of the EWS has been shown to be effective in preventing ICU admissions and reducing mortality and morbidity. It is recommended that all patients in acute settings should be monitored with the EWS as it improves the quality of patient observation and monitoring. There are, however, some limitations—it is not a comprehensive assessment tool, staff training in interpretation of the scores and when action is required takes time, baseline scores and management plans need to be clearly documented, and, as already stated, the EWS is not a replacement for clinical judgement.

Further reading

Royal College of Physicians (2017). National Early Warning Score (NEWS) 2: standardising assessment of acute illness severity in the NHS. ℘ https://www.rcplondon.ac.uk/projects/outputs/national-early-warning-score-news-2

Fractures

Fractures are a loss of continuity (or break) in the substance of a bone and may be either partial or complete. They range from a 'hairline' break to a fracture with many fragments. Fractures are also associated with injury to the soft tissues in the surrounding area.

Types of fracture

Fractures can be described as:
- *Closed*—skin is intact, no contact between the fracture and the outside air; low infection risk and minimal haemorrhage
- *Open/compound*—there is an external wound which connects with the fracture; there is a severe risk of infection; blood loss may be significant; open fractures can be classified according to their severity (see ➔ Open (compound) fractures, pp. 346–347)
- *Simple*—involving one fracture line and only two fragments
- *Comminuted*—involving more than one fracture line and more than two/ multiple fragments; usually unstable and caused by direct trauma
- *Complicated*—involving other vital structures, e.g. nerves, arteries, veins, organs
- *Pathological*—resulting from underlying disease which has caused weakness of the bone; the force required to produce a fracture is reduced
- *Avulsion*—normally produced by sudden muscular contraction, causing a fragment of bone to be torn away by the tendon or ligament
- *Fracture–dislocation*—associated with a dislocated joint or when the position of a fracture leaves the joint unstable.

Causes of fractures

- *Direct violence*—where fractures occur at the point of impact; the application of stress exceeds the limits of strength of the bone
- *Indirect violence*—a twisting or bending force is applied to the bone resulting in a fracture a distance from the casual force
- *Stress*—a bone is subjected to excessive and persistent stress.

Classification of fractures

- *Hairline*—difficult to detect on radiograph (X-ray) and often missed, but usually heal quickly
- *Transverse*—the fracture line runs at right angles to the long axis of a long bone and is usually caused by direct trauma
- *Oblique*—the fracture line runs at an angle <90° to the long bone; usually caused by indirect violence
- *Spiral*—the fracture runs in a spiral fashion around the bone, usually caused by an indirect rotational force
- *Impacted*—one fragment is driven into another, usually caused by indirect violence; is stable due to the interlocking of bone ends
- *Depressed*—a localized blow pushes a segment of bone below the level of surrounding bone; common in skull fractures
- *Crush*—when bone is compressed beyond the limits of tolerance; common in the spine and the heels (calcaneum)

- *Greenstick/incomplete*—the bone bends on one side and cracks on the other; common in children
- *Intra-articular*—involving a joint; the fracture line extends through articular cartilage; any irregularity in the surface may cause secondary OA.

Signs and symptoms

- *History*—the following questions will illuminate the likely nature of the fracture:
  - What was happening at the time? e.g. playing football, working at a height
  - What was the nature of the incident? e.g. a kick, a fall
  - What was the type of force? e.g. if falling from a height, was the fall broken? What surface did they land on?
  - What was the point of impact? Which way did the force go?
  - Was there any significance to the incident itself? e.g. did the person collapse? This requires separate investigation
- *Pain*—where is it? How severe or diffuse is it?
- *Loss of function*—e.g. inability to weight bear
- *Deformity*—if deformity is severe, there is usually a fracture
- *Swelling*—in the first few hours and days after injury there will be localized swelling which can become diffuse
- *Tenderness*—there is normally tenderness above the fracture on palpation
- *Crepitus*—when the patient is being moved, the sound of bone ends rubbing together may be heard. This must not be looked for on purpose as it is very painful.

Diagnosis

In some cases, diagnosis of a fracture is relatively simple because the bone is visible or there is severe deformity. If a fracture is suspected, it must always be confirmed by X-ray; taken from several angles (at least AP and lateral) so that an accurate picture of the fracture can be built up which will be used to help plan treatment.

Further reading

White TO, Mackenzie SP, Gray AJ (2015). *McRae's Orthopaedic Trauma and Emergency Fracture Management*, 3rd edn. Edinburgh: Elsevier.

Fracture healing

Different bones take different amounts of time to heal but generally follow five stages of repair (see Fig. 8.1).

1. *Fracture.* Fractures cause haemorrhage, inflammation, swelling, and destruction of the tissues and a blood clot forms.
2. *Formation of granulation tissue.* Fibroblasts and capillaries rapidly grow into the blood clot forming granulation tissue in response to cytokines (protein chemical messengers) instigated by the tissue damage; fibrovascular tissue replaces the clot, collagen fibres are laid down, and mineral salts are deposited at the site.
3. *Replacement of granulation tissue by callus.* At 2–3 weeks the swelling decreases and the fracture stiffens while new bone begins to form some distance from the fracture (this cannot yet be seen on X-ray).
4. *Replacement of callus by lamellar bone.* The cells capable of changing into bone cells (pluripotential mesenchymal cells) are induced to do so and the new bone (callus) begins to bridge the fracture (this can be seen on X-ray).
5. *Remodelling of the bone.* This stage can last several years and involves the fracture site remodelling itself—most deformities can also be rectified; any fragments of dead bone are reabsorbed by the osteoclasts; the cell density increases and the collagen that gives bones their strength positions itself along the lines of stress, increasing bone strength.

These stages do not occur independently and there is some overlapping. The rate of healing and the ability of the body to remodel a fracture vary from person to person and depend on several factors such as age, health, the kind of fracture and the bone involved.

Bone healing in children

Due to the increased density and porosity of children's bones, the thick periosteum helps to support the fracture and they heal much more quickly than adults. Table 8.3 gives an indication of the differences in the healing time of fractures between adults and children although many factors can extend healing times and the times given are an estimate.

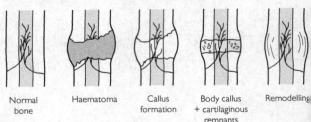

| Normal bone | Haematoma | Callus formation | Body callus + cartilaginous remnants | Remodelling |

Fig. 8.1 Bone healing.

Table 8.3 Comparison of healing times in adults and children

Type of fracture	Healing time for adult	Healing time for child
Upper limb fractures	6–8 weeks	4–6 weeks
Lower limb fractures	8–12 weeks	4–6 weeks
Shaft of femur fracture	8–10 weeks	4–6 weeks

Further reading

Marsell R, Einhorn TA (2011). The biology of fracture healing. *Injury* 42:551–5.

Open (compound) fractures

Fractures that are open and, therefore, provide a conduit between the bone injury and the outside atmosphere are of great concern. In some cases, the bone protrudes through the skin and, in others, there may only be a small wound or blister near to the site of the fracture. There is usually significant soft tissue damage and infection is a very high risk, potentially leading to osteomyelitis and/or non-union of the fracture. These injuries are particularly problematic for three main reasons:

- Significant damage to the soft tissues surrounding the fracture site because of the involvement of high-energy mechanisms in the injury
- Severe risk of early and late infection
- Difficulty in healing of the fracture.

Open fractures often have multiple fragments (comminuted), bone loss, and severe soft tissue damage as well as skin loss. Such injuries are most common in the distal lower limb—fractures of the tibia being a particular problem because the bone is very close to the surface at the shin, making it more prone to direct trauma, and the blood supply to the shin is poor. Injuries can be classified according to the severity of the soft tissue injury. One example of a classification system is that of Gustilo et al.[1] which helps practitioners to assess the severity of the injury (see Table 8.4).

Due to the challenges, there are very specific guidelines about the management of such fractures, such as those published by the British Orthopaedic Association (BOA)[2] that are based on a strong evidence base and include:

- Early administration of prophylactic IV antibiotics
- Initial and continuous assessment of the neurovascular status of the limb in the early weeks (see ⊃ Neurovascular compromise, pp. 196–197) while the soft tissue injury settles. The practitioner should be particularly vigilant for the signs of compartment syndrome (see ⊃ Compartment syndrome, pp. 198–199)
- Immediate surgery must take place to repair any vascular injury and perform excision and debridement of any devitalized bone and soft tissue such as muscle
- Specialist orthopaedic and plastic surgeons must work together to formulate a plan to manage the soft tissue injury. Primary wound

Table 8.4 Gustilo classification of open (compound) fractures

Type I	An open fracture with a wound which is (a) <1 cm and (b) clean
Type II	An open fracture with a wound which is (a) >1 cm long and (b) which is not associated with extensive soft tissue damage, avulsion, or flaps
Type III A	An open fracture where there is adequate soft tissue coverage of bone in spite of (a) extensive soft tissue lacerations or flaps or (b) high-energy trauma irrespective of the size of the wound
Type III B	An open fracture with extensive soft tissue loss, with periosteal stripping and exposure of bone. Massive contamination is usual
Type III C	An open fracture associated with an arterial injury which requires repair

Adapted from McRae and Esser.[1]

closure is nearly always impossible because of tissue loss and is not recommended if contamination of the wound is likely

- In the first few hours after injury the limb must be carefully splinted. Fracture stabilization may then be provided by applying an external fixation device (see ➲ Care and education of a patient with external fixation, pp. 392–393) which may be used to manage the fracture in the longer term, especially if reconstruction is needed. Internal fixation is usually not advised if there is extensive soft tissue damage. Long-term management of the fracture should take place in a specialist centre
- The wound and soft tissue damage should be managed in collaboration with a plastic surgeon and may involve vacuum-assisted closure of the wound using a negative pressure device as well as moist wound healing principles.

During the first few weeks following the injury, the most essential aspect of care is close observation of the limb for signs of neurovascular problems and infection. Careful elevation and support of the limb is also essential. The use of a Braun frame is essential (see ➲ Fig. 9.5, p. 385). The patient will be less mobile than normal for some time while the injury is stabilized. Severe open fractures with tissue loss require long-term treatment with lengthy recovery and rehabilitation. This will have a significant impact on the patient and their family, both psychologically and a great deal of support will be required.

References

1. McRae R, Esser S (2008). *Practical Fracture Treatment*, 5th edn, p. 24. Edinburgh: Churchill Livingstone.
2. BOA (2017). Open fractures. British Orthopaedic Associate and British Association of Plastic, Reconstructive and Aesthetic Surgeons. Standards for Trauma. ⌀ https://www.boa.ac.uk/wp-content/uploads/2017/12/BOAST-Open-Fractures.pdf

Fracture healing problems

There are several factors which contribute to fracture healing:

- *Age*—in children, fractures heal quickly. The speed of union decreases as skeletal maturity is reached. For example, a child with a fractured shaft of femur could heal in 4 weeks; in an adult this could be as much as 3 months or more. Children's bones remodel more effectively due to the cycle of bone cell production/reabsorption being much faster
- *Smoking and alcohol consumption*—these delay the rate and quality of fracture union due to the negative impact on osteoblastic activity
- *Fracture mobility*—any movement at the fracture delays union. This can be caused by insufficient stability at the fracture site
- *Separation of bone ends*—union will be delayed or prevented if bone ends are separated. This can occur because:
  - Soft tissue may interpose the fragments of bone
  - Excessive traction used in reduction may lead to separation of bone ends
  - Following internal fixation, the fixation device can prevent load bearing within the bone, leading to non- or delayed-union of the fracture
- *Infection*—bone tissue infection (osteomyelitis) (see ➲ Osteomyelitis, pp. 272–273) delays or prevents union
- *Disturbance of blood supply*—where blood supply is reduced or there is interference with circulation at the fracture site, there will be non–union; some bones are poorly vascularized and known to heal poorly, e.g. scaphoid, tibial shaft
- *Joint involvement*—when a joint is involved, union is often delayed because of the presence of synovial fluid and poorly vascularized joint surfaces
- *Underlying pathology*—diseased bone such as that with metabolic disorders or malignancy can delay or prevent union
- *Poor nutrition*—a lack of the nutrients required for bone healing can delay union
- *Ethnicity and gender*—women have lower bone mass than men, live longer, and have decreased oestrogen following the menopause which accelerates bone loss. People with darker skin have a higher PBD than white or Asian people and are less prone to osteoporotic fractures.

Each or a combination of these factors can lead to:

- *Non-union*—the fracture fails to heal; further surgery may be required to unite the fracture
- *Slow union*—the fracture takes longer than usual to heal; often healing will eventually occur if the fracture is well supported.
- *Delayed union*—the fracture does not heal in the expected time. This is different from slow union as X-rays will show abnormal changes in the bone. Differentiating between delayed union and slow union is important. If the fracture is still very mobile at 2 months or not healed at 4 months, there should be close assessment of the fixation as poor fixation is the commonest cause of delayed union and may need to be revised.

- *Malunion*—the fracture heals in the wrong anatomical position. If the limb looks unsightly or is not functional in the early stages of healing, the fracture can be re-manipulated, and a cast applied. In the later stages of healing, further surgery is needed. If the limb is functional and not unsightly, it may be accepted as it is
- *Shortening*—can occur following malunion. If the shortening of a lower limb is minimal, i.e. <1.5 cm, this may be tolerated. If the shortening is greater, a shoe raise will be needed.

Specific complications of fracture treatment

- *Complex regional pain syndrome*—chronic post-traumatic pain usually follows a fracture of the wrist but can follow any fracture. It is not noticed until the cast is removed. There is gross swelling, finger movement is restricted, and the skin is warm, pink, and shiny. The cause is unknown, but is believed to be an unusual sympathetic response to trauma.[1] It is usually self-limiting and resolves slowly over a period of 4–12 months, although restrictions in movement may be permanent.
- *Avascular necrosis*—death of bone due to disruption of the blood supply. In some cases the bone will slowly revascularize from the periphery, but secondary osteoarthritic changes in the affected joint are inevitable. The patient will be advised not to weight bear and surgery may be necessary.
- *Myositis ossificans*—a calcified mass appears in the tissues near a joint leading to restricted movement. Treatment involves excision of the mass. If this is done prematurely, it will reoccur and needs to be done at between 6–12 months. This is very rare.
- *Osteitis*—there is infection in a closed fracture, it is rare and seldom diagnosed until the infection is well established. There is often recurrent pyrexia, a raised ESR and WBC count, prolonged pain, local tenderness, and swelling:
  - Drainage may be required along with high-dose antibiotics and wound care. If well established, this may need excision with open wound healing.
- *Compartment syndrome*—see ➲ Compartment syndrome, pp. 198–199.
- *Fracture blisters*—blisters can appear on the skin surface over the fracture, especially in the region of the ankle, foot, lower leg, and elbow. These appear 24–48 hours after injury and result from traumatic oedema of the skin. They should be left intact if possible.
- *Fat embolism*—see ➲ Fat embolism syndrome, pp. 212–213.
- *VTE*—see ➲ Venous thromboembolism, pp. 194–195.

Observation of the patient is paramount following a fracture and recognition of fracture complications is key to prompt intervention.

Reference
1. Thurlow G, Gray B (2018). Complex regional pain syndrome. *Int J Orthop Trauma Nurs* 30:44–7.

Principles of fracture management

Aims of fracture management

- The attainment of a sound bony union without deformity[1]
- Restoration of function, so the patient can resume their former independence as quickly as possible without complications, although this cannot always be achieved.
- This is achieved through:
  - Reduction
  - Retention
  - Rehabilitation.

Reduction of the fracture

Displaced fractures need to be 'reduced' to put the fragments into proper alignment so that healing can occur in the correct position. Undisplaced fractures do not require reduction but those not in alignment will heal slowly or not at all. The main methods of fracture reduction are:

Manipulation

Often under local or general anaesthetic, the pulling or pushing of bones back into place.

Traction

Weights or splints are used as a force against the patient's own body weight to pull the bones into alignment.

Open reduction

Surgery is conducted to expose the fracture and manually bring the fragments into alignment. This may be followed by internal fixation:

- For compound fractures—debridement of the wound will mean an open wound remains
- Where other methods have failed or where the position is unstable
- Where the best method of holding the fracture is to internally fix it.

Retention of fracture position

Once a fracture has been reduced, it needs to be retained in that position until it is sufficiently healed to:

- Prevent angulation and displacement of fragments
- Prevent movement which might interfere with fracture and soft tissue healing
- Relieve pain.

Methods for support/immobilization during healing include:

- Cast application using plaster of Paris or synthetic casting materials
- Traction is used to hold the fracture in position, especially if the fracture is unstable and the patient is not medically fit for surgery. Traction can be applied via the skin (skin traction) or via bone, e.g. (skeletal traction) using a skeletal pin
- Internal fixation is used when reduction cannot be achieved by a closed method, or reduction can be achieved but not held by the closed

method. It is also indicated when perfect reduction and fixation is required e.g. when the fracture involves joint surfaces
- Advantages of internal fixation are:
  o Possibility of achieving and maintaining high-quality reduction
  o Early mobilization of joints resulting in less stiffness, etc.
  o Earlier discharge from hospital and earlier return to full function
- Disadvantages are:
  o The possibility of introducing infection
  o Technically difficult surgery to perform
  o Equipment, devices, and tools are costly
  o Time under anaesthetic can be lengthy
- External fixators—the bony fragments are held in alignment by skeletal pins or wires and an external frame (see ➲ Care and education of the patient with external fixation, pp. 392–393)
- Cast/functional bracing—the limb is contained in a hinged cast after the fracture has been reduced. The advantages of cast/functional bracing include:
  - Promotes bone healing as axial loading and micro-movement at the fracture site stimulates bone healing
  - Maintains mobility of the joint and muscle function
  - Allows early mobilization and independence.

Recovery and rehabilitation

This includes restoration of function of the injured part and the rehabilitation of the whole patient. Rehabilitation should commence as soon as possible following injury and should involve the whole MDT (see ➲ Rehabilitation, pp. 176–177).

The following are the main principles of care during fracture healing:
- Encourage active exercise of as much of the injured part as possible to improve circulation, reduce oedema, and prevent joint stiffness
- Encourage static exercises to prevent muscle wasting and improve venous circulation
- Encourage exercise of all movable joints
- Assist mobility by teaching the correct use of walking aids
- Encourage and motivate the patient to be as active as possible
- Aim to restore function required for the activities of daily living
- Ensure social and physical support is sought if not able to function as well as before
- Ensure the home is suitable for any functional limitations
- Ensure the individual and their family can cope.

Reference
1. McRae R, Esser S (2008). *Practical Fracture Treatment*, 5th edn. Edinburgh: Churchill Livingstone.

Dislocation and subluxation

Dislocation

Dislocation is the complete loss of congruity between the articulating surfaces of a joint caused by the joint being forced beyond its normal range of movement. The bones involved completely lose contact with each other.

The most commonly dislocated joint is the shoulder. Other joints prone to dislocation include the elbow, the joints of the foot and hand, the wrist, the knee, and the hip. Some fractures can also be associated with dislocation such as *fracture dislocation of the ankle* and *central fracture/dislocation of the hip* in which the femoral head is forced into and through the acetabulum resulting in fracture of the acetabulum.

Subluxation

Subluxation occurs when there is partial loss of congruity between the articulating surfaces of a joint. The loss of contact is incomplete. This may proceed to complete dislocation. In addition to other joints, subluxation can occur in the facet joints of the spine and can happen spontaneously in patients with RA. Subluxations can be just as painful as dislocations and require similar active treatment.

Assessment

Initial assessment of dislocation and subluxation should consider:
- The history of the injury with consideration of the mechanism of injury will help to identify joint dislocation
- Deformity of the joint is often obvious or can be felt on palpation
- The patient may have felt the joint come out of place
- The injury is often immediately extremely painful because of stretching or tearing of the joint capsule and surrounding ligaments, neurovascular structures, and other soft tissues
- There will usually be severe, acute swelling of the joint
- The patient will have lost most, or all, use of the joint
- There may be bruising and signs of inflammation such as redness and heat
- Dislocations can be associated with neurovascular damage so thorough neurovascular assessment is essential (see ➲ Neurovascular compromise pp. 196–197)
- X-rays will provide a clear picture of the injury and identify any fractures associated with it.

Care and management
- Immediately following the injury, adequate pain relief must be provided as soon as possible, but especially before examination of the joint
- Resting the joint in a splint or sling may be helpful while transport and assessment takes place
- Some dislocations may reduce spontaneously—especially if the joint has been dislocated frequently and/or recurrently and/or is lax

- Closed reduction of the dislocation will usually be required—depending on the nature of the injury, this may take place with pain relief and sedation or under anaesthesia. Hip dislocations usually require general anaesthesia. Open reduction may be necessary in some severe injuries where closed reduction cannot be achieved—this is relatively common in the knee
- Surgical repair may be needed if there are tears of, and need for repair to, the surrounding soft tissue structures such as muscles and ligaments
- Recurrent dislocation is common in the shoulder and this may need surgery to restabilize the joint with soft tissue repair (see ➜ Soft tissue injury 1 and 2, pp. 356–359)
- Where there is significant stretching and damage to ligaments supporting and stabilizing the joint, it may be necessary to rest the joint until the tissue has recovered. Activity restrictions may be needed to give the tissues the opportunity to recover
- Following dislocation of the hip, skin traction is sometimes used, along with bedrest, to reduce swelling and inflammation and promote soft tissue healing
- Physiotherapy-led exercise therapy will help the patient to achieve recovery of the joint.

Traumatic wound management

Traumatic wounds should always be treated as if they are contaminated from the outset. They carry a high risk of infection and loss of viability of the tissue involved. They are created under conditions that it is not possible to control and in an environment with many potential pathogens.

Wounds occur when the force involved is greater than the resistance of the skin. The trauma causing such wounds is often blunt and can, therefore, cause damage to the vascular structures in the tissues around the wound, resulting in diminished or lost blood supply to the tissue, affecting healing. Traumatic wounds include:

- *Lacerations*—due to both blunt and sharp trauma and varying in depth and amount of tissue damage
- *Contusions/bruising*—often caused by blunt trauma; closed wounds but further swelling and bleeding into the tissues can be minimized using ice and elevation
- *Crush injuries*—associated with significant trauma and are considered in detail in ➲ Crush injuries and traumatic amputation, pp. 362–363
- *Degloving injuries*—the upper levels of skin and other structures are sheared away from underlying tissues; these can range from pre-tibial lacerations to major injuries with significant areas of sheared tissue— they require specialist care with involvement of the plastic surgery team
- *Gunshot wounds*—require specific management because of the nature and depth of the tissue damage and the very high risk of infection and devitalized tissue
- *Thermal injuries/burns and chemical burns*—can be associated with musculoskeletal trauma and require specialized care
- *Compound fracture wounds*—traumatic wounds can be associated with fractures. Any wound or blister near a fracture site should raise suspicion that there is a connection between the wound and the fracture and the principles of caring for compound fractures must be obeyed (see ➲ Open (compound) fractures, pp. 346–347).

All wounds must be fully assessed as soon as possible after the injury. Each wound type requires specific consideration, but general principles of traumatic wound care must be adhered to in all cases. Once emergency management of any haemorrhage from the wound has been executed, the following must be conducted:

- *Exploration and debridement* of the wound to ascertain the depth and extent of the wound and any damage to underlying structures such as tendons. Any devitalized tissue must be debrided from the wound as soon as possible as this can act as a focus for infection, particularly with anaerobic organisms.
- *Irrigation* of the wound should be conducted to facilitate removal of foreign body particles. Thorough cleaning or irrigation of the wound with tap water, saline, or an antiseptic solution (depending on local policy) can reduce the rate of infection.

- *Protection* of the wound from infection should be provided by covering the wound with an appropriate sterile dressing until wound closure is achieved. Some highly contaminated wounds may require prophylactic antibiotics. The anti-tetanus status of all patients with traumatic wounds must be considered.
- *Closure* of the wound should only take place if the wound is very clean and is <6 hours old. Wounds >6 hours old or considered more heavily contaminated should not be closed until the risk of infection has passed. Wound closure can only then be achieved with the most appropriate available method such as sutures, clips, or adhesives.
- *Follow-up* assessment of the wound is essential so that any wound infection (see ➲ Wound infection, pp. 206–207) or problems with healing can be detected.

Where wounds are not closed, e.g. where there has been tissue loss, healing by secondary intention and the principles of moist wound healing need to be considered. Wound dressings should be chosen that do not adhere to the wound bed and maintain the optimum environment for healing. 'Tulle' dressings are often not the most appropriate in such instances as they often stick to the granulating tissue and several low- or non-adherent/silicone-coated dressings are now available which are more suitable. Granulating traumatic wounds should be disturbed as little as possible. All conditions required for wound healing, such as warmth and good nutrition, should be considered as part of the care plan.

Major traumatic wounds

Extensive wounds can result from severe trauma—including degloving injuries and burns. Such wounds present a challenge to the orthopaedic team, particularly where significant skin and other tissue have been lost. Such wounds are prone to infection and other issues such as fluid loss from wound exudate. Their management must involve the plastic surgery team—with potential for skin grafting and other procedures. Wound care will be provided in accordance with their recommendations while care continues in an orthopaedic setting for other aspects of their injuries.

Further reading

Bryant RA, Nix DP (2016). *Acute and Chronic Wounds: Current Management Concepts*, 5th edn. St. Louis, MO: Elsevier

Soft tissue injury 1: muscle and tendon

As described in ➔ Chapter 2 (pp. 50–53), the musculoskeletal system comprises soft tissue as well as bone. Soft tissues include muscles, tendons, ligaments, and cartilage that make up the boundaries and connections between bones and the muscles that facilitate bone and joint movement. The soft tissues covering the skeletal system are even more prone to injury than bone itself and frequently need medical attention. Skeletal injuries such as fractures and dislocations often include significant soft tissue injury which must be considered when planning treatment. Managing soft tissues may be more important than managing the fracture itself.

Muscle injury

Muscle injury, or strain, can occur during sport or exercise. Muscles provide the power for movement, placing them under considerable stress. Most acute injuries occur as a result of over-contraction or overstretch of muscle tissue which is particularly vulnerable to injury if it is stretched in a direction which is outside its normal plane of activity.

Varying degrees of damage can be caused to the muscle fibres, resulting in focal inflammation, pain, and swelling. Muscles have a very rich blood supply, so bleeding, contusion, and haematoma are common. The hamstring, quadriceps, and gastrocnemius muscles of the leg are particularly prone to injury. The severity of the injury can be classified by how much muscle fibre is damaged—varying from minor separation to full rupture of the entire muscle. Partial tears are the most common.

As with all soft tissue injuries, acute management, for at least the first 48 hours after the injury, should begin with 'RICE':

- *Rest*—until the inflammatory phase has subsided and pain is reduced. Crutches may be required to rest a lower limb injury. Lengthy immobilization of a muscle can, however, result in slow recovery. Consequently, as inflammation subsides, passive, and then active, use of the muscle should take place while gradually increasing in intensity. This will maintain the function of the associated joints
- *Ice*—use of ice (see ➔ Pain management, pp. 142–143) will help to reduce bleeding, inflammation, and associated swelling
- *Compression*—tubular bandages or compression garments are thought to be useful in preventing further bleeding at the site of injury and help to support the affected muscle/s. The value of support/compression bandaging, however, is debated as evidence is limited
- *Elevation*—of the affected area also helps to reduce bleeding and swelling during the acute phase of the injury.

Acute inflammation should subside after 3–4 days and the injury will take a further 2–3 weeks to heal, but may need further weeks or months to regain close to previous strength and flexibility, depending on the severity of the injury. Muscle fibres need to be stretched in order for new collagen to be laid down in the correct lines of function. Gradual rehabilitation of the muscle, especially in athletes, needs to be carefully planned and monitored. Once inflammation has subsided, the gradual active use of the injured muscle should be supervised by a physiotherapist. Athletes often need to be discouraged from returning to full activity too soon after the injury to avoid increasing the length of time inflammation takes to subside.

Tendon injury

Tendons are resistant to injury and acute strains and ruptures of tendons are unusual—they are more likely to avulse (pull away from the bone) under excessive strain.

A common site of tendon injury is the Achilles tendon which is under strain when the foot is in dorsiflexion or plantarflexion as it provides the attachment for the large muscle on the back of the calf to the calcaneum. The pathology of the injury and repair is like that of muscle described earlier. Patients with Achilles tendon rupture often say that they heard a snap at the time of injury, followed by intense acute pain and loss of function of the foot and ankle, resulting in a limp and including loss of plantar flexion of the foot. Again, swelling and pain are significant features and should be managed with 'RICE' particularly in the first few days after injury.

The treatment of Achilles tendon rupture may be either surgical repair or conservative management. Conservative management involves the use of immobilizing casts or splints followed by a period of serial casts or functional bracing for 8–10 weeks.

Care and support

As with many types of injury, patients with soft tissue injuries are likely to be immobile for varying periods of time and require information and psychosocial support as well as physical care, especially those who are athletes and/or whose livelihoods depend on good functional recovery.

Soft tissue injury 2: ligament and cartilage

Ligament and cartilage injuries are other types of soft tissue injury that, to some degree, behave in a similar way to muscle and tendon injury. Some specific additional issues need to be considered.

Ligament injury

When stretched beyond the boundaries of their elasticity, ligament fibres are unable to return to their original length and will remain stretched. They are also prone to tearing; the whole structure of the ligament can be torn. This can lead to adhesions, tissue degeneration, and loss of function with severe pain and disability. The most common site of ligament injury is around the ankle joint, followed by the knee, because of the strain placed on these joints. Ligament injuries should be taken seriously as they can be debilitating and affect an individual's activities of daily living for several weeks.

Ligament injuries are often termed 'sprains', 'strains', or 'ruptures' and are classified according to three grades of severity:

- *Grade 1*—a few fibres have been damaged; resulting in relatively mild pain and swelling over the affected ligament
- *Grade 2*—damage has occurred to a significant number of fibres; resulting in partial rupture of the ligament and there is intense pain and swelling which may affect the entire joint
- *Grade 3*—there is enough injury to fully rupture the ligament so function and stability of the joint may be affected and there will be severe pain and swelling.

Ligament strain can also cause avulsion fractures where the ligament pulls away from the site where it is attached to the bone—often pulling a fragment of bone with it.

Healing of ligaments follows a pattern of haematoma formation and inflammation followed by the proliferation of collagen fibres over a period of ±6 weeks. However, the remodelling and maturation phases of ligament repair may take a year or longer, resulting in a ligament that does not regain its previous strength, stretch, and flexibility. This results in a structure that will be prone to injury if placed under strain in the future. The collagen fibres of ligaments are not well vascularized but are designed to remodel themselves by making new fibres—the right conditions for this to take place must be facilitated. This includes the use of the RICE (see ➲ Soft tissue injury 1, p. 356) acute phase treatment plan. Severe ligament injuries, particularly full ruptures, may require surgical repair or replacement surgery particularly for the cruciate ligaments of the knee (see ➲ Soft tissue injuries of the knee, pp. 446–447).

Cartilage injury

Cartilage damage, tears, and ruptures are usually caused by indirect trauma. Cartilage, particularly hyaline/articular cartilage (see ➲ Ligaments, tendons, and cartilage, p. 52), can also be damaged by degenerative conditions such as arthritis and other arthropathies. Articular cartilage is sometimes damaged when underlying bone is fractured and this can lead to secondary OA

The most common site of cartilage injury is the menisci of the knee (see ➲ The knee, pp. 74–75).

Cartilage injuries are usually treated conservatively in the first instance. Initial treatment will involve rest and physiotherapy with a gradual return to activity. Surgical options may include repair, removal, transfer, or implantation. Healing is inhibited by the poor blood supply to cartilage.

Peripheral nerve injury

The peripheral nervous system includes all nervous tissue outside the CNS, (the brain and spinal cord). The peripheral nerves transmit impulses to and from the CNS.

Peripheral nerves are closely associated with bone and muscle and are made up of axons, nerve cell bodies, and dendrites. Dendrites are the input-receiving portion of a neuron; they are short and tapered with many branches. Axons propagate impulses towards another neuron, muscle fibre, or gland cell and are a long cylindrical projection.

Bundles of nerve fibres are bound by a sheath of connective tissue (perineurium) and several bundles are surrounded by a fibrous sheath (epineurium) along with a blood supply. All the nervous system can be subject to injury but the peripheral nerves, which supply the limbs, are very sensitive to damage. Disruption to their structure leads to degeneration of the fibre and faults in conduction of sensory and motor impulses along the nerve. The axons (the main conduction unit) can regenerate at a rate of 1–5 mm per day depending on the separation of the two damaged ends of the nerve.

There are three main grades of nerve injury:

Neurapraxia

Neurapraxia is the mildest grade of nerve injury. Often due to blunt trauma and compression, the ensuing inflammatory response causes transient loss of neural conductivity; the nerve generally recovers spontaneously within a few weeks.

Axonotmesis

Axonotmesis is a more severe grade of injury caused by compression which results in disruption and damage to the axons and surrounding myelin sheaths with degeneration of the nerve; regeneration of the axon is possible at a rate of 1 mm per day so may take months for healing to occur.

Neurotmesis

Neurotmesis is the severest grade of nerve injury and involves partial or complete severance of the nerve with disruption of the axon and myelin sheath; the nerve may be completely divided by penetrating trauma or severe traction injury. Nerve repair does not usually occur without surgical intervention which has variable success.

Nerves prone to injury include:
• Upper limb—axillary, brachial, radial, ulnar, and median nerves
• Lower limb—femoral, peroneal, tibial, and sciatic nerves.

Assessment

Peripheral nerve injuries are often associated with musculoskeletal injuries such as fractures, dislocations, or penetrating trauma. There is a need for full neurovascular assessment of the affected limb as many symptoms of peripheral nerve injury manifest distally to the site of injury. Depending on the nature and severity of the injury these symptoms may be transient or permanent and include:

• Pain—neuropathic in nature
• Weakness—muscle grading monitored
• Altered, or loss of, sensation
• Loss of function.

Investigations may include:

• X-ray—if there is associated skeletal injury
• Nerve conduction studies—to distinguish the severity of the nerve damage
• MRI—to visualize peripheral nerve structure.

Care and management

The grade of injury, the nerve involved, and the treatment choice of conservative or surgical management will all determine the ongoing care required by the patient.

With a severe injury (axonotmesis), it may be many months before the patient knows how much residual damage there is and how this will affect their function. They require sensitive support, involving a complete holistic approach to their care management. This will include full explanation and information of their injury and provide them with physical, psychological, emotional, spiritual, and socioeconomic support.

Patients with the severest peripheral nerve injury (neurotmesis) may face life-changing disability as a result of their injury; while it is important to encourage them to have a positive attitude, they should be advised on realistic expectations of future function.

Following nerve repair, a period of enforced immobilization with splints may be required to protect the nerve anastomosis and surrounding tissue from overstretching. Due to sensory impairment in the limb, it is important to carefully observe and care for the skin, as pressure ulcers can occur easily where the skin is insensate. Joint stiffness can be a significant problem if recovery takes many weeks or months, so patients need to be taught to perform passive joint exercises to prevent this.

Where dysfunction is permanent, patients may require an orthosis to be fitted to assist their daily living activity abilities. Patients may require sensory retraining, especially where sensory loss in a limb places them at risk from burns and other injuries.

Further reading

Wellington B (2014). Soft tissue, peripheral nerve and brachial plexus injury. In: Clarke S, Santy-Tomlinson J (eds) *Orthopaedic and Trauma Nursing*, pp. 265–75. Oxford: Wiley Blackwell.

Crush injuries and traumatic amputation

Pathophysiology of crush injury

Crush injury is damage caused by blunt trauma from compression and cavitation of the tissues under the area of impact. This may include soft tissue and skeletal injury along with damage to underlying organs and structures. Damage occurs, not only to the tissue structure, but to the microcirculation to that tissue and to the main blood and nerve supply traversing the area. Several issues must be considered:

- In severe injuries, large areas of tissue damage may occur and, because of the impact on the blood supply, necrosis often ensues and can result in the death (necrosis) of large areas of tissue. This can only occasionally be revitalized by repair of blood vessels.
- A significant problem is that large areas of necrotic tissue are attractive to anaerobic bacteria, leading to severe infection—including possible invasion by the organism responsible for gas gangrene (*Clostridium perfringens*).
- Crush injury can result in the release of toxins from damaged muscle tissue into the bloodstream, leading to a rare condition commonly known as 'crush syndrome' or *rhabdomyolysis* which can lead to acute kidney injury and other organ failure.
- A pattern of severe comminution is often seen in underlying fractures. Management of the skeletal injury, however, must be secondary to the soft tissue and organ injuries as these can lead to critical illness and death.

Assessment and management of crush injury

Prolonged extraction from the scene may result in a patient who is seriously ill—most often due to hypovolaemic shock. Many patients with crush injuries require major resuscitation and subsequent care in an intensive care unit, especially if there are multiple injuries (see ➔ Multiple injuries, pp. 330–331).

- Close observation of physiological signs along with assessment of the neurovascular status of the limb are essential. Crush injuries are extremely painful and the assessment and management of pain is essential—requiring opiate analgesia and PCA if the patient is well enough to cooperate (see ➔ Patient-controlled analgesia and epidural, pp. 146–147).
- Once physiological stability has been achieved, the definitive management of the injury itself can be considered. If the circulation to the limb cannot be restored, amputation may be the only surgical option.
- If the microcirculation to the limb is viable, or can be restored, the first priority is to manage the soft tissue injury—involving debridement of devitalized tissue, tissue repair, and skin and tissue grafting under the supervision of the plastic surgery team.
- Risk of infection is offset by meticulous aseptic cleansing and dressing of large wounds may need to take place in the operating theatre by a plastic surgeon. The wound must be continuously assessed for signs of infection (see ➔ Wound infection, pp. 206–207).

- Associated fractures must be managed in line with recommendations for other compound and comminuted fractures (see **➔** Open (compound) fractures, pp. 346–347). External fixation is often used until the soft tissue injury begins to improve (see **➔** Care and education of the patient with external fixation, pp. 392–393).
- Compartment syndrome is a significant potential complication in a limb with such severe tissue damage (see **➔** Compartment syndrome, pp. 198–199).

Traumatic amputation

Traumatic amputation can occur following both crush and blast injuries to a limb and can occur in four ways:
- The limb is totally or partially severed at the time of the incident due to the mechanism of injury and cannot be repaired
- The limb is trapped and has to be amputated in order to free the patient
- The limb is so severely damaged that it is not viable and the only course of action is amputation soon after arrival at the hospital
- The limb is amputated during the first few days or weeks following injury once the damage becomes more apparent

One problem with traumatic amputation is that the surgeon often has very little choice over the nature of the stump and wound, making wound healing and rehabilitation more difficult than following elective amputation. The fitting of prosthetic limbs is also more difficult.

Skilled psychological support from practitioners who have an in-depth understanding of the issues and can help the patient to deal with the sudden loss of a limb is needed. The patient and family have little time to prepare psychologically, so may have to deal with the amputation as a sudden event, adding to the already distressing trauma they have suffered. When they are ready, many patients benefit from talking to others who have adjusted to the loss of a limb in similar circumstances.

Further reading

Greaves I, Porter K (2004). Consensus statement on crush injury and crush injury syndrome. *Accid Emerg Nurs* 12:47–52.

Injury management

Casting: an overview

Casting has been used for several hundred years. It involves the use of different materials to immobilize injured and deformed limbs while they heal. Fracture management often still involves immobilization of the affected limb or body part in a rigid cast until enough bony union or healing allows mobilization. Plaster of Paris (POP) remains the most widely used material for constructing casts as it is relatively low cost in comparison to other casting materials. Synthetic materials were introduced from the 1970s onwards to supplement the already common use of POP. The mechanical properties of such materials have been studied and their benefits have been clearly shown. Despite this technological advancement, however, the techniques of applying casting materials have remained relatively unchanged for many years except for a few new practices.

Use of casts

A cast is a shell, made from POP or synthetic material, designed to encase a limb or, in some cases, larger sections of the body. This is used to hold a fracture, surgical site, or injury in position until healing is confirmed. Casts can also be used, serially, to correct joint deformities.

Some of the many functions of casts include:

• Supporting fractured bones, controlling movement of fragments, and resting damaged soft tissues
• Stabilizing and resting joints where there has been ligament damage
• Supporting and immobilizing joints and limbs postoperatively until healing has occurred, e.g. after nerve or tendon repair
• Correcting deformities by either wedging the cast or application of serial casts
• Providing pain relief by making sure tissues are rested
• Making removable splints to aid progressive mobility programmes or prevent deformity
• Preventing removal of or tampering with dressings or wounds
• Aiding the healing of pressure ulcers or foot ulcers
• Making negative moulds of body parts so that there can be accurate construction of orthotic or prosthetic appliances.

Casting materials

There are many types of casting materials. They fall into four distinct categories:

• *POP*—these bandages are made from gauze impregnated with POP, a powdered form of gypsum. When water is added, the gypsum recrystallizes and hardens in a heat-releasing reaction facilitating mouldability of the cast for a short period of time. POP takes between 2 and 8 minutes to set but is not fully set or at its maximum strength for 24 hours. Although POP is less expensive than alternatives, it is difficult to apply and becomes weak when wet
• *POP with melamine resins*—melamine resins set after being in contact with water, reinforcing the cast and producing a lighter and more radiographically translucent cast than those made only of POP

- *Materials which have undergone polymerization*—when resin undergoes polymerization, the small molecules of resin link to form long-chain polymers. This changes the resin's state from mouldable to rigid, a process usually activated by water but which can be activated by other agents
- *Low-temperature thermoplastics*—these materials contain plastic with properties that change with temperature; they are soft and mouldable when heated and harden when cool.

Selection of casting materials

There is much discussion about which casting materials are suitable and appropriate for what purpose, often depending on surgeon or applier preference. Despite its popularity, POP is not ideal as it has a poor strength-to-weight ratio. It also adversely affects the definition of radiographs, is difficult to apply, and takes a long time to fully dry. Some patients prefer POP as it is more supple at the edges than synthetic casts which feel rougher and can more easily damage the skin. POP also has the added advantage of being significantly cheaper and can easily be split or bivalved if swelling occurs. Synthetic casts, however, have a greater resistance to wear and tear are lighter, helping patients to maintain their activities of living. They cannot be used on patients who have a history of allergies and gloves must be worn by the person applying the cast.

Ideally, a casting material should be:
- Easy to mould to body contours but quick setting
- Non-toxic both to the patient and the user and clean to use
- Unaffected by fluids
- X-ray transparent
- Easy and safe to remove and easy to alter
- Permeable to air, odour, exudate, and water
- Safe and non-flammable
- Light and strong
- Cheap and available in several sizes.

The choice of the most suitable material for the individual patient should be made by the practitioner after careful assessment of the patient using evidence-based practice and working within the medical prescription.

Casting: safe application

The application of casts is a highly skilled activity and should only be conducted by those with the relevant training, education, skills, experience, and qualifications. Staff training should involve:

- The development of skills and knowledge in musculoskeletal injuries and their management
- The principles of fracture healing
- Musculoskeletal anatomy
- The properties and use of casting materials
- Application techniques
- Safe adaptation, revision, and removal of casts
- The complications of casts and cast aftercare.

If casts are poorly or inappropriately applied, the patient is placed at risk of injury and professional and legal action may ensue. Cast application involves manual dexterity and it is best done by those who are experienced and practise it daily. Those who do not practise casting, but care for individuals in a cast, also need to know how casts are applied to care for the patient effectively after application.

Application techniques

Casts should be applied considering the following principles:

- Reading and checking the medical cast prescription
- The provision of adequate pain relief prior to the application of the cast
- Correct and comfortable positioning of the patient to facilitate the cast application
- The patient's skin should be fully assessed before the cast is applied. Any sore areas or wounds should be carefully padded and a record made of their condition
- The colour, movement, and sensation of the limb should be checked and recorded
- Protection of the patient, cast applier, and environment from spillages of casting material and water
- All jewellery must be removed
- Availability of all the materials, staff, and equipment needed to apply the cast in the correct position
- Full preparation and consent of the patient so that they know exactly what will be happening and in what ways they will be expected to cooperate
- Stockinette and/or padding should be applied carefully without wrinkles and should neither be too thin nor too thick (stockinette should not be applied to a patient who is having a manipulation of a fracture or is having a full plaster cast applied). Extra attention should be paid to bony prominences such as the malleoli of the ankle and the tibial crest at the shin
- Casting materials should be applied according to the manufacturer's instructions using timings and water temperature as instructed. Water temperature is critical, as the curing of casting materials causes an exothermic reaction. Using water that is too warm may result in burns

- The cast should be applied quickly but carefully, ensuring that it is not too loose and not too tight
- The casting material should be moulded to the shape of the limb and according to the type of cast required
- The cast should also be carefully smoothed using the palm of the hand, not the fingers
- Particular care should be taken to ensure that the cast begins and ends at the right point so that the cast is not too close to areas such as the back of the knee and base of the toes and that important joints are left free to enable the patient to move them
- The edges of the cast should be as smooth as possible without sharp edges; the stockinette (if used) is turned over to ensure the edges are smooth
- Extra care must be taken to ensure that there are no undulations or dents in the surface of the cast—these will be reflected inside the cast and may cause pressure/cast sores.

Cast aftercare

Casting materials cure and set at different rates so it is important that the practitioner advises the patient how long their cast will take to set. During this period the patient should be advised to rest the limb or body part as much as possible. The colour, movement, and sensation of the limb should be checked, recorded, and any changes from pre-application of the cast reported. Usually the patient should not bear weight on the cast until it is set, even then only on medical staff instructions. Limbs should be elevated and rested on a pillow. Casts should be left uncovered for the first 48 hours to allow them to dry. They should be handled as little as possible until they are fully dry to avoid dents.

Patients should be advised not to get the cast wet. Although some casting materials are waterproof, the underlying padding is not and patients should be told that if they get the cast wet, the padding will become waterlogged and will cause sores under the cast.

Aftercare of the patient is extremely important and, as stressed in the following topics, the patient needs a full awareness of how to care for their cast, what complications may occur, and what to do and who to contact if they occur. This information must be given to them verbally and in writing to ensure that they comply.

Casting: potential complications

Application of an appropriate and good-quality cast should leave the patient comfortable and with a well-supported limb. There are several potential complications to consider:

Cracking, softening, or breakdown of the cast

This occurs if the cast is mishandled. Patients need verbal and written instructions on how they should treat their cast. Following initial application, practitioners (or the patient) must observe the cast hourly for any problems until it is dry. If problems occur, the cast may need to be reinforced or re-applied following medical review.

Bleeding through the cast

This may occur if a cast is applied over a traumatic or surgical wound. Initially, the cast should be observed hourly, reducing this as the patient condition dictates and the cast dries. If any seepage is seen through the cast, this should be marked and medical staff must be informed if the seepage is increasing, excessive, or smelly.

Circulatory and nerve impairment

This can occur due to a poorly applied cast or due to swelling of the limb. Swelling within a rigid cast rapidly leads to increased pressure within the limb (see ➋ Compartment syndrome, p. 198). This affects circulation and nerve conduction and prompt action is essential in preventing irreversible damage. Patients should know when to alert practitioners so that prompt action can be taken. Until risk of swelling has subsided, it is essential that the limb is observed for colour, movement, sensation, warmth, and capillary refill. Initially this should be hourly.

Arterial compression

Practitioners should check extremities to see if they are white, blue, or purple (black is a very late sign of arterial compromise). The toenail bed does not return to pink when pressed with the finger and movement of the digits will be limited and painful. Peripheral pulses should be observed if possible and any change should be reported. An absent pulse is also a very late sign.

Venous pressure

The patient's limb should be observed for redness pain and/or swelling. Any worries should be reported to medical staff immediately.

Nerve compression

Pins and needles, numbness, and limitation of movement must be reported immediately.

Fluid volume deficit (cast syndrome)

This is a condition that can occur in patients who have a body cast applied to the torso, pelvic area, or abdomen. It is sometimes called *superior mesenteric artery syndrome* but is usually known as *cast syndrome*. It can occur following prolonged supine positioning, spinal orthosis, or application of body casts. The practitioner must observe for vomiting or nausea and/or abdominal pain and inform medical staff immediately. Patients who go home in a body cast need to be aware of when to contact the hospital, as this can occur several weeks or months after cast application. It is believed to occur through hyperextension of the spine which causes compression of the duodenum between the superior mesenteric artery and the posterior aorta. This may lead to partial duodenal obstruction and then full obstruction. To avoid this, an abdominal window should be made in the cast to allow for distention after meals and on position changes. If the patient has nausea or vomits, they should be fasted and a nasogastric tube may be passed to enable recording of the type and quantity of the emesis. The patient should be repositioned onto their abdomen if possible and the cast may be bivalved or removed. If this condition is left untreated it can be fatal, as obstruction of the superior mesenteric vein can lead to gastrointestinal haemorrhage and necrosis.

Pressure/cast sores

Sores under the cast can occur either due to poor cast application, poor patient education or objects being used to relieve itching under the cast. Observations need to be made for:
• Pain and/or burning under the cast
• Localized heat on the cast
• Disturbed sleep and restlessness
• Swelling of the extremities after the initial swelling has subsided
• Discharge through or from the cast with or without an offensive smell.

The cast can be eased back or trimmed to observe the area, but extra padding should not be added as this will only increase pressure. A window can be cut in the cast to inspect the site, but this must be replaced to prevent pressure at the edges of the window. If the skin is broken, medical staff must be informed. If the area cannot be observed easily, then the cast may need to be bivalved to allow access. If a foreign object inside the cast is suspected an X-ray may confirm where this is and then a decision can be made as to whether the cast is removed and reapplied.

Stiffness of joints

The limb and joints immobilized by a cast can become stiff. This can be overcome once the cast has been removed by an adequate exercise programme. Patients need to be instructed to continue to move limbs not held by the cast, otherwise these will also become stiff.

Skin reactions

It is unusual for a cast to produce an allergic reaction. However, the padding that is used can be an allergen or irritant. Often the patient will have had a history of a previous reaction. The key things to observe for are complaints of itching, non-localized burning pains, blisters, and rashes on the skin. Medical staff must be informed, and the cast will need removal and reapplication with a different type of padding.

Care of casts

Following the application of a cast it is important that the patient is given the opportunity to take control and maintain their own care. Patients can usually self-care in their own homes with support from family and health professionals. However, the presence of a cast can make it difficult or impossible for patients to self-care and greater input from practitioners will be needed where patients do not have family or friends who can help to provide that care or their function is significantly affected.

Immediately following cast application

It is important that practitioners:
- Ensure the patient is comfortable and the limb is elevated on a pillow to prevent the cast being dented and allow it to dry
- Check the cast edges and trim, if necessary, to ensure the joints can move fully. Trimming can be done with scissors or a knife if the cast is not yet set. If it has set, shears or an electric cast cutter may be required. Once a cast has been trimmed, the trimmed edges must be padded, and the stockinet taped in place
- Areas of the cast that may come in contact with body fluids should have waterproof tape applied to the edges to help keep the cast clean and dry
- If there is swelling the cast may need to be bivalved, but this should only be done on the instructions of medical staff as bivalving may disturb the fracture position
- Full written and verbal instructions should be given to the patient and/ or carer
- Ensure the application of the cast and all other details have been documented in the care records.

Documentation

The following should be recorded:
- Date and time of application
- Name of patient
- Diagnosis and rationale for the cast and under whose instructions
- Cast type
- Cast instructions given and how given
- Cast check date
- Who applied the cast.

Every cast application must be recorded in the patient's care records, as should every check, adaptation, removal, and all complications/untoward incidents. This ensures that everyone involved in the patient's care receives adequate information to enable safe practice. As patient education and advice is crucial, it is important that all information given to the patient is documented.

Patient education and advice

Both verbal and written information should be given to patients in a way that they will be able to assimilate it. Any specific activities should be demonstrated to the patient. It is essential that patients understand their cast and why they have had it applied. Information should also be given to carers so that they can identify a potential problem and know when to contact or return to the hospital. Information about exercise should also be given to the patient and carers as appropriate. Mobilizing when in leg casts is crucial and instructions on how to use mobility aids is also very important; all patients must be assessed using this equipment prior to discharge (see → Aids to mobility, pp. 172–173).

Self-care deficit

Some patients in a cast may find that they are unable to carry out their usual activities of daily living. Some may take practice and some adaptation will be needed when any limb is immobilized. A comprehensive assessment by the MDT must take place to ensure the patient will be able to cope with the cast at home. This will depend on several factors:

• The patient's previous level of independence
• The patient being able to accept a different level of self-care than they had before
• Any assistance that can be offered by friends and/or relatives
• Practical advice given, e.g. how to maintain personal hygiene in a cast.

If activities of daily living are severely affected, short-term alternative accommodation may be required where a higher level of care can be provided.

Body image disturbance

Some patients find it difficult to cope with the fact that they must wear a cast and may be distressed by the image of their limb following the removal of the cast. A positive self-image concept can be promoted by the clear explanation of what the limb will look like following removal of the cast. Reassurance that the skin and hair on the limb will return to normal after several weeks will also help.

Casts: removal and bivalving

Removing a cast is a skilled task and should only be undertaken by practitioners with the skills and knowledge to undertake this safely. Removal is usually achieved by bivalving the cast (cutting the cast in half along both sides of its length). A cast must be fully bivalved so the patient's limb can be safely and easily lifted out. The technique and equipment used to remove and bivalve casts should always be safe for the patient and operator. The lines along which the cast is to be cut should be marked with a pen or pencil down the medial and lateral sides. The lines should avoid bony prominences to reduce the risk of skin damage.

When bivalving or removing casts, the following principles should be applied:

- Clear, written instructions should be obtained from medical staff
- The patient should be positioned appropriately for the type of cast to be removed and informed consent obtained
- A clear explanation and, if necessary, a demonstration of the procedure and how the equipment is used should be given to the patient
- Equipment and techniques used should not damage the patient's skin
- The patient should be comfortable and not subjected to any pain. Pain relief should be given if the patient requires it before the procedure
- The bivalved cast should be kept in place to support the limb until they are reviewed and it is decided by medical staff that it can be discarded.

Casts may be cut with shears or an electric cast cutter (oscillating saw). Synthetic casts require special shears and saws with tungsten hardened blades. Shears are usually used for children's, small, and upper limb casts. Electric cast cutters must not be used on unpadded casts as the skin beneath will be at risk—it is a myth that skin damage cannot happen. Using the electric cast cutter on children may frighten them due to the noise so shears may be preferable.

Using plaster shears

The blade of the shears passes between the cast and the padding. The hand nearest the cast should be kept parallel to the limb and kept still to prevent the point of the heel of the shears digging into the patient's skin and lacerating it. The shears are then pushed together with the other hand to cut the cast. After both sides have been cut, the plaster is eased open with spreaders and the padding cut with bandage scissors. The padding must be cut all the way through.

Using the electric cast cutter

The electric cast cutter has an oscillating circular blade; the blade does not rotate but vibrates back and forth at high speed, rubbing its way through the cast. It should be used only on dry, padded casts and is held at right angles to the cast, applying light pressure to make a cut. The blade is then removed and reapplied slightly higher or lower down the cast along the line to be cut. The blade must not be dragged along the cast as the skin may be cut; instead an in-and-out motion is used to create the cut.

As with all electrical appliances, the cast cutter should not be handled by someone with wet hands. The blade may become very hot and burn the skin if:

- It is used continuously for long periods of time, particularly on synthetic materials
- The blade is dragged along instead of using the in-and-out motion
- The padding is thin, and the patient can feel the heat.

The skin can be cut if:

- The cast is bloodstained as the padding may become hard and the saw may cut straight through it
- The limb is swollen as this makes the skin very taut and then it can be easily cut
- The blade is blunt or is damaged
- The cast is unpadded and due care is not taken.

As removing and bivalving a cast can produce fine dust particles, particularly if POP is used, there is a risk of inhalation. To prevent this and to comply with safety regulations, a vacuum removal system should be used.

Post-cast removal care

It is important that the practitioner informs the patient that, when the cast is removed, the limb will have a scaly, withered look. When a cast is worn for any length of time, the upper layers of skin cannot be shed as normal and so collect as flaky yellow scales. The muscles in the limb lose tone and bulk because they are not being used. The patient should be advised that the skin can be washed gently and patted dry. In no circumstances should the skin flakes be pulled off. Oil or moisturizing cream should be applied if the skin is dry.

Orthotics, appliances, and braces

Orthoses is a term used to describe splints, appliance, or braces. An orthosis or orthotic device is an externally applied device used to modify the structural or functional characteristics of the neuromuscular and skeletal systems.[1] Examples of orthotic devices range from a shoe-raise to compensate for leg length inequality to a knee brace worn to support an unstable joint. A prosthesis or prosthetic device is used to replace, wholly or in part, an absent or deficient limb segment,[1] e.g. an artificial lower leg following below-knee amputation. The orthotist is an important member of the MDT in trauma and orthopaedics and provides a specialist service in the assessment, fitting, and maintenance of orthoses. The role of the orthotist includes:

- Advising the team regarding appropriate prosthetic and orthotic prescription, specification, design, and sourcing
- Clinical assessment and examination of the patient
- Design, fitting, and evaluation of orthotic and prosthetic devices
- Providing information and ongoing support to patients with orthotic or prosthetic devices.[1]

The purpose of orthoses

Orthoses have several purposes including:

- To immobilize a limb to reduce pain and promote rest, e.g. a hand splint for repetitive strain injury or inflamed joints
- As part of fixed or balanced traction, e.g. a Thomas splint applied to a leg for a fractured femur
- To prevent and/or correct a deformity, e.g. a Hartshill splint to support the foot, ankle, and lower limb for a patient with a dropped foot
- To provide stability to unstable joints, e.g. a knee brace
- To maintain correct posture, e.g. insoles to correct inversion/eversion deformities.[2]

Care of the patient with an orthosis

If not correctly fitted, an orthosis may cause skin damage due to pressure and/or friction. The practitioner must check the skin frequently and make sure that any early signs of pressure, such as redness, are reported promptly to the orthotist so that adjustment or extra padding can be applied. If the limb becomes swollen with an orthotic device *in situ* this can lead to vessel and/or nerve damage. The practitioner must observe the limb and extremities for signs of impaired circulation and check both sensory and motor function. Patients will need to be given both verbal and written advice on how to care for their orthotic device and how to recognize complications such as pressure sores or circulatory or nerve impairment. Wearing an orthotic device will also impact the patient's body image and the practitioner has an important role in providing psychological support and helping them to adapt to wearing the device. For further details on altered body image, see ➜ Psychological aspects of care, pp. 168–169. It is important that adjustments to orthotic devices are only made by those with the competence and skill to do so as inappropriate adjustment can lead to injury to the patient.

References

1. British Association of Prosthetists and Orthotists (BAPA) (2008). *Guidelines for Best Practice.* https://www.bapo.com/wp-content/uploads/2019/06/BAPO-Standards-Best-Practice-2018-update.pdf
2. Kneale J, Davis P (2005). *Orthopaedic and Trauma Nursing*, 2nd edn. London: Churchill Livingstone.

Further reading

Royal Collage of Nursing (2015). Traction principles and application RCN guidance. London: RCN https://www.rcn.org.uk/professional-development/publications/pub-004721.

Traction: an overview

Traction is a pulling force applied using weights or other devices which aims to manage bone and muscle disorders or injuries. For this to happen, according to Newton's third law of motion—that for every action there is an equal and opposite reaction—traction (countertraction) in the opposite direction is also necessary. Traction allows control of the injured part, facilitating bone and soft tissue healing. Although it is based on simple mechanical principles, care must be taken as traction can lead to complications.

Uses of traction

Traction can be used to:
- Prevent/correct deformity due to contraction of soft tissues caused by injury or disease
- Rest diseased or injured joints, minimizing pain and maintaining them in a functional position
- Prevent contracture of healing soft tissues following joint surgery
- Allow movement of the joints during fracture healing
- Reduce, restore, and maintain alignment of bone following fractures or dislocations
- Control movement of an injured part of the body to facilitate bone healing
- Relieve pain caused by muscle spasm that occurs following fractures and dislocations.

Methods of applying traction

- *Manual traction*—the pulling force is applied manually, usually with the hands
- *Skin traction*—a traction force is applied over a large area of skin which is then transmitted through the soft tissues to the bone
- *Skeletal traction*—the force is applied directly to the bone through metal pins or wires. Skeletal traction is used if traction is to be maintained for long periods of time and when greater weights are required.

See → Figs. 9.1–9.3, p. 381, for examples of different methods of traction. Skin traction and skeletal traction have two mechanisms:
- *Fixed*—where there is a pull between two fixed points, i.e. with a Thomas splint
- *Balanced or sliding*—where the pull is between weights and the patient's own body weight, i.e. Hamilton Russell traction (see → Fig. 9.2).

There are several ways these two forms of traction can be applied:
- Fixed skin traction
- Sliding skin traction
- Fixed skeletal traction
- Sliding skeletal traction
- Combined fixed and balanced traction
- Modified skeletal traction.

The application is dependent on the condition or injury it is for.

Principles of applying traction

- The grip on the body must be secure
- There must be countertraction to balance the traction
- Any weights used should be prescribed and documented
- Cords and pulleys must be applied carefully so there is no friction
- Traction equipment and the patient must be checked every 2–4 hours to ensure:
  - The traction is functioning as planned and is safe
  - The patient is not suffering any adverse consequences of the treatment
  - The traction, once established, must be maintained.

Traction that is not applied correctly can cause considerable discomfort and even further injury to the patient and can delay rehabilitation. It is therefore extremely important that staff responsible for setting up, maintaining, and removing traction are familiar with the principles of applying the traction and that its mechanics are well understood.

Further reading

Newton-Triggs N, Pugh H, Rogers J, et al. (2014). Key musculoskeletal interventions. In: Clarke S, Santy-Tomlinson J (eds) *Orthopaedic and Trauma Nursing: An Evidence-Based Approach to Musculoskeletal Care*, pp. 80–95. Oxford: Wiley-Blackwell.

Royal Collage of Nursing (2015). *Traction Principles and Applications: RCN Guidance*. London: RCN https://www.rcn.org.uk/professional-development/publications/pub-004721.

Skin traction

Skin traction involves the application of traction to a large area of the skin using adhesive tape or strapping. This acts on the muscles in order to exert a pull (see Fig. 9.1) along with countertraction. It can be used in fixed traction (using a Thomas splint) or sliding traction (see Fig. 9.2). The aim of skin traction is to straighten and immobilize limbs and to assist in maintaining correct alignment. This allows bones, muscles, and joints to heal. The value of some types of skin traction has been questioned over the last few decades, but it is still uses in some settings. For example, the use of skin traction for the management of pain in preoperative pain in patients with proximal femoral fractures has been discredited. Skin traction is still, however, commonly used to treat femoral shaft fractures in children <2 years of age using Bryant's (or Gallows) traction (see Fig. 9.3). Dunlop's traction is occasionally used for upper arm fractures in children (see Fig. 9.4). Because traction is used less frequently, skills are being lost and traction should only be applied by practitioners who have the appropriate skills and knowledge.

Application of skin traction

Adhesive plaster or non-adhesive foam extensions are applied to each side of the limb below the level of the injury with a spreader bar about 10 cm from the base of the foot. This is attached to traction cord on which the pull is exerted either through a Thomas splint or sliding traction with a pulley and weight. Sometimes a sling is placed under the thigh and incorporated into sliding traction—this is known as Hamilton Russell traction (see Fig. 9.2). The extensions are secured with bandages. Adhesive extensions are most reliable and less likely to slip, but cannot be used for patients who are adhesive allergy/sensitivity. The skin should be checked regularly for signs of reaction and other skin breakdown. The following should be considered in the application of skin traction:

• Skin traction should be avoided in patients with fragile skin, ulcers and tears, eczema, and other dermatological conditions and poor circulation
• Bony prominences such as the malleoli and tibial crest should be protected with padding
• Bandages should be applied firmly but should not be too tight. In particular, the area at the back of the knee should not be tight as major nerves and blood vessels are close to the surface here
• The patella should not be covered with bandages so that passive exercise can be carried out during physiotherapy
• Care should be taken over the Achilles tendon at the back of the heel as this is prone to pressure from the bandages if they are not loose enough or padding has not been applied
• A full 10 cm of clearance should be left between the bottom of the foot and the spreader bar to allow foot exercises to be conducted to prevent dropped foot.

The principles of the care of skin traction are described on → Traction daily care, pp. 386–387.

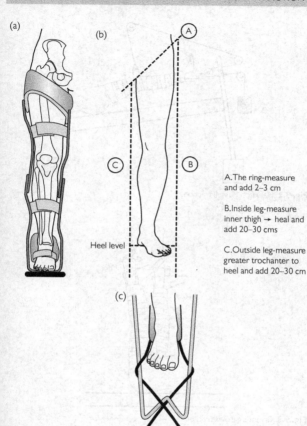

(a)

(b)

A. The ring-measure and add 2–3 cm

B. Inside leg-measure inner thigh → heal and add 20–30 cms

C. Outside leg-measure greater trochanter to heel and add 20–30 cm

Heel level

(c)

Fig. 9.1 (a) A leg fixed with a Thomas splint. Reproduced from the *Oxford Handbook of Clinical Specialties*, 8th edition, with permission from Oxford University Press. (b) Measuring for a Thomas splint. (c) Attachment of traction cord to a Thomas splint.

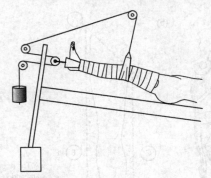

Fig. 9.2 Hamilton Russell traction.

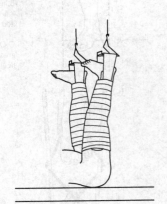

Fig. 9.3 Bryant's gallows traction.

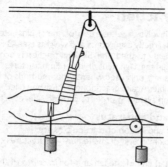

Fig. 9.4 Dunlop's traction.

Further reading

Duperouzel W, Gray B, Santy-Tomlinson J (2018). The principles of traction and the application of lower limb skin traction. *Int J Orthop Trauma Nurs* 29:54–7.

Skeletal traction

Skeletal traction involves the insertion of metal pins into bone to which traction is applied directly using cords and weights (see ➲ Fig. 9.5, p. 385) to exert traction directly to the bone. Skeletal traction is occasionally used to reduce and maintain the alignment of lower limb fractures. This, however, is now uncommon and is only used where other methods of fracture management are not feasible. Again, practitioners must be skilled in application and care of the traction system in order to provide safe, effective care.

Traction pins and apparatus

Common sites of application of traction pins are:

- The upper (proximal) end of the femur—for fractures of the pelvis and hip
- The lower (distal) end of the femur—for fractures of the upper or mid femur
- The upper end (proximal) of the tibia—for fractures of the lower femur and around the knee
- The calcaneum—for fractures of the of the tibia and ankle
- The skull—for the management of fractures of the cervical spine.

Two main types of pin are used: *Denham pins* are threaded in the centre where they are inserted into the bone, while *Steinman pins* have no thread. The ends of both pins are sharp so must be padded to provide protection from injury. Stirrups are usually applied to the pins to which the traction cord is attached. The amount of weight needed should be prescribed by the medical team in the patient's notes.

The traction may incorporate a Thomas splint (see ➲ Fig. 9.1, p. 381) or a Braun frame (Fig. 9.5) to support the limb. It is essential that countertraction is provided by either elevation of the foot of the bed or use of a suspended Thomas splint.

Management and care of skeletal traction

Skeletal traction must only be applied under medical instruction and guidance. The position of the fracture should be checked by weekly X-rays reviewed by the medical team. The traction should be continuous and not removed unless under medical instruction as this is likely to disrupt the fracture site.

The complication rates of skeletal traction are thought to be very high because of patient immobility and the invasive nature of the pin and traction apparatus. The general principles of traction care should be followed (see ➲ Traction daily care, pp. 386–387). Care of skeletal pins is described on ➲ Traction daily care, pp. 386–387. Daily care of skeletal traction is described on ➲ Traction daily care, pp. 386–387.

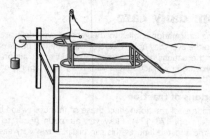

Fig. 9.5 Calcaneal traction supported on a Braun frame.

Traction: daily care

The following information applies to the general everyday care of traction in addition to the everyday holistic care of the patient. The care will depend on whether the patient has skin traction or skeletal traction and should always be provided by practitioners who have been appropriately trained and educated.

Complications of traction

The complications of traction reflect those of immobility and bedrest (see ⊃ Mobilization, pp. 170–171). However, attention needs to be paid to the skin on the affected limb as this can break down very easily. The following daily care principles reflect the need to maintain safety and prevent complications.

Care of skin traction

- All traction equipment, such as beams and hinged clamps, should be checked daily. This ensures that they remain tight and have not become loose with patient movement
- The traction should be checked at least every shift and whenever the patient is moved, particularly following physiotherapy or when the patient has been to radiography as the traction may have shifted
- Check the patient's skin at least 4-hourly to identify signs of pressure or friction
- Check the bandages to ensure they have not become loose or slipped
- The traction cords and knots should be checked to ensure no fraying or slippage—only non-slip knots should be used
- All cord ends should be short and tied back on themselves with adhesive tape to prevent fraying
- The alignment of the cords should be checked to ensure that the appropriate pulling forces are maintained
- Pulleys need to be checked at least each shift to ensure that they are free running as this minimizes friction and ensures the traction is working effectively. They may also need oiling to make sure they run freely and are not noisy at night
- The cords must rest in the pulley and there must only be one cord per pulley wheel to prevent friction
- Weights need to be checked to ensure the correct weight is maintained as documented in the nursing notes. They should not be resting on the floor or any other surface as this will compromise the traction's efficiency
- Weights should also be checked to ensure they hang free
- Observe for loss of fracture position, e.g. sagging
- Bed aids should be *in situ* such as bed cradles to keep the bed clothes away from the patient and ensure that the traction cords run freely
- Countertraction should always be checked and maintained to ensure the efficacy of the traction (see ⊃ Fig. 9.2, p. 382)
- Care should usually be given with the traction *in situ* and it should not be removed.

Care of skeletal traction

Skeletal traction requires the following additional care (see also ➲ Pin site care, p. 394):

- If pins are used to hold the traction, the pin sites need to be checked at least each shift for any signs of infection
- Pins also need to be checked each shift to ensure they have not become loose or moved
- Pointed ends of pins or wires need to be padded to prevent injury.

Care of Thomas splint traction

All the previously discussed principles apply to Thomas splint traction but with the following additional considerations:

- The Thomas splint should fit correctly
- Every shift, the patient's skin under the splint ring should be checked and gently moved to prevent pressure sores. The patient can be taught to do this if able. Light oiling of the ring and skin may be helpful to prevent friction. Talcum powder should not be used as it forms small balls when damp which cause pressure
- The skin should be kept clean and dry
- The splint ring should also be checked for increasing pressure due to swelling; elevating the foot of the bed a little more may help, but if the pressure is excessive the splint may need to be changed
- The groin should be checked for pressure—abducting the limb may help
- Observe the ring for soiling after bed pan use; the splint must be changed if soiled.

Thomas splint traction

A Thomas splint is a long leg splint that extends from a ring at the hip to beyond the foot (see ➔ Fig. 9.1a, p. 381). The Thomas splint, in conjunction with traction, is used to immobilize and position a fractured femur in a pre-operative or postoperative patient or for transportation and emergencies.

How to measure and prepare a Thomas splint

Selecting a Thomas splint

(See ➔ Fig. 9.1b, p. 381.) The most important decision to be made when selecting a Thomas splint is the ring size. The ring can be half, full, or split. To get the correct size, measure obliquely around the thigh of the patient at the highest point on the uninjured leg and add an extra 2 cm which will allow for any swelling. Thomas splints come in various lengths so, to obtain the correct length, the patient's inside leg from the perineum to the heel needs to be measured and 20–30 cm added to the measurement to allow for dorsi- and plantarflexion of the foot. The outside of the leg should then be measured from the greater trochanter to the heel and, again, 20–30 cm added. The Thomas splint can be for a left or right leg; look at the splint from the ring end and the medial side of the splint will be the shorter. This should give the correct splint size but when applying the splint, it is advisable to have available one size smaller and one size bigger just in case.

Preparing a Thomas splint

Calico slings should be used to cover the splint—or other fabric that provides sufficient rigidity to support the leg. The slings are looped over both sides and secured laterally using safety pins. Tubular elastic bandages should not be used as they do not provide enough support under the fracture site. A layer of wool should be placed on the covered splint and a pad to go under the fracture site to act as a fulcrum.

The Thomas splint can now be used with skin or skeletal traction.

Thomas splint with skin traction

The patient should be given adequate pain relief and then the skin traction extensions, adhesive or non-adhesive, should be applied while the limb is held using manual traction (see ➔ p. 378). When bandaging the traction in place, the knee should be left free to prevent pressure on the peroneal nerve. Once this is in position, the Thomas splint can then be applied. The patient needs to be warned that it may be painful, but this will just be for a short time. Two people are needed; one to support the leg and maintain traction and one to slide the splint into position. It should fit right up to the groin against the ischial tuberosity.

Finishing the traction

The traction cords should be attached to the splint and the cords guided over and under the lateral bar and under and over the medial bar (see ➔ Fig. 9.1c, p. 381) preventing lateral rotation. Spatulas can now be used to take up the slack and allow for maintenance and increase in traction force if it is required for fixed traction. If sliding traction in needed, the cords are attached to weights over the end of a bed that is elevated at the foot. The patient's comfort and pain levels should be checked. An X-ray will be needed to check the fracture position and the traction can be altered accordingly.

Thomas splint and skeletal traction

The patient should be fully informed and consent gained for all procedures. Once skeletal traction has been applied (see ➔ Fig. 9.5, p. 385), a metal loop (Tulloch Brown loop) may also be applied to allow direct pull in line with the limb. Either balanced or sliding skeletal traction will then be applied with the Thomas splint. A Pearson knee piece may also be used if there is to be flexion and controlled mobilization of the knee while the patient is in traction. X-rays should be performed to check the position of the fracture.

Care following application of a Thomas splint

The nursing care of the patient will be as for any patient who has had traction applied (see ➔ Traction daily care, pp. 386–387). The following additional issues need to be considered:

- *Ring care*—the ring on the Thomas splint needs checking every time patient care takes place but at least 2-hourly. The skin under the ring should be kept clean and dry and the ring gently moved away from the patient's skin. This relieves pressure and ensures no sores are forming. If the splint ring is not positioned correctly, or becomes too tight due to swelling of the patient's limb, then sores can develop; the ring may need to be removed and replaced or the splint removed completely so the sores can heal. Packing with dressings under the ring should not be done as this adds extra pressure.
- *Groin checks*—also observe for pressure in the groin region; abduction of the leg and splint may help with this.
- *Loss of fracture position*—the splint and the padding should be checked to ensure the fracture site continues to be well supported. If in any doubt, new X-rays may be required.
- *Swelling of the limb*—it is essential to check that the Thomas splint does not become too loose/tight following reduction/increase in swelling of the patient's leg. If this occurs, the splint may need to be changed for a smaller or larger one.

New types of splints are now available with rings that can be altered if the patient's leg swells or decreases in size. This avoids having to remove the splint to alter it.

Further reading

Gray B, Santy-Tomlinson J (2018). The Thomas' splint: application and patient care. *Int J Orthop Trauma Nurs* 30:20–2.
Royal Collage of Nursing (2015). *Traction Principles and Applications: RCN Guidance*. London: RCN https://www.rcn.org.uk/professional-development/publications/pub-004721.

External fixation

External fixation involves the surgical application of metal apparatus with pins and/or wires that penetrate both cortices of the bone and are attached to an external metal frame (see Fig. 9.6 and Fig. 9.7). It is used in the management of complex fractures, corrective surgery, limb reconstruction, and limb lengthening. The wires or pins allow fixation of the apparatus into the bone to provide skeletal support above and below the fracture or surgical site. Through the external frame, it allows manipulation of the position of fractures or osteotomy (incision of bone made surgically). Such apparatus allows access to wounds and damaged soft tissues as well as skeletal stability. This allows the patient to bear weight through the limb while the bone heals. As weight bearing is known to increase the rate of bone healing and growth, external fixation is often used where there are complex fractures that are difficult to manage and in the management of deformities.

There are two main types of fixator devices:
- Monolateral fixators involve the use of half-pins that penetrate the bone and stop in the second cortex (see Fig. 9.6)
- Circular fixators use finer-bore wires which penetrate through soft tissue and bone and are attached, under tension, to a circular frame with struts connecting the circles (see Fig. 9.7).

Complications

External fixation devices may remain *in situ* for many months while bone healing takes place. The main complication is pin site wound infection (see ➔ Pin site care, pp. 394–395). Pins, wires, and other parts of the fixator can become loose and it is important that the patient recognizes when this has happened and knows how to contact someone for help. Patients should be as active as possible in order to prevent the complications of immobility. On rare occasions pins or wires can break. Joint stiffness or contractures can occur where pins are close to a joint. Drop-foot can also occur in lower leg fixators where there are pins around the ankle or where wires have transfixed tendons or muscles. This can be avoided with good foot supports, exercise, and physiotherapy. Keeping joints flexed is often more comfortable for the patient, but this should be avoided. Pillows should not be placed behind knees as this causes flexion deformities. Joints, particularly the foot and knee, should be supported in a neutral position until mobilization takes place.

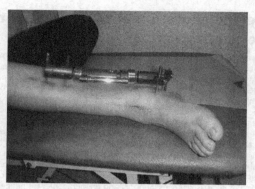

Fig. 9.6 Monolateral fixator. With permission. Hannah Pugh and Anna Timms, Barts and the London NHS Trust 2010.

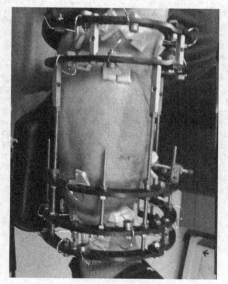

Fig. 9.7 Circular (Ilizarov) fixator. With permission. Hannah Pugh and Anna Timms, Barts and the London NHS Trust 2010.

Care and education of the patient with external fixation

Most care of the external fixator will take place in the patient's home. The patient and carer will need to be taught how to meet their own care needs, along with regular attendance at, and support from, the hospital team. Some patients will take longer than others to learn the skills required. Structured teaching sessions alongside clear, simple, information booklets are often helpful. Being able to contact someone within the team by telephone for advice and support is essential.

Part of the purpose of external fixation is for patients to mobilize with the external fixator *in situ*. The surgeon and the physiotherapist will be able to advise how much the patient should mobilize and how much weight they should bear on the affected limb. Initially, patients may be reluctant to weight bear as much as instructed and they will require assistance from walking aids such as crutches. Support and encouragement is needed from the MDT and regular visits to the hospital may be necessary until the patient is confident. Pain from the area around the pins can be a significant issue and good pain management with appropriate pain assessment, analgesia, rest, and elevation can help to manage the pain. This allows the patient to mobilize effectively. When limb reconstruction and limb lengthening are taking place, daily adjustment of the frame will be required. Patients and carers must be closely supervised while conducting this activity until they are confident with it.

Personal hygiene and clothing are important aspects of care. Patients must be encouraged to keep the fixator clean and dry. Although they can be allowed to shower before pin site care, the fixator should otherwise be protected from becoming wet. Sturdy shoes should be worn if possible when mobilizing. It is preferable for the fixator to be covered with clothing as this protects it from damage and from dust and other environmental contaminants and hazards which might lead to infection. Due to the bulky nature of the fixator, it may be necessary to adapt clothing and footwear and to provide padding in some circumstances to prevent the sharp parts of the fixator from damaging skin, bedding, furniture, etc. Many patients prefer to keep the fixator covered when in public places. Other adaptations to daily life are needed to maintain independence as for any patient with reduced mobility.

Psychological care

Both pre- and postoperatively, patients and their families need as much in-formation and support as possible. Living with an external fixator is not easy. Many patients benefit from sharing their experience with others who have, or have had, external fixation and need constant support from the healthcare team. The appearance of an external fixator and the associated pin site wounds can have a psychological effect on patients and those around them and body image will often be affected. Staff and carers need to be sensitive to this. In extreme cases patients can become depressed as a result of the impact of the fixator and the underlying condition on their lives.

Further reading

Newton-Triggs N, Pugh H, Rogers J, et al. (2014). Key musculo-skeletal interventions. In: Clarke S, Santy-Tomlinson J (eds) *Orthopaedic and Trauma Nursing: An Evidence-Based Approach to Musculoskeletal Care*, pp. 80–95. Oxford: Wiley-Blackwell.

Pin site care

External fixation, skeletal traction, and some forms of orthopaedic surgery require the use of externally protruding (percutaneous) pins or wires to enable fixation of apparatus to bone. Because of the presence of the pin or wire protruding through the skin, the wound is constantly subjected to an inflammatory foreign body reaction. This means that standard wound care aimed at wound healing is not necessarily relevant. Pin site infection is the most common complication of external fixation and its prevention is one of the most important aspects of care.

Guidelines for pin site wound care

Although there is only a small amount of reliable research evidence on which to base pin site care. It is important that practitioners keep abreast of the most recent research as well as established wound management principles. The following wound care principles must be followed:

• Pin sites should be disturbed as little as possible. Cleansing and
  redressing once a week (once the wounds have settled after surgery)
  should be sufficient
• Healthcare staff should maintain strict aseptic technique during wound
  care and patients/carers should be taught a clean dressing technique
• Each pin site should be cleansed gently using non-shedding gauze soaked
  in a solution of antiseptic and alcohol
• Crusts (crystals) and scabs should not be removed but may fall off, often
  as part of the gentle cleansing process discussed previously
• Wounds should be covered with a sterile, key-hole dressing of material
  which does not shed fibres
• The dressings should be secured with a device such as bandage, bung, or
  clip. This exerts gentle pressure on the area around the pin to prevent
  the skin from moving up and down the pin or 'tenting' around the pin.
  This prevents formation of a dead-space beneath the skin that will
  encourage bacterial growth.

Patient and carer education and support

Giving the patient responsibility for their own pin site care is both a good way to help them to maintain independence and helps to reduce infection by ensuring that there are as few people carrying out wound care as possible. Children and adults who are unwilling or unable to carry out their own wound care also benefit from having their wounds cared for by a family member or other carer. It is vital that the patient or carer fully engages with the practice of good wound care and understands the rationale for everything they need to do. This is most important with regard to hand hygiene and other aspects of infection control. A simple leaflet with clear diagrams or photographs should be used to supplement verbal information and demonstration. Patients also need to be aware of the potential consequences of wound infection as this may, ultimately, lead to the failure of the fixation if pins have to be removed due to severe infection. This can result in abandonment of the fixation. Deep pin site infections may lead to osteomyelitis (bone infection) which is very difficult to eradicate (see ➔ Osteomyelitis pp. 272–273).

Recognizing infection

One important aspect of education is ensuring that both patients and carers can recognize pin site infection when it occurs. This is so that it can be treated quickly and does not spread and become a major infection. It is also important to recognize the difference between the inflammatory reaction to infection and the milder, ongoing inflammatory reaction to the presence of the pin. The main symptoms of pin site infection which staff, patients, and carers need to be aware of are:

- Increasing pain around the pin—new, different to, and worse than the pain experienced previously related to the presence of the pin
- Redness which increases and spreads out from around the pin
- Purulent discharge—some clear, straw-coloured discharge is normal. However, when infection is present this may increase or become purulent (cloudy and creamy or brown). The absence of pus does not mean that there is no infection as not all organisms produce pus
- Some patients may feel generally unwell as if they have a cold or flu.

Taking a wound swab is of no use initially as it will often simply only identify commensal bacteria normally found on the skin and it may delay treatment.

Treating infection

Infection is often unavoidable, and many patients will suffer more than one infection over the period their pins are *in situ*. It is essential that any infection is treated as quickly as possible so that it does not deepen or spread. Most infections are caused by *Staphylococcus aureus* and it is, therefore, advisable that a suitable oral antibiotic is prescribed, and the course completed. Infections that do not respond may be caused by a less common organism and taking a wound swab for culture and sensitivity can be helpful so that the appropriate antibiotic can be prescribed. Increased frequency of wound care may be necessary while infection settles.

Further reading

Royal Collage of Nursing (2011). *Guidance on Pin Site Care*. London: RCN https://www.rcn.org.uk/professional-development/publications/pub-004137.

Regional musculoskeletal injuries

Spinal fractures

The bony spinal column can be injured following significant trauma such as falls from a height, blasts, extreme sports, or road traffic collisions. One exception is fractures that occur as a result of conditions such as osteoporosis: fragility fractures in which the vertebral bodies collapse following relatively minor trauma as a result of poor bone resistance to injury.

Types and mechanisms of injury

The spinal column protects the spinal cord from injury in all but the most severe incidents.

Common types of spinal fracture include:

- Burst, wedge, and compression fractures of the vertebral bodies
- Fracture dislocations of the vertebrae
- Seat-belt induced injuries causing hyperflexion/extension of the spine—usually at the neck.

Unstable and stable injuries

The spine is stabilized by interlinked bony structures. This is supported by a complex series of ligaments which bind the bony structures together and allow flexibility. Damage to a combination of these can lead to instability of the spine: fractures and dislocations can displace and cause trauma to the delicate spinal cord. Fractures of the spine are classified into stable or unstable injuries.

Fractures which are deemed 'stable' are those which are unlikely to displace and cause subsequent damage to the spinal cord. Unstable injuries are more likely to displace. Instability can be due to disruption of the spinal column either through bony injury or ligament damage—often both. The spinal column and each of its vertebrae are divided into three 'columns':

- *Anterior column*—this includes the anterior half of the vertebral body and the anterior longitudinal ligament
- *Middle column*—this includes the posterior wall of the spinal canal and the anterior part of the vertebral bodies, along with the posterior longitudinal ligament and posterior part of the annular ligament.
- *Posterior column*—this is vital for stability and comprises the neural arch, the pedicles, spinous processes, and the posterior ligaments.

Unstable injuries are most common when there is damage to the middle column along with involvement of either the anterior or posterior columns.

Management and care

If a spinal fracture is suspected, a full medical examination will take place in the emergency department (ED) (see ➔ Principles of assessment of the bony spine, pp. 96–97). Along with spinal X-rays, this will determine if the fracture is stable or unstable. An unstable spinal fracture should be assumed until proven otherwise. If patients are handled inappropriately, an unstable injury that is currently not impinging the spinal cord can move and cause spinal cord damage. Where there is an unstable injury that is impinging the spinal cord, further movement can result in worsening the damage (see ➔ Principles of physical assessment of the spinal cord, pp. 94–95).

Spinal 'immobilization' is essential until a full assessment of the injury has taken place and the senior medical practitioner gives permission ('clearance') for this to be removed. Immobilization involves the use of spinal boards, collars, braces, and strapping which prevent movement of the spine and maintain its anatomical alignment while assessment and care take place. Spinal immobilization must be carefully applied and checked for pressure on the skin. It is particularly important to 'clear' the cervical spine for injury—this is done by X-ray examination of the cervical spine in both AP and lateral views—prior to removing spinal immobilization. X-rays must include a clear view of C7 as this can be difficult to visualize because of the shoulder girdle.

To allow examination of all areas of the body, and to facilitate care, all patients with suspected or actual unstable spinal fractures should be log-rolled by a team of staff skilled in this procedure. Log-rolling involves moving the patient from side to side in a rolling motion in a very controlled manner which enables correct anatomical alignment of the spine to prevent injury to the spinal cord.[1] The procedure should be led by an experienced team member who should take the head of the patient. At least four other team members are required.

Stable fractures are usually managed with a short period of bedrest until the pain subsides and physiotherapist-guided remobilization can then gradually begin. A spinal brace may be applied until fracture healing takes place to assist with the management of pain and maintaining the correct posture. Surgery is occasionally required to correct spinal deformity.

Unstable fractures of the spine with or without spinal cord injury (SCI) require stabilization. This can be performed by open reduction and internal fixation of the fracture using rods, screws, or cages. Dislocation and subluxation require reduction under anaesthesia.

Conservative management of unstable fractures involves a longer period of 6–12 weeks of rest until the fracture heals. For lumbar and thoracic spine injuries, flat bedrest is required with log-rolling for nursing care. Specialist turning beds can assist in skin, hygiene, bowel, and bladder care. In all cases careful handling of the patient is essential—this must ensure that the spinal column always remains in correct alignment. In the case of cervical injuries, skeletal cervical traction may be applied with traction callipers attached to the skull. Neck movements must be carefully controlled. This may be followed by a period with a halo brace and jacket which allows the patient to mobilize while controlling neck movement.

References

1. da Cunha Rodrigues IF (2017). To log-roll or not to log-roll – that is the question! A review of the use of the log-roll for patients with pelvic fractures, *Int J Orthop Trauma Nurs* 27:36–40.

Spinal cord injury (SCI)

SCIs are caused by either direct force such as a penetrating injury from knife or gunshot wounds or compression from spinal tumours, but more commonly by indirect force including:

- Forced flexion injury (trauma)—rapid, unforeseen impact or deceleration (most common)
- Forced hyperextension injury—falling up or down stairs
- Compression injury—falling/jumping from height, diving into swimming pool
- Low falls—<6 metres
- Flexion and rotational movements—during deceleration.

The effect of SCI will depend on the level of injury, i.e. damage in the cervical area will have a more severe impact on sensation/movement than an injury of the lumbar spine. SCI can be classified as complete or incomplete. In complete injury there is no motor or sensory function below the level of the injury. With incomplete SCI there will be some motor and/or sensory function below the lesion. Patients may also have a spinal fracture or subluxation/dislocation without damage to the spinal cord (see ➲ Spinal fractures, pp. 398–399).

The incidence of SCI is estimated to be 500–700 people per year in the UK.[1] Young men between 20 and 30 years of age are the most commonly affected. SCI is a devastating injury for both the patient and their family and friends. Therefore, the practitioner has an important role in all stages of care and treatment, from initial assessment of suspected SCI through to rehabilitation and helping the patient adapt to their disability. The principles of good psychological support are essential (see ➲ Psychological aspect of care, pp. 168–169). Principles of care/treatment of the spinal cord injured patient include:

- All patients who have experienced multiple trauma and/or are unconscious should be treated as having SCI until it can be ruled out (see ➲ Multiple injuries, pp. 330–331)
- As soon as patients with a SCI have been diagnosed and stabilized they should be transferred to a specialist spinal injuries centre. Here specialist facilities and staff are available for both immediate care and rehabilitation. Recovery and rehabilitation can take many months depending on the level of injury
- A patient with suspected or confirmed SCI should not be moved unless the staff involved have received specialized training; the only exception to this is if the patient's life is in mortal danger if they are not moved
- The cervical spine should be immobilized using a semi-rigid collar while initial assessment and treatment take place.

The topic ➲ Emergency management of a suspected SCI, pp. 402–403 provides detail of emergency management and rehabilitation following a SCI.

Reference

1. Harrison P (2000). *Managing Spinal Cord Injury: Critical Care: The Initial Management of People with Actual or Suspected SCI in High Dependency and Intensive Care Units.* London: Spinal Injuries Association.

Further reading

Bellinger N (2007). Rehabilitation of patients with spinal cord injury. In: Jester RF (ed) *Advancing Rehabilitation in Nursing*, pp. 171–84. London: Blackwell Publishing.

Committee on Spinal Cord Injury and Board on Neuroscience and Behavioral Health (2005). *Spinal Cord Injury: Progress, Promise, and Priorities.* Washington, DC: National Academies Press.

Harrison P (2000). *HDU/ICU: Managing Spinal Injury: Critical Care.* London: Spinal Injuries Association.

Papathomas A, Robinson J (2017). *The Very Alternative Guide to Spinal Cord Injury.* Sheffield: Easy On The Eye Books.

Wang KW (ed) (2019). *Neurotrauma: A Comprehensive Textbook on Traumatic Brain and Spinal Cord Injury.* Oxford: Oxford University Press

Emergency management of suspected SCI

When SCI is suspected, emergency care involves assessment of the patient to ascertain the nature of the injury. This is known as 'clearance' (see ➲ Spinal fractures, pp. 398–399) as once the patient is 'cleared' of injury there is no further need for immobilization of the spine. Failure to clear the cervical spine can have severe consequences for the patient, leading to secondary SCI and even death. All trauma patients with the potential for SCI must have formal documented spinal clearance by a senior medical practitioner before any decisions about moving and positioning them can be made.

If the patient is unconscious, the practitioner must assume that there is a cervical spine injury unless it has been cleared by one of the following practitioners using spinal imaging:

- Consultant spinal or orthopaedic surgeon or neurosurgeon
- Consultant trauma team leader
- Consultant emergency physician.

Features which may indicate a spinal injury in the unconscious patient are:

- Flaccid areflexia (absence of reflexes), especially with flaccid rectal sphincter. Flaccid paralysis is a clinical manifestation characterized by weakness or paralysis and reduced muscle tone without other obvious causes such as trauma to the bowel
- Lack of neuromuscular reflexes
- Diaphragmatic breathing
- Ability to flex, but not extend, at the elbow
- Grimaces to pain above, but not below, the clavicle
- Hypotension with bradycardia, especially in the absence of hypovolaemia.

Assessment

- If the patient is conscious and can communicate, a full history should be taken to try and elicit the mechanism/cause of the suspected SCI. Alternatively, information about the mechanism of injury should be sought from any witnesses or prehospital care practitioners
- Examination should be conducted by a senior practitioner who has in-depth knowledge and experience of assessing patients with suspected SCI.

In examining the neck the practitioner should 'look, feel, but do not move the patient',[1] while checking for signs of trauma to the head and face which may have resulted in indirect force to the spine. The neck is then palpated for signs of deformity/tenderness. The full spine should be inspected and palpated, looking for injury/deformity/bruising and tenderness. To examine the spine, the patient must be log-rolled (with a semi-rigid collar in situ) by an experienced team with the most experienced member stabilizing the head and cervical spine. The patient will then require a full neurological examination to include:

- Ascertaining the level of consciousness using the GCS (see ➲ The Glasgow Coma Score, p. 333)
- Assessing motor and sensory function for each dermatome and myotome

- Testing the deep tendon reflexes
- Assessing cranial nerve function.

Clinical investigations

Clinical investigations will be decided by the senior specialist clinician based on findings from the history and patient examination, but are likely to include:

- Spinal imaging—see detail later in this topic
- FBC, U&Es, LFTs, ESR, CRP, blood glucose, and group and save
- A 12-lead ECG.

Imaging

The type of image needed to detect/exclude SCI in patients with multiple trauma will depend on two factors: the patient's GCS (see ⮕ The Glasgow Coma Score, p. 333) and their cardiorespiratory status.

Multiple trauma with cardiorespiratory instability? GCS <9

- CT entire cervical (C)-spine
- CT chest (incl. thoracic (T)-spine)
- CT abdomen/pelvis (incl. lumbar (L)-spine)
- CT abnormal/unclear areas.

Multiple trauma without cardiorespiratory instability? GCS <9

- Plain lateral T-spine
- Plain AP T-spine
- Plain lateral L-spine
- Plain AP L-spine
- CT entire C-spine
- CT abnormal/unclear areas.

Multiple trauma without cardiorespiratory instability? GCS >9

- Plain lateral C-spine
- Plain AP C-spine
- Plain lateral T-spine
- Plain AP T-spine
- Plain lateral L-spine
- Plain AP L-spine
- CT occiput to C3 only
- CT abnormal/unclear areas.

Reference

1. Blom A, Warwick D, Whitehouse MR (eds) (2017). *Apley's Concise Orthopaedics and Trauma*, 10th edn. London: Hodder Arnold.

Care and management of the patient with SCI 1

Once the patient has been assessed and a diagnosis of SCI has been made, the following principles of care should be followed:

- Transfer to the nearest spinal injury centre as soon as possible—the rehabilitation process can take from between 6 months to 1 year depending on the level of the injury, motivation of the patient, and incidence of any complications
- Effective interprofessional working to develop a collaborative rehabilitation plan with the patient and their family
- Surgery to stabilize any bony injury
- Early detection and treatment of complications
- Psychological support for the patient and their family.

There are several serious and life-threatening complications that can occur after SCI:

Neurogenic and spinal shock

Neurogenic and spinal shock following SCI is a common presenting feature of the injury. The practitioner must consider all forms of shock, particularly if the injury is a result of major trauma.

Neurogenic shock

This occurs from the impairment of the descending sympathetic pathways in the spinal cord.

Signs: loss of vasomotor tone and loss of sympathetic innervation to the heart. This causes pooling of intravascular blood and results in profound hypotension. Due to the loss of sympathetic tone the patient is unable to become tachycardic or even bradycardic. This is not a true hypovolaemia and requires judicious fluid management in order not to fluid overload the patient.

Spinal shock

This refers to the neurogenic condition which happens following injury and is due to bruising/swelling of the spinal cord. This can persist for up to 6 weeks post injury.

Signs: SCI patients can present with spinal shock which can compromise their cardiovascular status and stability. All patients with cervical and upper thoracic (above T6/7) injuries will have bradycardia and unopposed vaso-vagal reflex in response to tracheal innervation, i.e. T2–T4/5. Caution when undertaking tracheopharyngeal suctioning is required as overstimulating the vagal nerve during the procedure can lead to cardiac syncope and possible cardiac arrest. IV fluids should be administered judiciously. Careful use of diuretics may be required in early management.

Secondary SCI injury

Patients need to be carefully handled to prevent secondary spinal cord lesions and prevent pressure ulcers.

The North West Midlands Critical Care Network (NWMCCN) recommends:

- Patients are removed from the spinal board within 20 minutes of arrival at the ED
- All patients are transferred from surface to surface using a spinal board with a secure head device
- Spinal column alignment should be maintained throughout all turns, procedures, and transfer manoeuvres
- All patients must be assessed for pressure ulcer prevention needs
- All patients with a SCI and/or complex and multiple spinal column injuries should be managed on a spinal bed within 24 hours. Dynamic/airflow mattresses must not be used
- For ventilated patients, a maximum of 15° bed tilt should be maintained, and the patient must remain horizontal/flat
- *Exception*: patients with a head injury or respiratory compromise will require neurological or ventilation care as a priority.

Autonomic dysreflexia

Patients with SCI are at risk of *autonomic dysreflexia*. This is a life-threatening hypertensive response to noxious stimuli which may be precipitated by fundamental problems such as a full bladder. Close monitoring of the patient is essential:

- Assess the patient for risks or history of dysreflexia to include level of injury, time since injury, and previous symptoms
- Elevate/tilt the bed if appropriate on the advice of the leading clinician
- Administer glyceryl trinitrate spray or tablets.

Typical features of autonomic dysreflexia

Sudden uncontrolled rise in BP, with other signs of sympathetic overactivity:

- Systolic pressures reaching up to 250–300 mmHg
- Diastolic pressures reaching up to 200–220 mmHg.

Other features of autonomic imbalance vary, but may include:
Pounding headache

- Sweating or shivering
- Feelings of anxiety
- Chest tightness
- Blurred vision
- Nasal congestion
- Blotchy skin rash or flushed above the level of their spinal injury (due to parasympathetic activity)
- Coldness with goose bumps below the level of injury (due to the sympathetic activity).

Care and management of the patient with SCI 2

SCI can lead to complications within many of the body systems:

Cardiovascular protection

Patients with SCI can present with spinal shock which may compromise their cardiovascular status and stability. The underlying issue is the loss of functioning baroreceptor reflex and basal sympathetic tone in high spinal lesions. All injuries above T6/7 will have a problem with bradycardia and unopposed vasovagal reflex in response to tracheal stimulus. This applies to those without cardiac sympathetic innervation, i.e. injuries between T2 and T4/5. The following action is required:

• Ensure that a prescription of atropine has been written for use in the event of cardiac syncope or extreme bradycardia
• Fluids to be given judiciously—seek advice from senior colleagues
• Spinal cord injured patients are not able to internally regulate their body temperature (known as poikilothermia) and often are 1° cooler than non-injured patients—use warming devices cautiously.

Respiratory care

Pulmonary complications can have a significant impact for SCI patients:

• All cord- and column-injured patients should be cared for in a supine position. If ventilation is required, the bed should be tilted to an angle of 15° (or more following multidisciplinary case discussion)
• Monitor the patient closely for signs of respiratory distress/fatigue; monitor for hypoxia and hypercapnia
• Patients must be turned every 2–3 hours. Liaise with the physiotherapist regarding a specialized respiratory turning regimen
• Incentive spirometry and non-invasive ventilation as treatment intervention where appropriate. All patients should be referred for physiotherapy to initiate a preventative/prophylaxis regimen, e.g. assisted coughing.

Gastrointestinal protection

There is increased risk of mucosal ulceration due to vagal overactivity (in the high-lesion patient). There is also increased risk of abdominal distension resulting in 'splinting' of the diaphragm. Acute SCI patients present with a transient paralytic ileus. Gut peristalsis must be nurtured to avoid aspiration of gastric contents.

All SCI patients should have an H_2-receptor blocker on admission until discharge to a spinal cord injury centre.

Bowel care

Acute SCI patients will present with definitive neurological bowel dysfunction. Failure to appropriately care for bowel function may seriously affect the patient's bowel rehabilitation and quality of life.

A digital rectal examination must be performed on all SCI patients in the ED by the attending clinician and the findings recorded. A bowel care plan must be instigated on admission which can be modified according to individual response.

Bladder care

Acute spinal cord injured patients present with definitive neurological bladder dysfunction. The paralysed bladder is at significant risk of nosocomial infection. All spinal cord injured patients should be catheterized on admission with a size 14–16-gauge catheter.

Brachial plexus injuries

The brachial plexus is a network of nerves originating from the spinal cord in the cervical spine, formed from the cervical 5,6,7,8 and thoracic 1 nerves. The brachial plexus is responsible for control of movement and sensory innervations in the upper extremity.

Brachial plexus injuries are uncommon but awareness of them is important as they can lead to long-term disability, impacting all aspects of a patient's life.

An acute brachial plexus injury (ABPI) can occur following falls, road traffic collisions (especially motorcycle), contact sport, and penetrating trauma when the nerves may be stretched, crushed, or torn. Damage to the upper nerves happens when the shoulder is forced down and the neck stretched up and away from the injured shoulder. The lower nerves are injured when the arm is forced above the head. Injured nerves prevent signals to and from the brain, resulting in loss of function of the hand and arm. There are a few brachial plexus conditions that may be caused by benign or malignant tumour. There is also an obstetric (perinatal) condition associated with shoulder dystocia and resulting in palsy of the limb.

Assessment should include:

- History of injury and presenting symptoms including mechanism and associated injuries—note any bony injury, vascular disruption, and time of onset of any paralysis
- Observation of the face—Horner's sign affects the ipsilateral eye, causing a constricted pupil with drooping of the upper lid and is indicative of disruption to the sympathetic nerve supply to the head and neck
- Pain assessment—pain is a major feature of brachial plexus injury and is related to the extent and level of the nerve damage
- Neck and shoulder pain—exclude cervical spine injury
- Weakness and heaviness of the arm and hand—use the Medical Research Council (MRC) grading scale for muscle strength
- Sensory examination will show altered and diminished sensation of the hand and arm—perform dermatome examination
- Diminished pulses suggest a related vascular injury
- Swelling of the shoulder—exclude glenohumeral dislocation
- Radiographs will show any fractures and any increase in distance between the spinous processes and the clavicle
- MRI scan may show the location of any root avulsion with visible meningocele (sac filled with CSF leaking from spinal cord)
- Neurophysiological tests—these are performed to study nerve conduction but are a later investigation.

Management

- Conservative—depending on the severity of the injury, some injuries will heal over a period of time although this may be lengthy. Passive movements should be encouraged and an orthosis fitted to support a flail limb.
- Surgical—there is a wide choice of surgical intervention but there are no guaranteed outcomes. Open injuries to nerves from penetrating trauma should be surgically explored and repair of divided nerves performed.

Other surgery is usually performed within 2 weeks or after 2–3 months post-injury.

- Direct nerve suturing—minor damage to nerves with approximation of ends in the correct alignment to minimize cross-wiring can be micro-sutured or glued.
- Nerve grafts—nerves are taken from areas such as the sural nerves in the lower leg or cutaneous nerves of the forearm and grafted to bridge the injured segment directly. Regeneration and recovery time slow.
- Nerve transfers—the damaged nerve is reinnervated by connection to a functioning nerve that is expendable. There are many commonly used transfers and surgery is performed closer to the target muscles to enhance recovery.
- Following the results of spontaneous recovery and surgical intervention, there may be late reconstructive procedures possible including joint fusion (arthrodesis; commonly shoulder and wrist), functioning free muscle transfer, and tendon transfer.

Care

In the acute phase following a traumatic injury, advanced life support may be required until the patient is stable. Care will then vary depending on the type of injury. The aim is to help the patient achieve optimal physical and psychological health. The following should be considered:

- Following nerve grafting and nerve transfers the limb will be immobilized. Passive exercises should be conducted to reduce joint stiffness. Splints should be worn to maintain correct position of the arm and shoulder.
- Realistic explanation of the injury, treatment options, and prognosis.
- Patient information should explain nerve tissue grows slowly (at ~1 mm per day) and maximum recovery may take several years.
- Pain—chronic neuropathic pain commonly experienced; expert pain management advice should be sought; pharmacological and alternative therapies are considered such as mindfulness, TENS, and CBT. More complex options include a dorsal root entry zone (DREZ) procedure which may be performed as a late attempt to resolve intractable neuropathic pain.
- Holistic approaches to care must attend to physical, psychological, emotional, and socioeconomic needs, including an awareness of body image issues, self-worth, sexuality and relationships, and setting realistic future goals.

The success of treatment is often uncertain; the patient may be left with an arm that is relatively useless, being flail and swollen or contracted and muscle wasted. Amputation may be considered for a paralysed and in-sensate limb that is a hindrance to function but the patient must understand it is unlikely that neuropathic pain will improve following amputation.

Further reading

Gray B (2016). Quality of life following traumatic brachial plexus injury: a questionnaire study. *Int J Orthop Trauma Nurs* 22:29–35.

Hems TEJ (2015). Brachial plexus injuries. In: Shane Tubbs R, Rizk E, Shoja M, et al. (eds) *Nerves and Nerve Injuries*, Vol. 2, pp. 681–706. London: Elsevier.

Wellington B (2014). Soft tissue, peripheral nerve and brachial plexus injury. In: Clarke S, Santy-Tomlinson J (eds) *Orthopaedic and Trauma Nursing*, pp. 265–75. Oxford: Wiley-Blackwell.

Upper limb injuries

Assessment

Upper limb injuries include those to the shoulder, humerus, elbow, radius, ulna, wrist, and hand. While there are several possible mechanisms of injury, injuries to the arm are commonly caused by a fall on an outstretched hand (often known as 'FOOSH'), occurring when the patient has put out a hand to break the fall. Assessment of upper limb injuries must include an assessment of the whole limb. Patients may report significant pain in one part of the arm but also have sustained an injury elsewhere. The practitioner must examine the upper limb from the clavicle (see ➲ Principles of physical assessment of the shoulder, pp. 86–87) and shoulder to the wrist and hand—beginning away from the area where the most obvious injury is and moving towards it.

Immediate care

In the first few days following injury, swelling is the most significant problem. This should be managed as follows:
- The arm and hand should be elevated as high as possible during the first 24–48 hours
- Even if the hand is not affected and there is no or very little swelling, it is essential that finger rings and arm jewellery are removed as soon as possible. Swelling can increase and can affect parts of the limb not directly around the injury. Rings rapidly become too tight, restricting the circulation to the finger and resulting in neurovascular damage. If jewellery cannot be removed easily it may need to be cut off
- Frequent exercise ('wiggling') of the fingers will aid venous return—assisting in preventing and managing swelling in the hand and arm.

Arm slings

In the first few days following injury or surgery, slings may be helpful in supporting the limb and in reducing and preventing swelling as well as elevation on pillows the arm can be supported using:
- *Triangular bandages* provide simple means of elevation. There are two main types of slings:
  - The *high arm sling*—used for support and for higher elevation (see Fig. 10.1a)
  - The *broad arm sling*—used for support across the whole arm (see Fig. 10.1c)
- Some injuries benefit from a *collar and cuff* type sling (see Fig. 10.1b) which is used when support is only required at the wrist.

Several points need to be considered in caring for patients with slings:
- The sling should be applied with regard for patient comfort and safety
- The patient should be informed about care of the sling and how to reapply it if needed
- The part of the sling around the neck can become uncomfortable; soft padding can be used to combat this
- Slings should not be worn for any longer than necessary as they restrict movement of the joints

- Even with the sling in place, exercises of the fingers, wrist, elbow, and shoulder should be continued to prevent joint stiffness and reduce swelling
- The sling should be removed at least once daily to assess and care for the skin.

Subsequent care

- Fractures and dislocations of the upper limb can have a significant impact on activities of daily living and patient independence, particularly if the dominant arm/hand is affected
- Practitioners must make sure the impact of the injury on the patient's ability to cope at home is assessed. Older patients, living alone, for example, may need support with washing dressing, and preparing food until they are able to use the limb effectively again. The limb should be immobilized for the shortest time possible
- Even with a cast *in situ* many patients can use their hand and fingers to grip and perform activities such as cutting up food. This should be encouraged. This will help to maintain their independence and enhance recovery of the limb, including the muscles which become weak and wasted when not used.

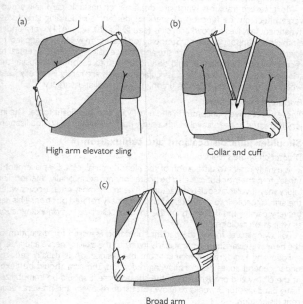

(a)

High arm elevator sling

(b)

Collar and cuff

(c)

Broad arm

Fig. 10.1 Types of sling. (a) High arm sling (triangular bandage). (b) Collar and cuff. (c) Broad arm sling (triangular bandage). Part (c) is reproduced from the *Oxford Handbook of Adult Nursing* with permission from Oxford University Press.

Shoulder injuries

The 'true' shoulder joint (the glenohumeral joint) includes the articulation of the head of the humerus with the glenoid fossa of the scapula. Skeletal injuries to the shoulder include those to the scapula, clavicle, and head of humerus. The shoulder is a very mobile joint with movement in almost all planes and is prone to soft tissue injury. The glenohumeral joint is unstable due to the relative shallowness of the glenoid fossa and there are a complex series of ligaments, tendons, and muscles surrounding the joint. The shoulder is frequently injured following a fall on an outstretched hand or a fall or blow directly to the tip of the shoulder.

Fractures around the shoulder

Clavicular fractures

These are very common and are usually cause by a direct blow to the shoulder—often during a fall. This should be considered when there is a fall on an outstretched hand.

The middle third of the clavicle is usually affected. Fractures are often undisplaced and stable and require little in the way of treatment other than pain management. The fracture tends to heal quickly without complications.

More severe fractures which are displaced or unstable can have an adverse effect on the function of the shoulder and surrounding structures. Treatment involves a broad arm sling (see → Fig. 10.1c, p. 411) worn under clothing to support the arm. Strapping or bracing may also be applied to exert pressure over the fracture site and reduce pain. Pain relief is central to recovery and the patient should be encouraged to recommence using the shoulder as soon as possible. Clavicular fractures are rarely internally fixed when acute but, if there is non-union, may require later surgery.[1]

Fractures of the scapula

These are relatively uncommon and usually involve significant force. The injury is treated conservatively with a sling, pain relief, and early mobilization.

Shoulder joint dislocations and subluxation

Dislocation of the shoulder

This usually refers to dislocation of the glenohumeral joint. Displacement is most often anterior but can also be posterior and, occasionally, inferior. The injury may involve associated fractures. The injury most often occurs when the arm is forced into an abducted and externally rotated position. This can be very painful and deformity of the shoulder can be seen on examination as well as on radiographs.

Following acute injury, the patient should be assessed for disruption of the neurovascular supply, particularly injury to the axillary nerve and artery

Following radiographic examination, the dislocation is usually reduced under general anaesthetic. Following reduction, the arm should be flexed at the elbow and brought across the chest where it should be immobilized using bandages for 3 weeks to allow soft tissue recovery and prevent recurrent dislocation.

Recurrent dislocation of the shoulder

This can occur because, during the first injury, the glenoid labrum is usually torn and leads to loss of stability of the joint. Relatively little force is required. The dislocation is usually reduced easily, and the patient can be advised to avoid activities resulting in dislocation. Where the recurrent dislocation becomes severe, surgery to stabilize the soft tissue structures may be conducted.

Acromioclavicular joint

This dislocation and subluxation may occur with damage to the associated ligaments. If the injury is stable, it will most likely be treated with a broad arm sling worn under clothing. Internal fixation is avoided.

Soft tissue injury to the shoulder

The rotator cuff muscles which surround the glenohumeral joint help to stabilize the joint. Acute tears of the rotator cuff can occur. Frequent minor injury and wear and tear to the shoulder may result in tears of the muscle/s and can lead to pain which may be severe and chronic. Symptoms can be relived with physiotherapy (exercise and heat) and with surgical repair of tears later date pain fails to resolve.

Because of the complex bony and soft tissue structures and the relative ease of injury to the shoulder, chronic pain can be a significant feature of later life so patients may need continued support and treatment from physiotherapy and pain services.

Reference

1. McRae R, Esser M (2008). *Practical Fracture Treatment*, 5th edn. Edinburgh: Churchill Livingstone.

Upper arm injuries

Injuries of the upper arm include various sections of the humerus. The humerus, a long bone, can be divided into the head (proximal), shaft (middle), and condylar (distal) regions. Fractures are usually a result of a fall on an outstretched hand—so the possibility of injury elsewhere in the upper limb or shoulder must be considered. A fall onto the side with the upper arm impacting the ground or by direct violence are also possibilities. Such fractures are most common in older people in the presence of osteoporosis—healing of the fracture may be protracted. Because of the amount of osteoporotic cancellous bone at the distal and proximal ends, fractures of the humerus are often impacted. Injuries around the elbow are considered in more detail on ➌ Elbow injuries, pp. 416–417. Injuries to the shoulder are considered in more detail on ➌ Shoulder injuries, pp. 412–413.

Upper arm soft tissues and other structures

The radial nerve winds around the distal humerus and the radial and ulnar nerves follow notches in the humerus towards the elbow. The brachial artery and its branches supply the arm and branch at the elbow into the radial and ulnar arteries. Elbow movement is brought about by the biceps and brachialis, anteriorly, and triceps, anteriorly. Contraction of these powerful muscles can lead to displacement of fracture fragments, especially when these fragments are sharp; there is a danger of damage to neurovascular structures.

Skeletal injuries of the upper arm

Two regions of the humerus are most prone to fractures with different implications (the distal humerus is considered on ➌ Elbow injuries, pp. 416–417):

Fractures of the head and neck of humerus (proximal)

The head and neck of the humerus are constructed largely of cancellous bone. This is particularly prone to fragility fractures where there is bone weakened due to osteoporosis. Such fractures often have several fragments and may be impacted, meaning that the fracture can be relatively stable and may respond well to conservative management. A broad arm sling or collar and cuff may be employed for this (see Fig. 10.1c, p. 411) where the fracture is complex and there is severe deformity that impacts on potential function. However, an MRI or CT scan may be done for a clearer picture of the fracture and open reduction and internal fixation may be performed.

Fractures of the shaft of humerus

Humeral shaft fractures are often unstable and easily displaced because of the action of the large biceps muscles and lack of support and protection of the arm in this area. Neurological damage is a significant potential complication because of this. The arm, distal to the injury, should be assessed for this throughout the course of treatment. Where there is minimal displacement/angulation and fragmentation of the fracture, some fractures of the humerus can be treated conservatively with a collar and cuff. The weight of the arm allows the humerus to 'hang', producing the effect of traction.

U-slab casts are usually applied. Displaced and comminuted fractures are more often treated by internal fixation or external fixation.

Several nursing factors must be considered:
- Humeral fractures can be very painful
- Bruising of the arm following humeral shaft fractures increases rapidly and early management with ice and elevation to reduce the bleeding into the tissues is essential
- Following fracture reduction, casting, or surgery, it is important to continue to observe for neurovascular compromise
- Humeral fractures and their treatment often make it difficult for patients to lift their arm. This can have a severe impact on activities of living and older people may need assistance
- Care of the skin in the underarm/axillary area is important to avoid skin damage from moisture and pressure.

Elbow injuries

The elbow joint is relatively stable due to the arrangement of its skeletal and soft tissue structures. It is a hinge joint with additional rotation ability. It is commonly injured by twisting forces, falls on an outstretched hand, or directly onto the elbow, and to chronic overuse injuries.

The median, radial, and ulnar nerves and brachial artery all cross the elbow joint so there is considerable potential for fractures (particularly those that are displaced) to cause damage to these structures.

Supracondylar fracture of the humerus

Fractures of the lower third of the humerus, close to the elbow joint, can be difficult to manage. These fractures are particularly common in children and usually result from a fall on an outstretched hand. The fracture is often displaced because of the mechanism of injury and the action of biceps muscles on the anterior aspect of the upper arm. Recognizing displacement is critical to effective management.

The brachial artery runs close to the condyles of the humerus near the elbow and, if the fracture is displaced, disruption of or damage to the blood supply can be caused by the sharp fragment of bone (see Fig. 10.2). The related nerve bundle may also be involved. Damage to the artery can lead to *Volkmann's ischaemic contracture*, a severe complication that may cause permanent flexion contracture of the hand and wrist.

Practitioners should frequently check the radial pulse and note any loss of colour, warmth, sensation, or movement of the limb distal to the injury (particularly the hand and wrist), pain, and/or tingling of the forearm.

Management of supracondylar fractures without neurovascular problems usually involves manipulation and reduction under anaesthesia. Once neurovascular status has been checked, a long arm POP slab with the elbow in flexion can be applied (this allows the triceps muscle to maintain the reduction of the fracture). The radial pulse and neurovascular status of the limb must be rechecked following application of the cast. Swelling is very common, hence the use of a slab rather than a complete cast. A sling should be applied.

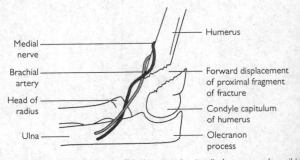

Fig. 10.2 Supracondylar fracture of the humerus showing displacement and possible impingement on neurovascular supply.

If reduction of the fracture cannot be maintained, Dunlop's traction (see ➔ Fig. 9.4, p. 383) may be used. Internal fixation is only used as a last resort but, in extreme cases, wiring of the fracture may be necessary. During and after these procedures the neurovascular status of the arm must be constantly monitored.

Other injuries around the elbow

Other fractures around the elbow include the distal humerus and proximal radius and ulna. The elbow can become very stiff if immobilized, so this is avoided wherever possible. Internal fixation using wires and plates is often required when fractures are unstable. In all cases, physiotherapy is often needed once healing has been achieved to improve elbow function. A stiff joint and/or OA may be a longer-term complication.

Dislocation

Dislocation of the elbow is also most common following a fall on an outstretched hand. Neurovascular impairment is also a potential complication. Reduction is usually carried out under general anaesthesia. A padded bandage and collar and cuff sling should be worn for approximately 2 weeks.

Olecranon bursitis

This is a common example of a chronic condition of the elbow. The olecranon process is the part of the elbow formed by the proximal ulna. It is protected by a fluid-filled sac known as the olecranon bursa. This structure can become inflamed, usually as a result of repetitive pressure. It can also become infected. Immobilization of the joint is not advised. Anti-inflammatory medication may be used. If conservative treatment is unsuccessful, the bursa may be surgically removed.

The elbow is a critical joint for the function of the upper limb and loss of range of movement seriously impedes activities of daily living, particularly in older people.

Lower arm (forearm) injuries

The forearm is made up of the radius and ulna. Both these bones are central in elbow and wrist joint movements, particularly in supination and prona- tion of the arm. These two bones are very commonly injured—particularly during falls on an outstretched hand. The two bones are linked together by a series of ligaments and membranes and move in unison so they are fre- quently fractured at the same time. Associated dislocation of the elbow is common. In children, 'greenstick'/incomplete fractures are frequent in this area—these tend to heal more quickly than other types of fracture.

Assessment

Assessment of forearm injuries is often relatively straightforward as the swelling and pain as well as deformity can usually be clearly seen. It is es- sential that assessment includes a full neurovascular assessment of the arm and hand distal to the injury both immediately after the injury and during treatment as neurovascular damage and compartment syndrome (see ➲ Compartment syndrome, pp. 198–199) are always a risk. Close observation and elevation of the arm are central to preventing and identifying these.

Care and management

Treatment of forearm fractures generally follows the following principles:

Undisplaced stable fractures

Undisplaced stable fractures, particularly those where only one of the two forearms bones is fractured (usually following a direct blow to the arm), are usually treated with a back-slab, then a full cast until union occurs. Simple fractures are sometimes managed using 'focused' rigidity casts which can be removed at night.

Angulated and displaced fractures

These fractures are usually reduced under general anaesthetic. Following reduction, a backslab is applied. The elbow and wrist are included with the elbow usually at 90° flexion and the wrist in a neutral position. A broad arm sling should be used to elevate the arm for the first 48 hours until swelling has subsided. Patients should elevate the arm on a pillow or several pil- lows (depending on sleeping position) at night. Once swelling has subsided, the cast can be completed. Adult fractures usually take 6 weeks to unite. The sling can be discarded once the risk of swelling has subsided (after 2–3 weeks). It is important that the patient conducts frequent exercises to those joints, not included in the cast, such as the elbow and fingers to prevent stiff- ness and avoid further swelling.

Unstable fractures

These are usually treated with internal fixation using plate/s and screws. If the fracture is caused by high-energy trauma/crush injury, is severely com- minuted, and there is an associated wound and severe soft tissue involve- ment, external fixation may be chosen. Angulated and displaced fractures sometimes displace following conservative treatment. The more severe the injury, the more likely forearm compartment syndrome and neurovascula compromise is likely to be.

Follow-up

Simple forearm fractures cause few problems for patients who are usually fit and manage well with most activities of daily living. It is important to remember, however, that frail older patients and those with other physical disabilities can significantly lose independence as a result of these relatively simple fractures. Practitioners working with patients with seemingly 'minor' injuries need to remember that social support/services may be required—particularly by those debilitated by the injury—until the cast is removed.

Fragility fractures

Fractures of the forearm are relatively common as a result of osteoporotic bone (see ➲ Osteoporosis, pp. 252–253). One fracture places an older person at risk of further fractures and patients should be referred for BMD assessment and treatment should osteoporosis be suspected.

Wrist injuries

Injuries at the wrist include sprains, strains, dislocations, and fractures. The wrist is made up of several bones that join to form large and small joints. Following an injury to the wrist, the amount of pain and ability to move the wrist does not reliably determine whether the wrist is sprained or has a bony injury.

Sprains and strains

Sprains occur when ligaments are either stretched or torn. They are usually caused by twisting or pulling and often occur during leisure activity. Symptoms include pain, muscle spasms, swelling, and difficulty moving the joint.

Assessment should include careful history taking to determine the mechanism of injury, examination and palpation to determine areas of tenderness, and X-rays to identify or rule out any bony injury.

Treatment for any injury is dependent on the severity, but all injuries will be eased with RICE. If injuries are more severe, the treatment may include:
• Velcro splints—these can be taken on and off and permit exercises
• Casting—for 2–4 weeks with repeat X-rays after a week.

In either case, the practitioner must ensure the patient receives verbal and written instructions.

Dislocations

Dislocations of the wrist are treated like any other dislocation by being reduced and then held in optimal position (see ➜ Principles of fracture management, pp. 350–351). Aftercare includes reduction and splinting or casting (see ➜ Orthotics, appliances, and braces, pp. 376–377 and Casting: safe application, pp. 368–369).

Fractures

Common wrist fractures are classified as follows:

Distal radial fracture (Colles' fracture)

Fracture of the distal radius is one of the most common injuries to the wrist and is suspected based on the reported mechanism of injury. The symptoms include wrist pain, swelling, and deformity, although not always. X-rays will confirm the diagnosis and determine the treatment required. If the fracture is in alignment, treatment will be a cast in a neutral position for 6–8 weeks with regular checks and X-rays to ensure the position is maintained. Patients will need verbal and written instructions on care of the cast and exercising the arm to prevent stiffness.

If the fracture is displaced, local anaesthetic will be given and the fracture is reduced by manipulating it into alignment. The position will then be held in a cast for 6–8 weeks with regular checks and X-rays to ensure the position is maintained. Patients will need verbal and written instructions on care of the cast and exercising the arm to prevent stiffness.

If the fracture is unstable or severely displaced, surgery may be required. Pins or plates and screws are usually used to hold the fragments in place. This allows for early use of the wrist. Postoperatively, the practitioner should observe the neurovascular status of the hand affected and report any concerns. The patient will need advice on wound care and follow-up on discharge.

Occasionally, an external fixator may be required to hold the fracture (see ➲ Care and education of the patient with external fixator, pp. 392–393).

Scaphoid fractures

The scaphoid bone allows complex and delicate movements of the hand. The bone lies under what is normally called the 'anatomical snuff box', the small indent at the junction of the thumb and the wrist. It has a tenuous blood supply which can make the scaphoid slow or fail to heal. Scaphoid fractures will be diagnosed from the history and mechanism of injury. Symptoms include pain and swelling on the thumb side of the wrist, along with difficulty gripping objects. X-rays will be taken but may not be conclusive as scaphoid fractures often cannot be seen until healing has commenced at 2–3 weeks. Consequently, the patient may be treated in a cast and reviewed at 2 weeks with further X-rays. A CT or MRI scan can be performed to give a diagnosis but is not usually necessary. If the scaphoid is displaced or is not healing, surgery will be considered; this will involve pins or screws and then a cast to maintain the position. Bone grafting may also be used to assist the healing process. Postoperatively, the practitioner must observe the neurovascular status of the affected hand. The patient will need written and verbal advice on cast care, exercises to prevent stiffness, and follow-up on discharge.

There are several other types of fracture of the wrist which may or may not involve radioulnar joint dislocation. Some of these can easily be missed. Many can lead to joint pain, swelling, and deformity if not treated correctly, often requiring open reduction and internal fixation. The nursing management remains similar. The wrist is important in a patient's daily life as we use it in almost everything we do and any injury to the wrist can make everyday tasks difficult to perform.

Hand injuries

The hand is a functional tool that we would have difficulty functioning without. Even what appears to be a relatively minor injury has the potential for a serious loss of function. Most hand injuries will heal well and with little significant loss of function if they are assessed in a systematic manner and treated appropriately as soon as possible. How well the injury heals will depend on the type of injury, the severity of the injury, delays in treatment, and compliance of the patient to a treatment plan.

Fractures of the hand

Fractures of the hand are common and can occur in any of the small bones within the hand. The signs and symptoms of a fractured hand will include:

- Pain
- Swelling and tenderness
- In some fractures there is obvious deformity
- Difficulty moving the fingers
- Shortened fingers
- Depressed knuckle
- Lacerations—if it is an open fracture.

The hand needs close assessment (see ➲ Principles of physical assessment of the hand, pp. 92–93) along with a history of the injury and its mechanism. If a hand fracture is suspected, X-rays will confirm it. Most hand fractures (if they are not displaced) can be treated conservatively in a cast or splint for 3–6 weeks. If the fracture is angulated or rotated, surgical intervention may be necessary. This may involve pins, metal plates and screws, or external fixation (see ➲ Care and education of the patient with external fixation, pp. 392–393). If pins are used, they will remain *in situ* for several weeks so the fracture can heal before removal. Open fractures are treated in the same way, but a dressing will be used over the wound.

Dislocations of the hand

Dislocations of the hand often occur following a fall, a blow, or by being involved in contact sports. The most common dislocations are of the lunate which dislocates anteriorly and can then press on the median nerve giving the patient paraesthesia and weakness of the thumb. The hand may appear deformed, but close examination is required (see ➲ Principles of physical assessment of the hand, pp. 92–93) and an X-ray will confirm the dislocation and rule out any fractures (which are often missed). The dislocation is usually manually reduced: traction is applied with the hand in dorsiflexion and the lunate is pushed back into position and the hand then splinted in neutral position. If the dislocation is missed at first, the delay in reducing it may require open reduction. The aim is always to preserve the function of the hand and stability of the joints.

Amputation of the hand

Amputation of the hand is similar to any other traumatic amputation (see ➲ Crush injuries and traumatic amputation, pp. 362–363). Replantation will be considered if the hand has viable circulation and the patient will gain as much use of their hand as possible. In some cases, replantation may no be possible if the hand is too damaged and amputation and a prosthesis will be the only remaining option.

Care following hand surgery

- Neurovascular compromise—following surgery, regular assessment of the hand must be undertaken, and any deficit reported immediately
- Pain—adequate pain relief is essential
- Swelling—elevation of the arm and the application of ice will help
- MDT assessment—this is important if the patient is struggling with the activities of daily living
- Splints/casts—verbal and written instructions will need to be given to the patient prior to discharge
- Exercises—specific exercises for the hand and fingers will be prescribed by the surgeon and/or physiotherapist; verbal and written instructions and follow-up will be needed
- Wound dressings—both verbal and written instructions will need to be given about dressing changes.

Complications

- Finger stiffness—due to immobilization and insufficient exercising of the hand infection
- Failure to heal—the function of the hand will be affected by non-union of fractures. Bone may need to be excised with or without a prosthetic replacement. As a last resort the hand may need to be amputated
- Avascular necrosis—the bone affected may need to be excised with or without a prosthetic replacement
- Secondary OA—can occur when a fracture or dislocation involves a joint.

Further reading

Schoen DC (2009). The hand. *Orthop Nurs* 28:194–8.

Finger injuries

The fingers are important for fine coordinated movements. Injuries can have a major impact on everyday function, particularly if the dominant hand is affected. Finger fractures are usually caused by a direct blow or indirect stress to the fingers—the finger has been hit, jammed, or crushed. Fractures can also occur when the finger has been pulled or twisted suddenly and forcefully. Amputation of the finger ends is relatively common (see ⊃ Crush injuries and traumatic amputation, pp. 362–363).

Assessment and initial treatment

Symptoms include those of soft tissue injuries or fractures generally. Visible deformity and numb or cold fingers may be evident if the blood supply is impaired. Diagnosis is confirmed by X-ray.

- If a fracture is undisplaced and closed, splinting to the adjacent finger (neighbour strapping) is the first line of treatment
- If a fracture is displaced, it will usually be reduced under local anaesthetic. The finger will need splinting to maintain position. The patient should be advised both verbally and in writing to keep the fingers like this for a week then to take the strapping off
- If the fracture is unstable or cannot be reduced, surgery may be needed (pins, plates, and/or screws). The practitioner must regularly check the neurovascular status of the hand and report any changes.

Verbal and written information needs to be given to the patient about wound care, the use of ice and high elevation to reduce swelling, and exercises following removal of the splint or bandage to prevent stiffness.

Specific fractures

There are two fractures of the fingers which require special consideration:

Bennett's fracture

A fracture at the base of the thumb. This is problematic as there is involvement of the joint between the wrist and the thumb. Common symptoms are swelling and pain at the base of the thumb, usually following a punch injury. If the joint surfaces are still in contact with each other, a cast will be applied. Alternatively, surgery will be needed to align and fix the bones fracture fragments.

Boxer's fracture

A fracture at the base of the little finger near the knuckle which usually occurs following punching a person or object. Symptoms include pain and swelling at the base of the little finger and a bump over the back of the hand just below the knuckle. Management is similar to that for Bennett's fractures.

Finger dislocations

Finger dislocations can disrupt tendons and ligaments. There will be visible deformity and swelling. X-rays will confirm the diagnosis. Most finger dislocations are straightforward and will be reduced under local anaesthetic and then splinted into position. Post-reduction neurovascular checks are essential and should be included in patient instructions.

Tendon injuries

There are several particularly common tendon injuries:

Mallet finger (baseball finger)

Injury to the extensor tendons of the fingers which are torn away from the bone at the end of the finger (distal phalanx). The finger droops and will not straighten fully. There will also be swelling and tenderness around the fingertip. A splint (stack splint) is applied with the finger in neutral position or slight hyperextension for 6 weeks. This should not be removed as this will delay healing.

Skier's thumb (gamekeeper's thumb)

Caused when, for example, skiers fall with an open hand onto their pole, tearing the ligament between the thumb and the palm of the hand (ulnar collateral ligament). There is pain and swelling at the base of the thumb and difficulty holding objects firmly. If the tear is partial it will be treated in a thumb spica for 4–6 weeks. Complete or unstable tears may need surgery with the hand placed in a cast for 4–6 weeks followed by physiotherapy to regain full movement.

Boutonniere deformity

The extensor tendon is torn between the proximal phalanx and the middle phalanx, usually caused by a blow to a bent finger. The middle of the finger droops and will not fully straighten either straight away or 7–21 days later. If not treated, the deformity will be permanent. Early treatment is with a splint for 3–6 weeks followed by physiotherapy-led exercises to improve the stretching and flexibility of the fingers. If the tendon is completely severed, surgery may be needed to improve pain and function, but may not correct the deformity fully.

Ligament injuries

Ligament injuries to the hand include:

Swan neck deformities

Occurring when the ligament responsible finger flexion (volar ligament) is torn between the proximal and middle phalanx. As it heals the ligament becomes slack and the finger bends into a 'swan neck'. A progressive extension splint is applied for 2–4 weeks; slowly increasing the extension, starting at 30°.

Further reading

Wieschhoff GG, Sheehan SE, Wortman JR, et al. (2016). Traumatic finger injuries: what the orthopedic surgeon wants to know. Radio Graphics 36:1106–28.

Skeletal chest injuries

Injuries to the chest wall include fractures of the ribs and sternum which may or may not be part of a severe injury to the chest organs. Major injury to the chest wall can be associated with potentially life-threatening damage to the lungs, heart, and associated structures. Respiratory and cardiac problems must be ruled out when injury is severe. The management of associated and potentially life-threatening injuries within the chest is considered on → Chest trauma, pp. 336–337. This section will consider the assessment and management of uncomplicated skeletal injury to the chest.

Rib fractures

Rib fractures are a common result of a blunt trauma caused by a direct blow to the chest, e.g. from a steering wheel in a road traffic collision, following a fall, or, sometimes, severe coughing. Injuries to a single or small number of ribs are generally uncomplicated and are not dangerous in fit active individuals. If more than three ribs are fractured and the patient has underlying respiratory difficulties, or there are signs of respiratory difficulty, they may be admitted to hospital for observation. Fracture of a significant number of ribs in high-energy trauma may lead to severe respiratory problems such as flail chest and pneumothorax (see → Chest trauma, pp. 336–337) which may be life-threatening.

Older people with osteoporotic bone can be particularly prone to rib fractures.

Assessment of patients with suspected fractures of the ribs should include:

- The mechanism of injury—this may include significant trauma to the chest wall
- Complaint of chest pain; particularly on movement and when breathing. There is often severe and acute pain, particularly on deep inspiration and there is localized tenderness on palpation at the fracture site
- Swelling or deformity of the chest wall. It is important to observe chest movement from both the front and the back
- AP and lateral radiographs can confirm which ribs are affected and the region of the rib, but are not always useful in diagnosis as the fracture may be difficult to see. False negatives are common.

Practitioners need to consider several issues when caring for patients with rib fractures:

- The most significant problem is pain. This can have an impact on respiration. Painful rib fractures can lead to respiratory problems if the patient is reluctant to breathe deeply, particularly on expiration or cough and can lead to a vulnerability to chest infection particularly if the patient has an underlying respiratory disease such as chronic obstructive pulmonary disease or asthma. Ensuring that pain is well managed can help to ensure that chest wall movement is relatively uninhibited.
- The focus of care should be on pain relief and prevention of respiratory problems. If pain relief is adequate, the patient should be able to undertake deep breathing exercises. They should also be encouraged to maintain normal mobility as this assists in breathing. Many patients feel more comfortable sleeping in an upright position, supported by pillows.

- Oral analgesia is usually sufficient. NSAIDs may be helpful in the first 24–48 hours or so, but should not be used in the longer term as they inhibit bone healing and cause abdominal problems.
- Patients with rib fractures often find it difficult to lift their arms, so may find it difficult to wash and care for their hair until the pain subsides. Older people with mobility problems or who are frail may need additional social support.
- Strapping or bandaging of rib fractures is not helpful and is more likely to restrict respiratory function, so should be avoided.

Sternal fractures

Fractures of the sternum are relatively uncommon but occur when there is significant blunt chest trauma—often involving road traffic collisions in which the chest hits the steering wheel or other part of the vehicle. Cardiac contusion is a rare but potentially fatal complication as the heart is at risk of cardiac shock and/or decreased output and arrhythmias due to trauma.

In common with rib fractures, respiratory and cardiac complications must be considered, and the most significant issues are pain, upper arm use, and breathing difficulty because of the pain. Again, pain relief and deep breathing exercises are central to care and recovery. Displaced fractures of the sternum may require internal fixation.

Pelvic injuries

The pelvis is a ring of bone with a series of rings within it. The parts of the ring are joined together by strong ligaments at the sacroiliac joint and the symphysis pubis. The pelvis is a very robust structure which acts as a weight-spreading device from the upper body to the limbs; it also acts as a bony bowl designed to protect the organs sitting within it. For the pelvis to be fractured, significant high-energy trauma is usually required. Mechanisms of injury can vary from a fall from standing (e.g. in older people with osteoporosis) to road traffic collisions and falls from significant heights. Many pelvic injuries are crushing injuries—particularly those of a pedestrian following road traffic trauma.

If the pelvis is only fractured in one place (without damage to the symphysis pubis or sacroiliac joints (Figs. 10.3a,b, p. 428)) then the injury is likely to be stable and the fragments will not move. If there is a fracture in more than one place within the ring of bone and/or there is damage to the symphysis pubis or sacroiliac ligaments, the fracture may be unstable (see Fig. 10.3). The ring may open out or displace or a section of the ring move backwards.[1]

The pelvis contains several of pelvic organs including the bladder, ureters, urethra, and uterus, and the pelvis and surrounding area is well supplied with blood vessels. In unstable injuries there is a significant risk of injury to these organs as well as the major blood vessels and nerves which run through the pelvis to supply the lower limbs. This presents a significant possibility of major haemorrhage and is an important factor in emergency care.

Assessment

Assessment of pelvic injuries involves careful consideration of the injury and its potential effects on internal organs and blood vessels. Radiographic (X-ray) imaging of pelvic injuries is central to understanding the extent and stability/instability of the damage. As far as is practically possible the team requires clear views of the injury to be able to build up a three-dimensional picture. This will enable effective decision-making and management of all aspects of the injury. Initially, a supine AP image of the pelvis may be enough to diagnose factures of the pelvis and inform an early management plan. Further imaging can take place once the resuscitation phase is complete, often involving CT and MRI scans to provide a clearer picture of the extent of bony injury as well as damage to internal organs and other structures.

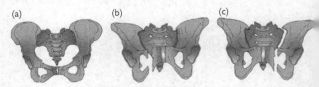

(a)   (b)   (c)

Fig. 10.3 (a) A vertically and rotationally stable pelvic fracture. (b) A vertically stable, rotationally unstable pelvic fracture. (c) A vertically and rotationally unstable pelvic fracture. Reproduced from the *Oxford Handbook of Clinical Specialties*, 8th edition, with permission from Oxford University Press.

Reference

1. McRae R, Esser M (2008). *Practical Fracture Treatment*, 5th edn. Edinburgh: Elsevier/Churchill Livingstone.

Further reading

British Orthopaedic Association (2018). *BOAST – The Management of Patients with Pelvic Fractures*. London: BOA. https://www.boa.ac.uk/resources/boast-3-pdf.html
Slater S, Barron D (2010). Pelvic fractures—a guide to classification and management. *Eur J Radiol* 74:16–23.

Unstable pelvic injuries

Unstable pelvic fractures are those in which there are multiple bone fragments, which may be displaced and/or in which there is disruption to the ligaments of the symphysis pubis and sacroiliac joints. High-energy, unstable pelvic fractures can be life-threatening—partly because of the high-energy mechanism of trauma involved as well as potential damage to major blood vessels and organs resulting in significant haemorrhage and associated shock.

Recommendations for the management of pelvic fractures[1] follow the following principles:

- Early stabilization of the fracture to prevent further haemorrhage and facilitate resuscitation and assessment
- Urgent treatment of haemorrhage and bleeding
- Early CT scanning to assess the extent of injuries
- Early urological input to assess and manage any genitourinary injuries and early ultrasound-guided suprapubic catheterization
- Referral to a pelvic surgery specialist to carry out pelvic reconstruction surgery if required.

Reduction and stabilization of the fracture/s helps to prevent further haemorrhage and shock. Emergency care includes the use of pelvic binding, pelvic slings with weights, or a crossed sheet—to exert side-to-side compression on the pelvis to bring the fragments towards normal alignment. Once general resuscitation has taken place, a pelvic external fixation device will be applied. This will enable stabilization of the fracture and associated injury and facilitate movement of the patient in bed.

Because of the risk of haemorrhage from internal organs, assessment for signs of internal organ damage is essential including consideration and investigation for urological, intestinal, vascular, and reproductive system damage. The most common site of internal injury is the bladder and/or urethra. Ultrasonography and cystoscopy can be used to gain a greater understanding of the nature of any injury.

If injury to the bladder or urethra is suspected, a suprapubic catheter will be inserted to enable urine to bypass a damaged urethra and enable drainage of the bladder while injury is assessed and repaired.

Subsequent care of the patient must consider the following:

- The nature of unstable pelvic injuries often means that the patient is immobilized in bed for many weeks with a very significant risk of complications of bedrest and immobility. All measures much be taken to manage such risks (see ➋ Chapter 5).
- The prevention of the development of pressure ulcers (especially in the sacral area) is a particularly important issue. The nature of the patient's injuries and the use of management strategies such as pelvic slings and external fixation devices mean that the patient will be unable to move independently and is likely to be most comfortable lying supine. Significant pain is likely to add to the patient's reluctance to move. Support surfaces designed for patients at very high risk of pressure ulcer development can be helpful in preventing pressure ulcers and such devices should be chosen and used carefully.

- Manual handling of the patient needs to be carefully planned and executed using appropriate assistance devices such as hoists and sliding boards.
- The care of suprapubic catheters is aimed at the prevention of infection both at the insertion site and through the catheter itself. Strict aseptic technique must be used at all times when handling the catheter or drainage bags. The insertion site may require cleansing and dressing if there is serous drainage. Signs of infection include pain, spreading redness, and purulent discharge from the site.
- Effective pain management is a central aspect of care. Well-managed pain will decrease the chances of complications because the patient is better able to move or be moved.
- Rehabilitation of the patient following significant unstable pelvic fractures will often involve management of chronic pain as well as residual physical, urological, and sexual problems. This requires a team approach to rehabilitation in a setting where the consequences of severe pelvic fractures are fully understood.

The practitioner requires an understanding of the anatomy of the pelvic region—including soft tissue structures and pelvic organs. This is in order to inform care which is initially aimed at saving life and later facilitating recovery and rehabilitation following one of the most significant and debilitating injuries.

Reference

1. British Orthopaedic Association (2018). *BOAST 3: Pelvic and Acetabular Fracture Management. The Management of Patients with Pelvic Fractures*. London: BOA. ℅ https://www.boa.ac.uk/resources/boast-3-pdf.html

Further reading

Rodrigues I (2017). To log-roll or not to log-roll – that is the question! A review of the use of the log-roll for patients with pelvic fractures. *Int J Orthop Trauma Nurs* 27:36–40.

Stable pelvic injuries

Stable pelvic injuries are those in which the ring of the pelvis and the stabilizing ligaments are intact to the degree that external forces will not deform the pelvic ring. Such injuries are usually the result of lower-impact forces such as falls from standing in older people.

Stable injuries are treated conservatively with analgesia and initial bed rest. Pain management is central to the management of such injuries and gradual weight bearing commences after 2–3 weeks, once the pain has begun to subside and the fracture begins to heal.

Fractures of the pubic rami

The most common fractures of the pelvis are fractures of a pubic ramus. It is often sustained by older people with osteoporosis following a fall onto one side of the body. Pain is usually felt in the groin. Sometimes fractures can occur to both sides of the ramus and/or to both rami. Conservative treatment may initially involve skin traction until the pain begins to subside. See Fig. 10.4.

Central fracture dislocation of the hip/acetabular fractures

The acetabulum is the part of the pelvis that forms the socket of the hip joint. It is a smooth depression lined with articular cartilage forming part of the hip. Disturbance of the acetabulum may involve the displacement of the head of the femur into or through the acetabulum. The mechanism of injury is usually forcing of the head of the femur into the pelvis when in a seated position in a motor vehicle during head-on collision where the knee is in contact with the dashboard. Indirect injuries may also involve falls onto the feet from a height. The injury may also form part of a more complex series of pelvic fractures as described on ➲ Pelvic injuries, pp. 428–429.

Immediate treatment will involve assessment for and management of haemorrhage and shock. Initially, the injury will be treated with bedrest and skin traction until the fracture has been fully assessed.

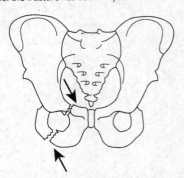

Fig. 10.4 Stable fracture of right pubic ramus without displacement.

Depending on the amount of force and the direction of the mechanism of injury, damage to the acetabular cup will vary from a crack to many fragments of bone pushed thought into the pelvic cavity (known as central fracture dislocation of the hip). The more severe the injury, the more likely there will be damage to the pelvic organs and the patient must be assessed very carefully to ascertain the full extent of the injury. Conservative treatment is usually recommended although internal fixation of fractures in which the floor of the acetabulum is not significantly fragmented may be considered. Conservative treatment usually involves traction for a period of up to 6 weeks followed by a period of NWB mobilization with crutches—followed by partial and then gradual full weight bearing. During the period of immobility, physiotherapy is necessary to guide active hip movements to prevent stiffness.

Lower limb injuries

General overview

The lower limb (the upper and lower leg, knee, ankle, and foot) is placed under significant stress during ambulation and other activities. It carries the weight of the rest of the body when standing and walking and is subjected to forces from all directions. Injuries are, therefore, relatively common and can have a severe effect on mobility, often leading to hospitalization.

The femur and tibia are the two largest long bones in the body and there are several important issues when there is a fracture. Specific injuries are considered in more detail in the following sections. The ankle and knee joint also present challenges as they are so instrumental in ambulation. Even so, it is important to consider that any injury to the lower limb presents specific care needs.

Potential complications

- Swelling of an injured limb can be a significant problem. Unresolved, it increases the rate of complications. Measures to reduce and resolve swelling must be considered as early as possible after the injury. Rest, elevation, ice, and compressions (RICE) are recommended (see ➔ Soft tissue injury 1: muscle and tendon, p. 356). Where the lower part of the leg is injured, a Böhler–Braun frame (or equivalent) is an essential tool for achieving sufficient elevation (see ➔ p. 385)
- Severe injury to the lower limb may require a period of bedrest, depending on the mode of treatment
- A high risk of complications including fat embolism, compartment syndrome, and VTE is associated with lower limb injuries. Close neurovascular observation for up to 72 hours after the injury is essential.

Immobility and aids to mobility

A bony or soft tissue injury to the lower limb may mean that the patient is unable—or advised not to—bear weight on at least one limb. This has an automatic impact on mobility. Even for fit, active patients this can severely restrict their ability to self-care with an impact on their independence. Many patients, however, will be able to cope after a few days with their altered mobility status. There may be more significant difficulties for patients who are older, less able, or frailer. Coping with the temporary loss of use of a limb can lead to increased care needs.

- Applying a cast to a lower limb may restrict mobility. Following drying or curing of the cast, a period of adjustment to PWB or NWB on the affected limb will be needed. Incorporation of the ankle and/or knee in a cast will have a significant impact on mobility
- Patients who are NWB following lower limb injury will require aids to mobility to enable them to move around. A full assessment of the patient's ability to use aids to mobility is needed to ensure the most suitable aid is recommended. Crutches are the most common form of mobility aid in lower limb injuries but must be carefully selected to meet the patient's needs and the patient must be taught how to use the crutches correctly. A period of supervised mobility may be needed (see ➔ Aids to mobility, pp. 172–173)

- Patients' social circumstances and living conditions must be carefully considered. Older people who live alone often find it difficult to cope with the mobility problems created by injury of the lower limb. General safety and falls risk must be considered. Assistance from physiotherapists, occupational therapists, and social care practitioners is essential.

Rehabilitation

Recovery time from injuries to the lower limb can be lengthy—in the case of long-bone fractures, healing will take a minimum of 12 weeks in most adults—increasing for frailer older people. Following a period of relative inactivity and immobilization of one or more joints, patients need physiotherapy support to help joint mobility and muscle strength improve.

Femoral shaft fractures

Fractures of the femoral shaft normally occur within the area between the trochanter and the condyles which is divided into proximal, middle, and distal thirds for description purposes.

As the femur is the largest bone in the skeleton, it is subjected to significant forces during normal daily life, particularly during ambulation. It requires significant force for it to be fractured and patients with such an injury may have been subjected to considerable trauma. In younger patients, femoral shaft fractures tend to be the result of high-energy trauma while in older people the trauma is usually relatively low energy.

The femur is also surrounded by the large muscle groups that surround the thigh. Muscle activity and spasm following femoral shaft fracture often results in displacement of the fracture; compound fractures are less common as a result, although they do occur in high-energy trauma.

Potential complications

The risk of complications related to the injury and associated soft tissue damage are high, even where there are no other injuries involved. Blood loss from the fracture itself and surrounding damaged soft tissue can be up to 2 litres in volume. Hypovolaemic shock is, therefore, a significant risk. IV access should be achieved as soon as possible after the injury and replacement fluids administered accordingly.

Apart from the complications of the injury and the immobility that results from it, fat embolism is most common specific complication following femoral shaft fractures (and of internal fixation) because of the amount of marrow within the bone. (See ➔ Fat embolism syndrome, pp. 212–213.) VTE (see ➔ Venous thromboembolism, pp. 194–195) and other complications of immobility are also a significant issue.

Initial care and management

- The injured limb should be carefully splinted at the scene and during assessment. Further movement of the fracture increases the risk of haemorrhage and fat embolism. Splintage should be maintained until the fracture has been stabilized by other means. It is important to assess the skin and circulation regularly during this period and take measures to prevent pressure/friction ulcers around the splint.
- An IV infusion should be commenced, preferably within the first hour after the injury, to facilitate replacement of fluid lost through bleeding and help prevent hypovolaemic shock.
- Fractures of the femoral shaft are painful, not only because of the fracture itself, but also from surrounding soft tissue injury and swelling. Spasm of the large muscles attached to the femur is common. Fractures are often displaced. It is essential that the patient is provided with adequate pain relief at the scene of the injury and during the acute phase of management.
- AP and lateral X-ray images of the fracture will be needed to facilitate a treatment plan. Any splints must remain *in situ* while X-rays are taken and pain relief must be provided during the radiographic procedure.

Subsequent care and management

Femoral shaft fractures in adults are usually internally fixed with an interlocking femoral nail. Surgery is performed under image intensification using a procedure that involves reaming of the femur and avoids exposing the fracture. This usually allows the patient to be mobilized early. Immediately following surgery, the limb should be elevated using a Böhler–Braun frame. The timing of mobilization following surgery will depend on the stability of the internal fixation and will be prescribed by the surgeon. Infection and non-union of the fracture are the most significant complications along with subsequent fractures around the nail.

Fractures of the femoral shaft can also be managed using external fixation—the stresses at the fracture site make circular (Ilizarov) fixation more likely to be most effective (see ⮞ Fig. 9.7, p. 391). The advantage of external fixation is that it allows early mobilization and the patient can weight bear on the affected leg soon afterwards; this increases the rate of fracture healing.

In some patients (particularly children and older people), conservative management of the fracture using skin or skeletal traction may be the most appropriate option. Although this is only used if other options such as internal or external fixation are not suitable, or the patient has concurrent health problems that make major orthopaedic surgery too much of a risk. Traction helps to overcome the displacement and shortening caused by the contraction of the thigh muscles (see ⮞ Traction: an overview, pp. 378–379). A Thomas splint can be used in conjunction with traction for femoral shaft fractures.

A functional cast brace may be applied after 4–8 weeks of traction, allowing weight bearing but preventing rotation of the limb.

Fractures of the shaft of the femur are major injuries that require careful and skilled nursing both in the immediate period and during the recovery and rehabilitation phases.

Fragility hip fracture: presentation

Fragility hip fracture is a general term applied to fractures of the proximal femur which includes the trochanteric region and femoral neck (see Fig. 10.5) in patients with fragile bone. The term 'fractured neck of femur' is often used inappropriately to include fractures outside of the neck region.

Although they are not exclusively a problem of old age, most patients who sustain this injury are >60 years of age and the incidence rises dramatically with increasing age. In most developed countries, hip fracture is the most significant reason for orthopaedic hospital admission. The rate of complications is high and many older patients who suffer a hip fracture die within 6 months of the injury due to the complications of the fracture, surgery, and immobility—particularly if the patient is frail and suffers from multiple medical conditions. A fractured hip often results in significant loss of independence and can be the event which leads to admission to residential or nursing home care.

Causes

Fragility hip fractures usually occur after a fall in which the mechanism of injury may seem relatively minor in comparison to the severity of the injury. The fracture is often a 'fragility fracture' as the bone involved is weakened due to osteoporosis. The proximal third of the femur and the femoral neck are weakened by loss of bone mass and are easily fractured following either a fall directly onto the hip or by an indirect injury. The injury is at least 4× more common in women than men because of the link between osteoporosis and oestrogen depletion following the menopause (see ➋ Osteoporosis, pp. 252–253).

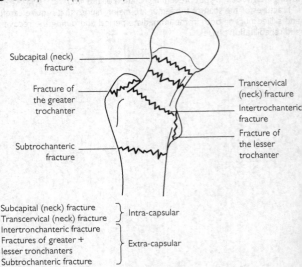

Subcapital (neck) fracture

Fracture of the greater trochanter

Subtrochanteric fracture

Transcervical (neck) fracture

Intertrochanteric fracture

Fracture of the lesser trochanter

Subcapital (neck) fracture
Transcervical (neck) fracture } Intra-capsular

Intertronchanteric fracture
Fractures of greater + lesser tronchanters
Subtrochanteric fracture } Extra-capsular

Fig. 10.5 Types of fracture of the hip/proximal fracture.

The causes of the fall and the resultant fracture must be fully assessed (see → Principles of fracture management, pp. 350–351) as soon as possible after admission to help identify risk factors for further falls and fractures which can be taken into account during the recovery and rehabilitation phases.

Anatomy and classification

Hip fractures are classified according to the region of the proximal femur affected and according to their severity. The hip is a synovial joint (see → Joints 1, pp. 56–57). Some fractures (e.g. capsular fractures and fractures of the femoral neck) occur within the synovial capsule. Others (e.g. intertrochanteric fractures) occur outside the capsule. The position of the fracture affects the type of surgery performed (see Fig. 10.5) to stabilize the fracture.

- Intertrochanteric fractures (extracapsular) are more likely to be fixed with a screw and plate (e.g. dynamic hip screw)
- Fractures of the neck and subcapital region of the femur can cause disruption to the blood supply to the head of the femur and are more likely to require a hemiarthroplasty involving replacement of the head of the femur with a metal prosthesis (e.g. Austin Moore prosthesis) or total hip arthroplasty if the patient is fit enough for longer surgery.

The fracture may be displaced and may also be impacted.

Initial presentation and emergency care

Most patients who attend the ED following a hip fracture are elderly and frail. The most common presentation is an inability to weight bear after a fall. Sometimes there is shortening and/or external rotation of the limb (but not always). The presence of a fracture and its nature is assessed using X-ray examination.

Emergency care may follow a significant period lying on the floor (sometimes overnight) before help arrives, affecting the patient's general physical and mental state. Immediate care should include the following:

- Rapid assessment and diagnosis of the fracture so that transfer from the ED to a hospital bed can take place as quickly as possible with transfer to an appropriate unit within a maximum of 2 hours of arrival in the ED
- Urgent assessment and treatment for any hypothermia
- Careful assessment of health status, pre-existing medical conditions, and medication
- Identification and management of dehydration and electrolyte imbalance with insertion of an IV cannula for hydration therapy
- All patients with a fracture of the hip are at high risk of pressure ulcer development. Immediate transfer to an alternating pressure mattress is essential along with fundamental skin care
- Careful management of acute pain so that the patient can be repositioned regularly—femoral nerve block may be conducted in pre-hospital care or the ED
- Assessment of urinary function and mental status.

Reference

1. van Oostwaard M (2017). Osteoporosis and the nature of fragility fracture: an overview. In: Hertz K, Santy-Tomlinson J (eds) *Fragility Fracture Nursing*, pp. 1–13. Cham: Springer. ℗ https://www.springer.com/gb/book/9783319766805

Fragility hip fracture: principles of care

In almost all cases of hip fracture surgical intervention is unavoidable and is the best option for managing pain, even if the patient is frail. It would take more than 12 weeks for the fracture to heal by conservative treatment and many older people may not survive the complications of the immobility involved. The care of older people who have suffered a fracture of the hip presents many challenges and requires specialist nursing care from practitioners who understand, and can meet the needs of, older people as well as those with a fracture and undergoing orthopaedic surgery.

Sustaining a hip fracture and undergoing major surgery is a high-risk event for older people and their recovery can be enhanced by careful specialized care. Based on growing evidence from research studies, the BOA[1] identified eight key elements of high-quality care for patients with hip fracture and other fragility fractures. These are the foundations on which all care of the patient with a hip fracture should be based:

- Prompt admission to orthopaedic care
- Rapid comprehensive assessment—medical, surgical, and anaesthetic
- Minimal delay to surgery
- Accurate and well-performed surgery
- Prompt mobilization after surgery
- Early multidisciplinary rehabilitation
- Early supported discharge and ongoing community rehabilitation
- Secondary prevention, combining bone protection and falls assessment.

Involvement of a physician/geriatrician in the medical management of the patient with a hip fracture is seen as beneficial as it helps the orthopaedic team to focus on the multiple medical problems and frailty that often accompany advanced age.

Preoperative care

Management of risk is central to the preoperative care of the patient with a hip fracture. Complication rates are high due to the age, frailty, and coexisting medical conditions of many patients (see Table 10.1). Preoperatively, the risk of these complications can be minimized by:

- Preoperative hydration and nutrition—including IV fluids and nutritional supplementation
- Preoperative fasting should be kept to a minimum and surgery should take place within 24 hours of hospital admission

Table 10.1 Potential complications of hip fracture

Confusional states/delirium	Chest infection and pneumonia
Dehydration	Urinary retention, infection, and incontinence
VTE	Loss of independence
Wound breakdown and infection	Further falls
Pressure ulcers	

- Pain assessment and adequate pain relief so that the patient can move around
- All possible measures to prevent pressure ulcers
- Use of correct fitting antiembolic stockings and other measures to prevent VTE
- Careful observation of urinary output—the reasons for any urinary incontinence should be assessed and it should never be assumed that incontinence is normal for the patient. Urinary catheterization should be avoided as much as possible (or used for a very short period) as it leads to bacteraemia which can result in infection transferred to the orthopaedic implant site.

It is essential that the patient undergoes surgery in the most favourable physical and mental state possible in order to support postoperative recovery.

Reference

1. BOA and British Geriatrics Society (2007). *The Care of Patients with Fragility Fracture*. London: BOA.
℗ https://www.bgs.org.uk/resources/care-of-patients-with-fragility-fracture-blue-book

Fragility hip fracture: postoperative care

Surgery should be performed as soon as possible after admission—within 24–48 hours of admission provides the best conditions for recovery. Depending on the type of surgery performed, specialized moving and handling of the patient may be required postoperatively:

- *Hemiarthroplasty*—replacement of the femoral head carries with it a risk of dislocation, particularly in the early stages of recovery. Flexion and internal rotation of the hip should be avoided. A wedge or pillows should be placed between the legs while in bed and high chairs and raised toilet seats should be used when sitting. When patients are in bed they may be turned onto either side, but it is essential that the legs remain abducted. Side-to-side movement can be painful and it is essential that this is supported by adequate pain management
- *Internal fixation*—although the positioning of patients following internal fixation is less problematic because dislocation is not a risk, there remains a risk of failure of the fixation because of the fragility of the bone. Careful observation of pain levels is needed to identify any problems with the fixation.

Commencement of remobilization within 24–48 hours of surgery results in the least risk of postoperative complications.

Surgery for a hip fracture carries great risk for frail elderly people. Some of these risks can be minimized by:

- Good postoperative pain assessment and management
- Careful observation for signs of postoperative delirium—often related to electrolyte imbalance and dehydration
- Hydration and nutritional support
- Careful observation and management of the surgical wound
- The patient should begin to remobilize on the first postoperative day and gradually increase their activity each day.

Models of care

It is well recognized that involvement of an orthogeriatrician in the care of patient with hip fracture ensures that medical conditions are managed appropriately. In many trauma units both specialized wards and nurses with specialist and advanced roles are working towards ensuring that care for patients with hip fracture is provided with their specialist needs in mind. Care pathways can help streamline and improve the effectiveness of care.

Rehabilitation and discharge

The aim of rehabilitation is to return the patient to as close to their previous level of independence as possible. Once postoperative recovery is complete, many patients need intensive rehabilitation. This includes:

- The involvement of all members of the MDT in recovery and rehabilitation
- A thorough assessment of social circumstances and previous level of independence and mobility

- Gradual remobilization based on achievable goals with the ultimate aim of returning to full independence. It is essential that remobilization occurs at a pace that meets the needs of the patient. In frail, older people, energy and motivation levels can be severely depleted
- Daily engagement in and practice with ADLs such as preparing drinks and food so that there is a focus on a return to independent living as early as possible
- Because depression and low mood can severely impact motivation for rehabilitation, the patient's mental health status must be carefully considered.

Further reading

Hertz K, Santy-Tomlinson J (2014). Fractures in the older person. In: Clarke S, Santy-Tomlinson J (eds) *Orthopaedic and Trauma Nursing*, pp. 236–50. Oxford: Wiley-Blackwell.

Hertz K, Santy-Tomlinson J (eds) (2018). *Fragility Fracture Nursing*. Cham: Springer. ✆ https://www.springer.com/gb/book/9783319766805

Fractures around the knee

The knee is a complex structure made up of the articulations of the condyles of the femur, the tibia, and the patella (see ➔ Fig. 2.10, p. 57). The joint is under a great deal of stress during many activities and is, therefore, prone to injury. As a major weight-bearing joint, injuries can be debilitating.

Knee stiffness and secondary OA can be a problem when fractures are close to the joint, especially those occurring within the joint itself. Physiotherapists always need to be involved from the outset so that stiffness can be minimized with careful exercise of the joint and mobilization of the patella.

Where there is a fracture within the joint capsule, particularly where there is displacement, reduction of the fracture is very important as secondary OA of the joint is likely to occur. This is particularly an issue in the knee because of its central role in ambulation.

It is important to acknowledge that any bony injury to the knee will also include varying degrees of soft tissue injury (see ➔ Soft tissue injury 1 and 2, pp. 356–359). It is important that, in the early period following injury, every effort is made to reduce the impact of such injury by managing pain and swelling. As a result of associated soft tissue injury, the knee joint may also be unstable and require splinting until a definitive diagnosis is made and treatment has commenced.

Fractures of the distal femur/femoral condyles

Fracture of the femur usually involves considerable force and immediate care should be the same as that for other femoral shaft fractures. The distal segment of the femur, which includes the femoral condyles, can be fractured when there is a severe blow to the knee with it in a bent position, such as when a dashboard is forced inwards during a vehicle collision. Where the fracture is even minimally displaced, this can result in disrupted function of the knee. As with all fractures close to joints, it is difficult for surgeons to achieve stable internal fixation of fractures; using an intermedullary nail for internal fixation, for example, is impossible because there is too little bone distal to the fracture to give the fixation hold in the bone. For this reason, traction may be used (often with the knee in flexion) and the fracture initially treated conservatively. Internal fixation may be conducted using screws and, a plate or intermedullary nail or screws. The closer the fracture is to the knee joint, the more technically difficult this can be, as there may be only a small amount of bone available at the distal side of the fracture to enable sufficient stability of the fixation.

Fractures of the patella

The commonest patellar fractures occur due to an indirect force on the knee, creating two separate pieces with disruption of the soft tissue structures of the knee. Such fractures require fixation. Fractures occurring as a result of a direct impact to the knee are often comminuted but, because the soft tissue structures are intact, they can be treated conservatively. Patellar fractures can be associated with painful haemarthrosis and are frequently comminuted. This can lead to OA in later life and the patella may be removed to prevent this. Internal fixation of the patella usually involves wiring of the fragments together. This is associated with significant postoperative pain.

Fractures of the tibial plateau

The upper surface of the tibia is prone to injury in violent lateral trauma to the knee. The condyles of the femur can be forced into the tibial plateau causing problematic intra-articular fractures. Fractures may be depressed (with the fragment/s impacted into the tibia) and are often comminuted. Reduction and internal fixation can be difficult because of the proximity to the joint. Conservative treatment with traction or external fixation bridging the knee are other options. Unfortunately, tibial plateau fractures are associated with a significant risk of secondary OA.

Recovery and rehabilitation

Remobilization of the joint is extremely important following injuries to the knee. Initially, the knee will be stiff and painful to move, resulting in a reluctance to undertake exercise. An exercise and remobilization programme will be supervised by the physiotherapist and may involve early use of a continuous passive motion machine to enable the joint to become more mobile before active exercises are commenced. Regaining strength in the quadriceps muscle is particularly important as well as gradually regaining flexion of the knee. For some patients, full flexion may never be possible. It is essential that pain assessment and management are conducted from the early stages of rehabilitation to assist in the goal of achieving as much mobility of the knee as possible. Hydrotherapy can be helpful. Recovery can take many months and may have a significant impact on the patient's social circumstances as they try to regain mobility and manage the pain.

Soft tissue injuries of the knee

Internal derangement of the knee is a term applied to disruption of normal functioning of the knee caused by damage to the ligaments and cartilages responsible for its stability (see ➔ Fig. 2.10, p. 57). This can include the following either in isolation or in combination:
- Sprain or tear of the medial or lateral collateral ligaments
- Rupture of the anterior or posterior cruciate ligaments
- Tear of the medial or lateral 'menisci' (semilunar cartilages).

Mechanisms of injury tend to involve twisting of the knee along with a lateral blow to the knee. The stability provided by the soft tissue structures of the knee is under considerable pressure, especially during some sporting activities such as contact sports (e.g. football/soccer/rugby) and in some field and track sports. Ligaments and cartilages, particularly those within the joint capsule which are bathed in synovial fluid, sometimes heal poorly; consequently, such injuries rarely recover without treatment and are at risk of chronic problems.

Assessment and investigation

Depending on the nature and severity of the injury, symptoms may vary but commonly include:
- Sudden acute pain in the knee
- Severe swelling of the joint—aspiration of the knee may demonstrate haemarthrosis
- Difficulty in weight bearing.

Bony injury of the knee can be ruled out using the Ottawa knee rules (see ➔ Principles of physical assessment of the knee, pp. 100–101). In severe soft tissue injuries, examination of the knee may indicate instability caused by disruption to one or more soft tissue structures. Arthroscopy is still sometimes used for investigating the nature and extent of the injury but MRI scanning is now also considered an effective non-invasive option.

Management

Where there is no evidence of significant soft tissue tears or bony injury, acute knee sprain can be assumed and treated with compression, elevation, ice therapy, and gentle remobilization until the symptoms subside.
- *Medial ligament injuries* not associated with damage to other structures are usually treated conservatively until the symptoms subside; they usually heal without problems.
- *Lateral ligament injuries* require operative repair.
- *Anterior cruciate* ligament tears may require reconstruction.
- *Posterior cruciate* ligament tears do not usually need repair; however, significant tears may lead to instability of the joint and are less likely to heal because of their position within the joint capsule so surgical repair may be necessary. This may involve reconstruction of the ligament using autograft material. Alternatively, a brace may be used for some activities.
- *Menisci tears* are often characterized by locking of the knee in addition to the other symptoms described earlier; early surgical treatment is needed by arthroscopic surgical removal or resection of the section of the structure causing the symptoms.

Surgery

Most surgery to the soft tissues of the knee is carried out arthroscopically (minimally invasive). The practitioner must recognize, however, that, although visible wounds may be small, surgery itself is not minor and can be extremely painful and effective pain assessment is an essential part of postoperative care. PCA may be used (see ➲ Patient-controlled analgesia and epidural, pp. 146–147) and pain can also be managed using nerve blocks and/or IA analgesia.

Recovery and rehabilitation

Following conservative treatment or surgical repair, patients undergo a lengthy period of recovery and rehabilitation. This involves exercise programmes which help to strengthen the musculature around the knee—particularly the quadriceps muscles as these are so central in providing support to and stabilize the knee joint. Rehabilitation is usually overseen by a specialist physiotherapist.

Many patients who sustain significant soft tissue injuries to the knee are often involved in high-level amateur or professional sport. While this can be helpful to the individual's motivation towards their recovery and rehabilitation, there can also be significant worries about being able to return to their previous level of fitness and sport performance.

Further reading

Clark N (2015). The role of physiotherapy in rehabilitation of soft tissue injuries of the knee. *Orthop Trauma* 29:48–56.

Memarzadeh A, Melton J (2019). Medial collateral ligament of the knee: anatomy, management and surgical techniques for reconstruction, *Orthop Trauma* 33:91–9.

Tibial fractures

The tibia is the main weight-bearing bone in the lower leg and fractures are common reason for trauma care. Injures to the fibula are usually relatively unimportant, unless the injury involves the ankle joint itself. The 'sharp' anterior tibial crest (the shin) lies just below the skin increasing the risk of compound fractures. Rotational injury (due to twisting forces) is common in the lower leg. These factors make the tibia prone to complicated injuries.

In adults, most tibial fractures are spiral or oblique and comminution is common, so injuries are usually unstable. The thinness of the soft tissues covering the anterior aspect of the tibia means that open/compound fractures often occur due to either external penetrating/lacerating injury or due to the fracture pushing through the skin from within. Soft tissue damage can be severe. Due to the relatively poor blood supply in this region, management of injuries is often not straightforward and healing can be slow, leading to delayed or non-union. Due to the anatomy of the lower limb, tibial fractures are associated with compartment syndrome (see ➲ Compartment syndrome, pp. 198–199), whether open or closed.

Fractures involving the tibial plateau (the articulating surfaces of the proximal tibia at the knee) or the tibial plafond (near the ankle) and which are intra-articular (associated with the joint) are prone to significant long-term problems such as secondary OA, even with the most careful management. The distal tibial plafond injury, known as a 'pilon' injury, is a potentially devastating peripheral fracture, and carries with it severe short- and long-term problems.

Management

In children, and in (rare) undisplaced and stable fractures, long leg casting is an option for the management of tibial shaft injuries. Depending on the nature of the fracture, weight bearing may be commenced early, and the use of a 'Sarmiento' (patellar tendon bearing) cast can help prevent knee stiffness. Most tibial fractures, however, are displaced and unstable. Except for children, simple manipulation and casting is inadequate, and surgical stabilization is necessary.

There are three main ways of stabilizing tibial fractures: internal fixation with plates and screws; intramedullary nails; and circular external fixation. Orthopaedic surgeons often prefer to internally fix tibial fractures with a nail, but there is a growing trend towards circular (Ilizarov) fixation as an approach to preventing deep infection and avoiding non-union (see ➲ Fracture healing problems, pp. 348–349). Open plating of the tibia is now uncommon because of the high risk of infection and wound healing problems.

Healing time of tibial fractures is often far longer than anticipated. It is uncommon for any tibial fracture in an adult to be healed before 3 months, and for a displaced or open fracture, time to bony union may be up to 18 months. Surgical stabilization or external fixation can enable weight bearing at an earlier stage, but union of the fracture most commonly occurs between 6–9 months.

Care

Tibial fractures are very painful. Pain assessment and adequate analgesia are essential, particularly following intramedullary nailing.

Swelling is always to be expected following tibial injury and fixation, and high elevation is essential in preventing further complications. This is best achieved using a Böhler–Braun frame, or similar device, as pillows are usually insufficient to provide enough support or high enough elevation. Vigilance for compartment syndrome is vital, and the limb must be frequently inspected. 'Dropped foot' (a plantar-flexed position of the foot) is common and care must be taken to ensure that the patient works with the physiotherapist to prevent a permanent flexion contracture which will significantly affect future mobility.

The patient will commonly be NWB on the affected leg, and will require significant support and education about correct usage of crutches or a walking frame as rehabilitation progresses. Ensuring that the patient can mobilize safely is an essential aspect of discharge planning. A period of supervised practice will be needed that includes ensuring that stairs can be managed safely if needed.

Ankle injuries

The ankle is a complex hinge joint (which also allows some degree of rotation) made up of the distal ends (malleoli) of the tibia and fibula in articulation with talus. The joint is stabilized by a series of strong ligament structures (see ⊃ The ankle and foot, pp. 76–77). Because of its significant weight-bearing function and its flexibility, the ankle is particularly prone to both bony and soft tissue injury from twisting forces. Injuries are usually caused by severe inversion or eversion of the foot and ankle while weight bearing. Both bony injuries and soft tissue injuries can occur at the same time. Severe forces are often involved and, when more than one part of this complex structure is damaged, the ankle joint can become unstable.

Soft tissue injuries

Ligament injuries of the ankle are one of the most common musculoskeletal injuries as the ankle is very vulnerable to soft tissue injury. See ⊃ Physical assessment of the ankle, pp. 102–103, and soft tissue injury 2, pp. 358–359 for further discussion of ligament injuries of the ankle.

Bony injuries

Fractures of the ankle (sometimes still termed 'Potts' fractures) are classified according to the complexity of the injury (see Fig. 10.6 and Fig. 10.7). Either the lateral or medial malleoli (distal ends of the tibia and fibula) may be fractured in isolation. Where both malleoli are fractured this is known as a bimalleolar fracture. There may be additional loss of congruity between the talus and the articular surface of the tibia. This is known as 'talar shift' and is crucial in the management of ankle fractures. An additional fracture of the posterior aspect of the tibia at the ankle joint is known as a Volkmann fragment—often termed (incorrectly) a 'trimalleolar' fracture. Injuries may also be associated with spiral fracture of the fibula or tibia (see Fig. 10.7).

Symptoms and assessment

Injuries to the ankle are usually accompanied by severe swelling and bruising. Initially swelling is likely to be close to the site of injury, becoming more diffuse over time. The joint may be swollen on one side only, while significant injury tends to lead to swelling of both sides.

Radiographs should be taken in all suspected cases of fracture—the need for this can be determined by use of the Ottawa ankle rules (see ⊃ Ottawa ankle rules, p. 103). There may be significant deformity if there is an unstable bony injury (see Fig. 10.6). There may also be tenderness at specific bony sites. It is essential that the neurovascular status of the limb distal to the site of the injury is constantly assessed.

Management and care

Treatment for ankle injuries is dictated by the structures involved and the stability of the bony injury. Stable injuries (and some unstable injuries) can usually be treated with either a below-knee or above-knee cast that extends to the base of the toes. Where casts are used for fractures that are unstable, they must be closely observed for loosening once swelling subsides and action taken to change the cast under medical supervision. Fractures that are easily displaced require reduction and stabilization through internal or external fixation (see ➲ Care and education of the patient with external fixation, pp. 392–393).

The care of patients with ankle injuries must consider the following:

- *Swelling*—this is a significant issue in most ankle injuries. It is essential that the ankle is kept elevated above the level of the heart until swelling has subsided. In hospital settings, the Böhler–Braun frame (see ➲ Tibial fractures, p. 448) is the most useful piece of equipment for this. At home, the patient can use pillows
- *Neurovascular compromise*—as with many lower limb injuries, damage to neurovascular structures is a major risk. This can be worsened by swelling. Close observation of the limb should continue for the first few days following injury (see ➲ Neurovascular compromise, p. 196) with

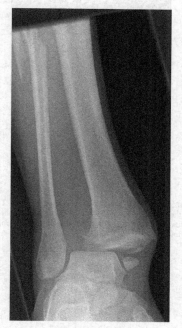

Fig. 10.6 AP radiograph of the right ankle in a patient with a pronation/lateral rotation injury showing a severe fracture–dislocation. There has been avulsion of the medial malleolus and the tibial attachment of the posterior tibiofibular ligament, a fracture through the distal fibular shaft, and complete rupture of the interosseous membrane resulting in diastasis. Image courtesy of the Nottingham University Hospitals Radiology Department.

a focus on the area distal to the injury—this will be the toes if there is a cast
- *Pain*—pain is likely to be severe in injuries where there is significant soft tissue involvement and swelling. Adequate pain management is essential.

Recovery of the ankle joint from severe injury can be lengthy. Patients need to be warned that their ankle is likely to be stiff for some time and will require exercise to regain mobility. Following severe injuries, the joint may never regain its previous flexibility.

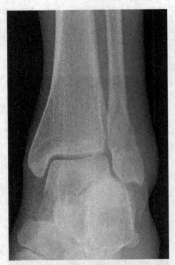

Fig. 10.7 AP radiograph of the left ankle after a traumatic injury. There is a spiral fracture through the lateral malleolus at the level of the joint (Weber B) with overlying soft tissue swelling. Image courtesy of the Nottingham University Hospitals Radiology Department.

Foot injuries

The vulnerability of the foot makes it prone to injury. The normal foot should have no pain or contractures, have good muscle balance, straight toes that are mobile, and three sites of weight bearing (the toes, the midfoot, and the hindfoot). Injury to the foot is usually due to trauma or overuse/misuse often associated with inappropriate footwear.

Soft tissue injuries

The foot can sustain serious injury without a fracture because the bones are very small. In the elderly and those with neurological problems and/or diabetes, soft tissue injuries can be particularly significant, especially if involving the sole of the foot as there is increased risk of neurovascular problems and infection. The patient with a soft tissue injury, unless it is very minor, will need neurovascular observation and, if the skin is broken, wound care is essential with prompt plastic surgery if there is a degloving or severe injury.

Hindfoot injuries

- *Talus dislocation*—the talus dislocates and loses all connection with the navicular and calcaneus. Closed reduction may be used but this is a serious injury and avascular necrosis often occurs
- *Peritalar dislocation*—this is a rare injury resulting from severe inversion stress, leaving the talus fixed and the rest of the foot hanging medially beneath it. The blood supply to the talus is not interrupted, so there should not be necrosis, but the joint will suffer from OA in the future. Closed reduction often fails, so open reduction is the only course of action.

Midfoot injuries

- *Midtarsal dislocation*—if a force is applied to the forefoot in either adduction or abduction, dislocation may occur. The dislocation may be less stable if there are fractures of the navicular and cuboid. If the injury is unstable, Kirschner wires (K wires) may be inserted, but screw fixation is sometimes the only course of action
- *Tarsometatarsal dislocations (Lis Franc injuries)*—this injury is caused by forced plantarflexion of the forefoot. It can result in fractures, but not always. There is always severe swelling and the injury is usually unstable. The circulation can be disrupted as there are links between the plantar arteries and the dorsalis pedis. Reduction of fractures is crucial to preserve the circulation and surgery with K wires is usually needed.

Forefoot injuries

- *MCP dislocations of the toes*—toe dislocations are common and can be single or multiple. Treatment is relatively simple and includes reduction and neighbour-strapping to the adjacent toe. The injury is rarely unstable, but if it is, K wires are used
- *Fractures of the fifth base of metatarsal*—this is a very common injury often caused by walking on uneven ground; the base of the fifth metatarsal (the styloid process) can be torn off when the foot is very suddenly inverted and the muscles contract to try and reposition

the foot. It is often missed as is usually mistaken for a sprained ankle. Treatment often involves a walking cast for 5–7 weeks
  • A Jones fracture (fracture distal to the fifth metatarsal distal to its joint and the fourth metatarsal) is usually caused by stress or direct violence and is common in athletes. The usual treatment is 7 weeks in a cast, but internal fixation with screws may be performed
• *Metatarsal neck and shaft fractures*—usually occur after crush injuries. If the displacement is minimal, a cast is applied, otherwise K wire fixation is needed
• *March fractures*—usually involve the second metatarsal and commonly occur in army personnel who are on their feet continually when marching. The fracture is not always visible on X-ray at first, but a large amount of callus formation usually makes diagnosis possible. It is treated by 'neighbour-strapping' to adjacent toes
• *Fractures of the toes*—usually caused by large objects being dropped on the toes. Treatment is usually by 'neighbour strapping' to adjacent toes. Open fractures need careful observation for infection.

Partial/full traumatic amputation of the foot

Traumatic amputation can occur either as a result of severe sharp trauma to the foot or as a result of a crush injury. Surgery will be required to tidy up the foot bones and the soft tissue.

Diagnosis

• Examination of the foot—the foot will be tender, swollen, and sometimes bruised over the area affected
• X-ray—may show fractures or dislocations
• CT scan—will pinpoint the fracture or dislocation and any displaced bones or fragments of bone that may need removing.

Nursing care of people with foot injuries

- *Pain*—pain assessment is required to ensure adequate titration of analgesia
- *Swelling*—requires elevation above the level of the sacrum and ice to reduce the swelling (RICE)
- *Dressings*—open fractures require sterile dressings and close observation for any signs of infection which will need prompt treatment
- *Wires*—verbal and written advice on how the patient should look after protruding wires and how to pad them adequately
- *Cast*—if casts are used, verbal and written advice needs to be given to the patient
- *Crutches/walking frame*—mobility practice with the physiotherapist to ensure safety and ability to cope; verbal and written advice will need to be given
- *Footwear*—advice will be required about footwear when discharged.

Complications

- *Foot stiffness*—due to lack of moving the foot and toes
- *Late secondary OA*—this is a complication that can occur after any foot dislocation or fracture. It may require fusion of the joint in the future
- *Avascular necrosis*—loss of blood supply to the bone may result in arthrodesis of the foot or even amputation
- *Delayed union*—this may occur particularly if the patient has an underlying medical condition which could slow down healing, i.e. diabetes
- *Non-union*—the fracture does not heal and may need bone grafting.

Measuring for compression stockings

- Measure circumference of the patient's calf while they are standing using a flexible tape measure. Place the flexible tape measure around the widest area of the patient's calf and write down the measurement on a notepad.
- Measure from the base of the patient's heel to the fold of the patient's knee, placing the flexible tape measure along the back of the calf. Write down the measurement on a notepad. This is for proper sizing of knee-high compression stockings only.
- Measure from the base of the patient's heel to the bottom of the patient's buttocks, placing the flexible tape measure along the back of the leg. This is for proper sizing of thigh-high compressions stockings only.
- Compare your measurements to the sizing chart provided by the compression stocking manufacturer you use. Select the proper size according to your measurements.
- Useful website: ℰ http://www.supporthosestore.com/pages/education

Index

Tables, figures, and boxes are indicated by an italic t, f, and b following the page/paragraph number